Stopping AIDS

AIDS/HIV education and the mass media in Europe

Kaye Wellings and Becky Field

LONGMAN

London and New York

Addison Wesley Longman Ltd,
Longman House, Edinburgh Gate,
Harlow, Essex CM20 2JE, England
and Associated Companies throughout the world.

Published in the United States of America
by Longman Publishing, New York

First published 1996

ISBN 0582 29227 1

British Library Cataloguing-in-Publication Data
A catalogue record for this book is available from the British Library

Library of Congress Cataloging-in-Publication Data
Also available

Produced by Longman Asia Limited, Hong Kong

Stopping AIDS

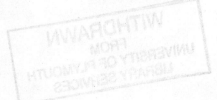

Contents

Preface

The advent of the AIDS epidemic in Europe saw the use of the mass media in health promotion on a scale unprecedented in the sphere of public health. The nature of the epidemic and the behaviours implicated in HIV transmission presented particular challenges for mass media work. Difficult messages had to be transmitted, to wide and heterogeneous audiences, using images generally regarded as more appropriate to private than public domains. This book attempts to document key features of European AIDS campaigns in order that lessons may be drawn from them. The first part of the book organizes the material into themes especially relevant to the AIDS epidemic in general; the country reports give the background to and information about individual countries' AIDS public education campaigns in particular.

The choice of illustrations and examples is still inevitably selective. The campaign materials featured are drawn from a large and growing collection but there are gaps, most notably in eastern and central Europe. In these countries AIDS public education was still in its infancy when this text was written. Furthermore, there are other possible ways of organizing the material and many other themes which might have been included – but books have finite lengths and their authors have their own particular perspectives. Suggestions for additional areas of interest would be welcomed by the compilers of the AIDS Public Education in Europe newsletter.

The collection of materials forming the basis for this book is housed in the AIDS Public Education resource centre in the Health Promotion Sciences Unit, which is part of the Department of Public Health and Policy at the London School of Hygiene and Tropical Medicine (LSHTM). It has grown out of a number of activities supported by the Commission of the European Union. One of the earliest of these was developed out of a European Commission (EC) 'Concerted Action' entitled 'Assessing HIV/AIDS Preventive Strategies'; it was coordinated from the University Institute for Social and Preventive Medicine (IUMSP) in Lausanne and funded by the EC BioMed I programme. One component of this project was concerned with the documentation of AIDS/HIV preventive initiatives directed towards the general population in different European countries. This part of the Concerted Action was extended and expanded through the EC

'Europe Against AIDS' programme in the form of the 'HIV/AIDS Public Education Information Exchange'. This was based at the LSHTM; its main aim was to allow participants in different European countries to share and learn from one another's experience in this previously uncharted area of public health.

Although the projects were funded from large EC programmes, certain key individuals played a major role in initiating and providing the impetus for these efforts. Among these were Dr André Baert at the EC, who steered the original project through the various procedures, and Professor Fred Paccaud and Dr Françoise Dubois-Arber at IUMSP in Lausanne, who managed the Concerted Action. Dr Bernard Merkel from the EC 'Europe Against AIDS' programme was instrumental in providing a great deal of help and encouragement and, indeed, invited the earliest application for funding for the AIDS Public Education Information Exchange. Subsequently Bernard LeGoff and Jasper Voss have continued to steer this project through the procedures necessary to maintain financial support.

Our greatest debt is to the many country collaborators who supplied us with information and materials, hosted our visits, and answered our questions relating to their AIDS campaigns. There are many others to whom we owe thanks. Carol Morgan acted as coordinator to the project and carried out the unwieldy task of processing and cataloguing all the materials. Bob Brookes and colleagues in the Visual Aids Department of the LSHTM were responsible for all the photographic work. Maya Matthews undertook the considerable task of collecting and collating the knowledge, attitude and behaviour surveys that were carried out to assess response to the AIDS epidemic in some European countries; selected chapters of this book draw substantially on this work. Joanna Goodrich from the UK Health Education Authority collected the condom sales data featured in Chapter 5. Lola Martinez provided day-to-day help in translation, and a large number of students and colleagues at the LSHTM assisted in the translation of documents and acted as consultants to the project; they are mentioned at the appropriate places in the text. Professor Frits van Griensven of the GGGD in Amsterdam, William Stewart at LSHTM, and Dominic McVey at the UK Health Education Authority read the manuscript and offered helpful comments. Last but by no means least, a very sincere thanks goes to our copy-editor David Williams for his patient, painstaking and unfailingly professional preparation of the book from start to completion.

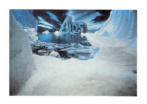

1

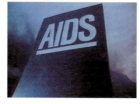

2

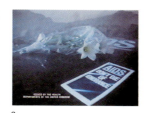

3

1–3 UK, 1987, Department of Health, TBWA agency, posters. **Voice-over:** *There is now a danger which has become a threat to us all. It is a deadly disease and there is no known* *cure. The virus can be passed during sexual intercourse with an infected person. Anyone can get it, man or woman. So far it's been confined to small groups. But it's spreading. So* *protect yourself and read this leaflet when it arrives. If you ignore AIDS it could be the death of you. So don't die of ignorance.*

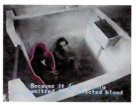

4

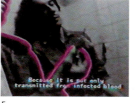

5

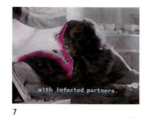

6

7

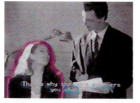

8

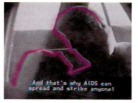

9

10

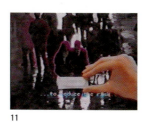

11

12

AIDS
SE LO CONOSCI LO EVITI
SE LO CONOSCI NON TI UCCIDE

AIDS. IF YOU KNOW IT.
YOU AVOID IT.

4–12 Italy, 1990–91, Ministry of Health, Armando Testa agency, TV.
This Italian TV spot featured several scenarios in which infection could occur, each linked in a continuing sequence. **Voice-over:** *AIDS. You can't see it but it's growing. Because it is not only transmitted from* *infected blood, by using the same syringe, for example. It is also transmitted by having sexual relations with infected partners. That's why the more you change partners, the greater the risk you run. And that's why AIDS can spread and strike anyone. AIDS may be closer than you imagine. Let's* *think about that before we have occasional sexual relations with different people. And if we really have to, let's always use a condom...to reduce the risk. AIDS. If you know about it, you can avoid it. If you know about it, it won't kill you.*

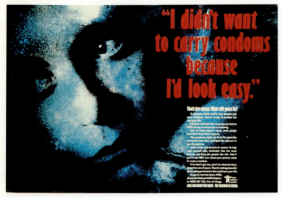

13

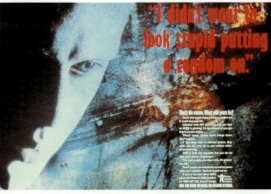

14

UK, 1988, HEA, TBWA agency, press, magazines.

13 '*I didn't want to carry condoms because I'd look easy*' That's her excuse. What will yours be?

If someone thinks you're easy because you carry condoms, they're wrong. A condom can save your life. Infection with HIV (the virus that can lead to AIDS) among heterosexuals is increasing. And to make matters worse, most people don't even know they've got it. The symptoms might not show for years but during this time they could pass the virus on to you through sex. AIDS is fatal with no cure or vaccine. To help keep yourself safe, remember that the more partners you have the greater the risk. And if you're not 100% sure about your partner, insist he wears a condom. If he hasn't got one, don't be ashamed of giving him one of yours. There's nothing shameful about taking precautions that could save your life. If you're worried about AIDS, phone the National AIDS Helpline on 0800 567 123. AIDS. You know the risks. The decision is yours

14 '*I didn't want to look stupid putting a condom on*' That's his excuse. What will yours be?

Don't feel stupid about putting a condom on. It could save your life. Infection with HIV (the virus that can lead to AIDS) is growing. So the chances of you getting it are now higher. What's worse, people don't always know they've got it. If you sleep with an infected person, they could pass the virus on to you through sex without either of you knowing. AIDS is fatal and incurable but you can reduce your chances of getting it. The more people you sleep with, the greater the risk. And if you're not completely sure about somebody, use a condom. You'd be stupid not to. If you're worried about AIDS, phone the National AIDS Helpline on 0800 567 123. AIDS. You know the risks. The decision is yours

15 UK, 1990, HEA, BMP DDB Needham agency, posters.

The brighter colours of this 1990 advertisement contrast with the sombre 1988 'excuses' campaign. The punitive tone of the earlier ads has given way to simple acknowledgement of human fallibility and advice on how to reduce the adverse consequences. A change of advertising agency has helped ease the transition.

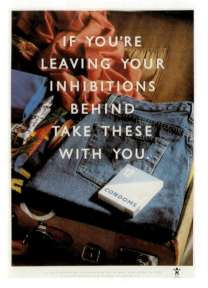

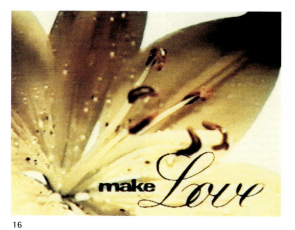

16

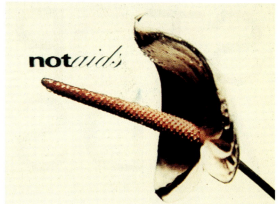

17

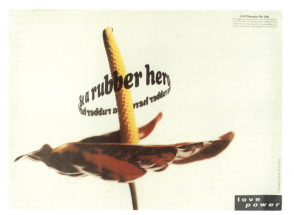

18

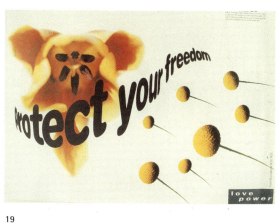

19

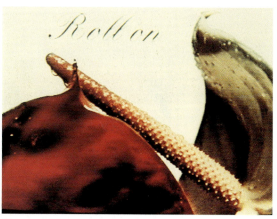

20

16–20 Sweden, 1991, RFSU,
RFSL, Folkhälsoinstitut, posters,
brochures, postcards, TV,
cinema.

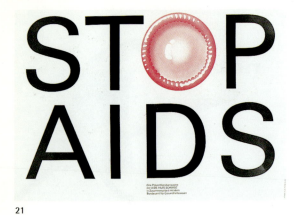

21

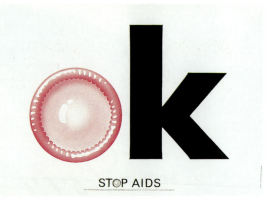

22

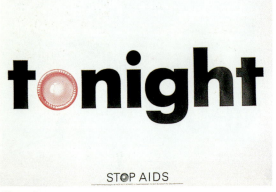

23

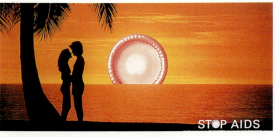

24

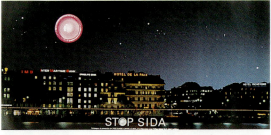

25

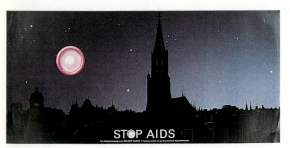

26

27

21–7 Switzerland, FOPH, 1987, 1988, 1989, 1992, all media. The condom image has been a strong and integral part of the Swiss 'Stop AIDS' campaign from the start, serving as the O in 'Stop AIDS', in 'OK', in 'Tonight', and as the moon above Geneva, Zurich, Berne or Montreux, etc.

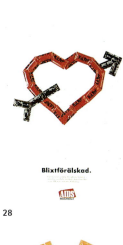

Blixtförälskad.

28

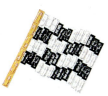
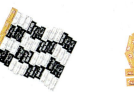

Målgång.

29

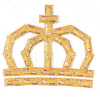

I slott och koja.

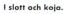

AIDS

30

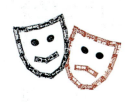

Att vara eller inte vara.

AIDS

31

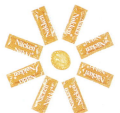

Semesteräventyr.

AIDS

32

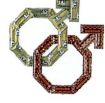

Man till man.

AIDS

33

Rock'n'Roll.

AIDS

34

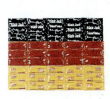

När tu blir ett.

AIDS

35

Kör försiktigt i kväll.

36

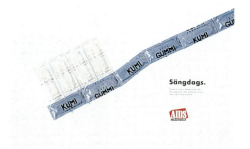

Sängdags.

AIDS

37

HIV syns inte.

38

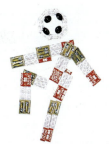

Nya spelregler.

39

Sweden, 1990, AIDS Delegation, BRO agency, posters.

28 *Head over heels*

29 *Reaching goal*

30 *In castle and hut*

31 *To be or not to be*

32 *Holiday adventure*

33 *Man to man*

34 *Rock 'n' Roll*

35 *When two become one*

36 *Drive carefully tonight*

37 *Bedtime*

38 *HIV can't be seen*

39 *New rules*

The use of the condom is the unifying theme in the Swedish 'Black Jack' campaign.

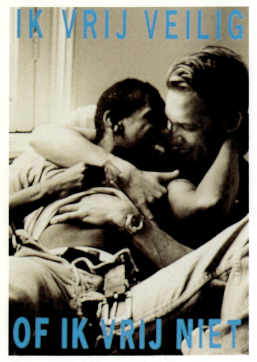

40

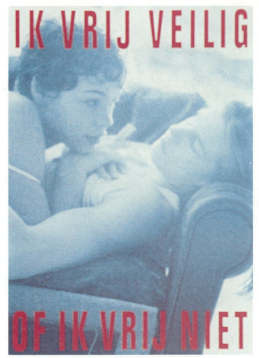

41

40–2 The Netherlands, 1993–94, Ministry of Health, Welfare and Culture Working Group, posters, booklet, postcards, TV.

In this Dutch campaign, the integration of AIDS with other sexual health issues is achieved by focusing on the risk-reduction practice and by making reference to prevention of unplanned pregnancy, HIV and other STDs.

The message 'Have safe sex or no sex' provides the option of choosing not to have sex at all. The campaign extended the message to both gay and heterosexual couples.

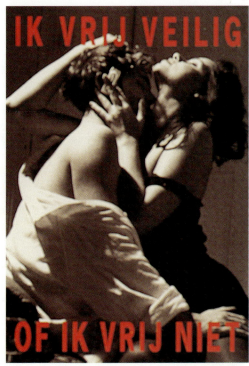

42

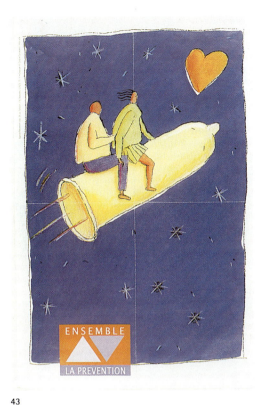

Stop and go.

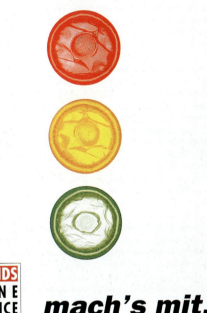

GIB **AIDS** KEINE CHANCE

mach's mit.

43

44

45

On a tous un vêtement Chouchou

3 SUISSES

AIDES
Association de lutte contre le sida.

LE PRESERVATIF: POUR NOUS PROTEGER DU SIDA

43 Belgium, summer
1992/1993, INFORSIDA, Agence
Prévention SIDA, posters,
postcards, video.

44 Germany, 1993, BZgA,
posters, press, postcards,
stickers, notepads.
Do it with one

45 France, summer 1993,
AIDES (NGO), Joker/Benetton
agencies, posters.
*One always has a favourite
garment*

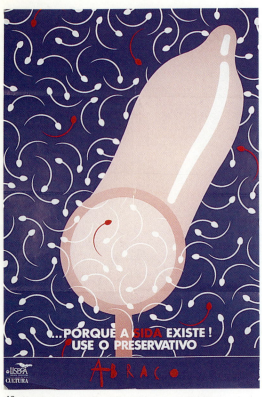

46

46 Portugal, 1993, Abraço
(NGO), Antonio agency, posters,
leaflets, press, TV.
*... Because AIDS exists! Use a
condom*

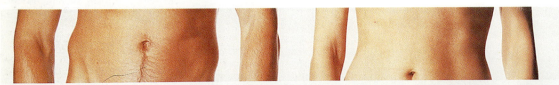

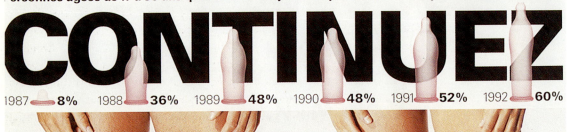

47

47 Switzerland, 1993, FOPH/SAF, posters.
In this Swiss initiative, evaluation data on the increase in condom
use are used to show how much progress has been made and so
encourage continued efforts.

1 Introduction

A European approach

Defining the limits of the region which lies within the scope of this project was not easy. Today there are many Europes. There is the European economic space, the geographical Europe, the European Union and, if we extend this to the European region of the World Health Organization (WHO), the 850 million people living on a land mass of 50 countries stretching from Greenland to the Mediterranean and eastwards to the Pacific shores of the Russian Federation. The extraordinary political events of the past decade have made us reconsider what we mean by the term 'Europe' and to accept that for the immediate future the boundaries will be difficult to define. This is a healthy perspective in the context of disease prevention. Political frontiers are not recognized by viruses. Human mobility and population mixing have enabled previously restricted viruses like the Human Immuno-deficiency virus (HIV) to cross vast geographic regions into new susceptible populations. The movement of people which stirred this virus into action now makes it impossible to treat the disease at a national level. We live in an age which has seen the contraction of the world in terms of communicable diseases, and AIDS/HIV is clearly a global problem.

Just as it is difficult to pin Europe down geographically and politically, it is also difficult to define it epidemically. There is no single Acquired Immune Deficiency Syndrome (AIDS) epidemic in Europe. Data from the European Centre for the Epidemiological Monitoring of AIDS show that prevalence generally increases to the South-East of the region. But within that broad configuration, a number of different characteristics can be identified. A concentration of homosexually acquired AIDS characterizes a swathe of northern Europe covering Britain, Scandinavia, Belgium, the Netherlands, Germany and northern France. Mapping AIDS cases attributable to injecting drug use produces a distinctive Mediterranean crescent consisting of Spain, southern France and Italy in which injecting drug users account for a larger proportion of the total AIDS cases. Charting heterosexually acquired AIDS cases, a further band of morbidity can be seen in eastern and central Europe.

The origin of these patterns is behavioural. Both the pattern of the epidemic and the response to it have been profoundly affected by social norms surrounding sexuality and drug use, by attitudes towards populations at risk, by different conceptions of the role of the state in protecting the public health, by systems of health care, and by pre-existing patterns of policy concerning infections and sexually transmitted diseases.

This complex web of factors is reflected in the huge variation of national responses. European traditions in health policy have evolved in an extraordinarily independent manner, and the search for a common response to the epidemic is frustrated by the wealth of anomalies to be found within Europe. The UK, for example, has shown relatively high tolerance of measures such as needle exchange schemes but has been less at ease with matters relating to sex. In Germany, the opposite is probably true. In Italy and Spain, the Catholic church has been vociferous in condemning condom promotion. Yet in France some of the most candidly erotic prevention campaigns in Europe have met with only minimal resistance from the church. Nor can we make any generalized statement about drugs policy in response to HIV. Some countries – Britain and the Netherlands, for example – have softened their line; others – Italy and Spain, for example – have hardened it since the start of the epidemic.

It is clearly impossible to identify an approach which is unique to Europe, or universal across Europe. Yet there are some common characteristics. Certain options have been open to western Europe, by virtue of its being an economically advanced region with a commitment to liberal democratic values. And by the same token, there are certain risks from which the region has been exempt, particularly those contingent on high poverty levels and inadequate medical infrastructure. In many poorer nations, the cost of an HIV test exceeds the per capita health budget.

Public health traditions: classic epidemic control vs. social persuasion

Ultimately, political and economic factors may prove to have been less significant in shaping the epidemic than established traditions of public health. At the start of the AIDS epidemic, the foundations were laid for two distinct approaches, each representing a very different approach to public health (Kirp and Bayer 1992). Route one, the control and isolation strategy, derived from the classic tradition of public health which developed in the context of the control of epidemic diseases a century ago. This strategy had recourse to legal and statutory intervention. The key words are control and isolation, and in the context of HIV the measures used would include compulsory measures to identify those with HIV infection, i.e. mandatory testing and screening, notification, and reliance on contact tracing, isolation and even internment as a way of preventing infection.

Route two reflects a newer tradition in public health. The key words here are cooperation, inclusion and harm-reduction, with the emphasis on the role of persuasion in modifying lifestyles linked to disease. This approach relies on engaging those most vulnerable to HIV through education, voluntary testing and counselling, protecting their privacy and social interests; it uses information and education to assist the healthy avoid infection and be supportive to those affected.

Each of the industrial democracies has had to decide which elements of each tradition would be drawn upon to contain the spread of HIV. The choice was by no

Table 1.1 Two contrasting approaches to the prevention of AIDS/HIV

Strategy	Control and isolation	Cooperation and inclusion
Mechanisms	Government control	Professional intervention
	Legal sanctions	Health service provision
Measures	Mandatory testing and notification	Anonymous testing (surveillance) and voluntary confidential testing
	Contact tracing	Personal counselling
	Controls on behaviour: Prohibition of intercourse Quarantine Internment Control of immigration	Harm reduction: Provision of condoms Needle exchange schemes

means automatic. The answers reflect the balance of political forces in each nation: the importance placed on matters of privacy, the commitment to personal liberty, the value placed on voluntarism, the role of medicine and scientific expertise and, of course, the changing face of the disease. At the outset there was disagreement and prevarication, and in some cases this resulted in a delay in official response. In 1984, for example, Germany was toying with the idea of a stern new Act for the Control of Diseases Transmitted by Sexual Contacts. Particular political interest groups in Europe lobbied for the use of the hardline approach – the National Front in France favoured, among other things, a prohibition on air travel for those with HIV, and the Danish right-wing Progress Party attempted to incorporate AIDS into the punitive Venereal Diseases Act of 1973, without success.

Overall, though, such classic epidemic strategies have been rejected in favour of the liberal, behavioural approach, relying on persuasion and social learning. Only in very few countries or parts of countries, notably Sweden and Bavaria, were elements of the hardline strategy implemented, and even then with difficulty. The Swedish government brought AIDS within the ambit of pre-existing harsh laws on venereal disease, which permitted isolation of infected persons, but they have been little used. Even in Bavaria only those most accessible were tested – civil servants, foreigners, prison inmates.

There has been no mandatory screening, except in the case of blood, organ or sperm donation. There are no requirements for quarantine. Testing has been unlinked and anonymous for the purposes of surveillance, or else voluntary and confidential. While gay bathhouses were closed or regulated in New York City and San Francisco, in the Netherlands, Spain, Germany and Denmark they stayed open. Needle exchange schemes, which have been a source of bitter controversy in the US, have been relatively uncontroversial in the Netherlands and Britain. So the strategy for preventing this epidemic in Europe, with a few exceptions, has relied on understanding and informing human behaviour rather than restraining and controlling it.

An appropriate medium for persuasion: the role of the mass media

The focus of this book is on the use of the mass media in AIDS public education. The social learning approach depends almost entirely on education, information and motivation, and the mass media occupy a major role in these tasks. The past decade has seen the use of this communicational means on a scale unprecedented in health education. Some maintain that the use of the mass media in health promotion is expensive, largely cosmetic and has little proven effect on health behaviour (Wallack 1981; Flay 1987; Redman *et al.* 1990). Yet research indicates that, in the absence of visible signs of the disease, high levels of media activity act as an indicator of the potential scale of the problem. A mass media presence helps to ensure that AIDS continues to be seen as an important issue.

Much debate on the subject of the cost-effectiveness of mass media in educating young people has been fuelled by findings that despite improvements in awareness and knowledge such interventions have little demonstrable effect on behaviour. Nevertheless, the evidence is that television programmes and advertisements (i.e. both free and paid-for media coverage) have been the main sources of AIDS information for all age groups. The general public claim to receive more of their health educational information from media coverage than from any other source. Leaflets and the print media are a secondary source of information, and family and friends very much a subsidiary source, although professionals rank higher than all media as reliable sources of information.

A major advantage of the broad-spectrum approach is that it reaches a wide variety of people. Campaigns involving high exposure advertising have the potential to reach hidden groups within the general population (Chapter 3). Gay men, ethnic minorities, prostitutes, injecting drug users and their partners, travellers, etc. may not identify with targeted approaches but they are likely to be at least occasional consumers of the mass media.

Major achievements and advances have been made in achieving universal awareness of AIDS. In most European countries, at least in those in which evaluative data have been collected, awareness of AIDS/HIV is perhaps higher than for almost any other disease. In addition, great progress has been made in shifting some of the old shibboleths – the taboo on condom advertising, on sexual explicitness, etc.

Legitimating action at other levels

Although the effectiveness of mass media interventions in raising awareness is well recognized there are nevertheless more doubts over their capacity to produce changes in behaviour. The most effective way of motivating behaviour change would seem to be by face-to-face communication and counselling, when messages can be tailored to the specific needs of individuals. A concern that mass media campaigns may be less effective in changing behaviour has resulted in a discernible shift from high profile television and mass media work to in-depth efforts with certain target groups, together with individual counselling. This shi.. has already begun in almost all European countries.

Yet the recognition that mass media campaigns may have limitations in changing behaviour should not prompt their abandonment. Mass media campaigns perform a valuable function in providing legitimacy to interventions at other levels (Palmer 1988). The media can create contexts of acceptability and agenda setting which are essential for those working at grassroot level (McCombs and Shaw 1972). There is a strong need for a national voice, to maintain global campaigns aimed at the general population in order to reinforce and provide' credibility to community activities, particularly initiatives related to the general public. Regular reinforcement of messages via the mass media and central (government or government-associated) agencies of communication are necessary to those working in the field with high risk behaviours, legitimizing the position of AIDS on the social and political agenda. Public recognition of AIDS as a major problem for the whole population is an important precondition for mobilization against AIDS and the emergence and stabilization of community-based work. The necessity of continuing a steady AIDS public education campaign is stressed by those charged with conducting local campaigns. It is difficult to assert a continual need for preventive initiatives at local or community level when there is no longer a presence initiated from the centre. Thus in relation to the possible shift towards working with specific target audiences and community level approaches, many are of the opinion that this could only take place hand in hand with the continuation of broad-spectrum programmes.

The relationship between mass media and more personal communication is mutually beneficial; issues are flagged up at a national level and acted on at a local level. Personal communication depends on AIDS being recognized officially as a continuing issue, just as the broad-spectrum approach depends on messages being picked up and worked on through more interpersonal communication. In order for this symbiosis to be exploited, a strong link is needed between national campaigns and community work, to ensure continuity and harmony between the two.

The individual vs. the social context

There is a constant tension in health promotion between individualistic approaches to prevention emphasizing lifestyle changes, and structural approaches emphasizing the importance of social and economic forces in determining health status. Conflict between the two is more in evidence in areas of health promotion in which there are strong and powerful lobbies from the tobacco and food industries, and in which socio-economic factors play a more prominent role in determining patterns of disease. But while these are less in evidence in the area of sexual behaviour (since it requires no material products and access is relatively equitably distributed), there are nevertheless areas in which social constraints do impinge on behaviour: cultural barriers to sexual explicitness, availability of condoms, social attitudes towards non-penetrative sex, the power relations between the sexes, etc.

While their role in changing health behaviour is uncertain, mass media campaigns:

- remain an important source of AIDS information
- act as an indicator of the seriousness of the problem
- help to reach hidden groups within the population
- validate and legitimate community interventions
- keep AIDS on the social and political agenda.

There is no doubt where the advertising industry locates itself in this dichotomy. Its skills are very much in the area of personal persuasion. Advertisers, because of their individualistic orientation, consider it generally acceptable to place responsibility squarely on the shoulders of the individual if he or she gets sick. There is now a gradual recognition that public education efforts to date have been marked by an overreliance on individual behaviour change and an insufficient emphasis on creating a favourable social context. As the numbers of those affected increase, this will be an increasingly important focus of attention.

More is likely to be achieved in this respect by exchange of information relating to efforts addressed at opinion formers, including free media coverage. A helpful bishop, a sympathetic editorial, a concerned comment from a politician cannot be paid for, but are invaluable in legitimating AIDS prevention efforts, and every effort needs to be made to exploit such opportunities nationally and to share the experience internationally. Major progress has been made by social marketing in creating a more accepting climate in which condoms could be discussed. This social advocacy function is as yet underexploited. In the long term, changing the social environment as opposed to changing individual behaviour may be the principal contribution social marketing can make in AIDS public education (Wellings 1992).

Countering the effects of free media coverage

The use of the mass media has the potential to fulfil a further function in countering the effects of free media coverage. The quality of unpaid-for reporting of AIDS issues, particularly by the print media, was initially poor in many countries. Representation of the scale of the problem was inconsistent, people with AIDS were stigmatized, the threat to heterosexuals was refuted, treatment of issues surrounding AIDS/HIV was victim blaming, homophobic and sensationalist. Efforts have been made to counter these forces and are now well established, as is evident in the campaigns aimed at encouraging solidarity (Chapter 5). The mass media work has been underpinned by local and community initiatives.

The social learning approach depends for its success on raising the awareness of individuals, informing them of the threat of the epidemic, the means of protecting themselves, and on motivating them to adopt risk-reduction strategies where appropriate. In addition, it depends on changing the social environment to one which supports and facilitates such modification. As a result, outcome indicators used in evaluation of mass media campaigns are often related to changes in individual attitudes, knowledge and behaviours. Again, although a broad-based spectrum approach is not the most efficient means of changing behaviour, there is evidence that some behaviour change has occurred (Matthews *et al.* 1995). It is easier to demonstrate that mass media campaigns can be successful in changing the social context, and it is in this sense that mass media has played the most significant role. It is a role which has not been sufficiently considered in evaluation. If a major aim of broad-spectrum communication is to change the social context then appropriate outcome indicators must be chosen which reflect this goal.

Much has been made in recent years of the advantages of extending marketing principles from consumer products to social ideas and behaviour (Hastings and Hayward 1990). AIDS is the most recent and serious health problem on the public health agenda to which social marketing principles have been applied, and one to which they have been applied energetically with generous allocation of resources, so it provides some useful illustrations of the strengths and weaknesses of the approach. Social marketing in health promotion has been on trial in the context of the AIDS epidemic. There are inherent weaknesses in the approach as far as health promotion is concerned, yet there is also much to be gained from its adoption. Objective-setting is all-important – goals should be set in terms of the social context as well as individual behaviour, for it is here that social marketing comes into its own. It should also be recognized and acknowledged that however useful the social marketing approach, it will not in itself be enough. Creating awareness may be achieved purely through mass communication but changing behaviour requires a mix of approaches, using more direct types of intervention alongside broad-spectrum approaches.

The end of the first decade

At the end of the first decade, the worst possible scenarios predicted for the spread of HIV in the general population have fortunately not happened in many parts of Europe, yet the threat of HIV infection remains an intractable problem, requiring long-term vigilance. The phrase 'low prevalence region in a high prevalence world' (Rubery 1993) effectively summarizes the position in Europe today, and could be used to good effect in maintaining risk-reduction behaviour.

In the 1990s, new challenges face those responsible for AIDS public education in Europe. Not least among these is the crisis of funding from which few European countries have been exempt. The transition in the epidemic, from acute crisis to chronic public health problem, has imposed fresh demands in terms of approaches and solutions needed. While early attempts at AIDS public education were conducted in an atmosphere charged with fear and apprehension, the mood in some countries is now increasingly one of complacency and lack of interest. Distrust of official advice continues and is perhaps heightened by the non-arrival of the much-heralded epidemic of AIDS in the general population in some European countries. The diminished sense of urgency reinforces the views of those who would see AIDS education as an unnecessary rather than a necessary evil. More positively, media attention to the disease is now more measured and circumspect than was previously the case; much has been achieved in terms of eroding barriers to the free flow of reliable information, and estimates of the future spread of the virus can now be made with increased confidence.

In times of diminishing resources the use of the mass media in AIDS prevention is likely to come under increasingly rigorous scrutiny. In this climate there is much to be gained from a comprehensive documentation of AIDS public education campaigns, and their evaluation, in European countries. Despite differences in epidemiological, political, economic and cultural factors, a crossnational comparison of the effectiveness of health promotion initiatives allows us to assess the extent to which interventions transfer from one context to another, and what relevance innovative or successful approaches developed in one country have for another.

This need is enhanced by current developments in Europe. The move towards a united Europe makes it no longer practicable to assess health promotional activity solely on a national basis. Crossnational broadcasting results in populations of one country being exposed to mass media interventions designed and executed in another. The opening up of eastern and central Europe has further implications for health education, creating a fresh demand for health promotion expertise and experience.

The situation in eastern and central Europe bears similarities with that in the West a decade ago, and these are likely to increase. The convergence of lifestyle in Europe in recent times is likely to continue with the removal of the barriers between East and West and the growth of satellite-based mass media serving to increase the flow of people, goods, ideas and services across national boundaries. Since equity is a goal shared by both the WHO and European Union (EU) we can expect to see a reduction in differences in health status between countries. The EU's execution of the Maastricht mandate can be expected to increase harmonization of health reporting systems throughout the region.

Clearly there are also essential differences. The pattern of HIV transmission in eastern Europe has initially been different from that seen in western Europe; the cause of infection has often been iatrogenic, a consequence of the failure to institute adequate health care procedures to prevent infection. The situation is made worse by political instability, by the desperate economic situation, and by an absence of a network of appropriate non-governmental organizations (NGOs). Some of the problems of western European countries – crime, drug abuse, prostitution – may be superimposed upon, and will further aggravate, the situation. Eastern and central Europe have not shared the democratic tradition of western Europe. Many disadvantages and failures of the strictly state-controlled health care system are becoming apparent: underdeveloped health promotion, overdeveloped medicalization of public health problems, overreliance on testing and screening. Compared with western Europe, prevention of HIV in the eastern and central European countries is in its infancy, and there is an opportunity for informing policy with the lessons learnt in the West.

Just as the spread of HIV infection was facilitated by the technological and economic advancement that made worldwide travel so easy, so is knowledge and expertise relating to transmission of the virus and its prevention. This book is part of that exchange. In times of diminishing budgets, crossnational comparisons of AIDS public education that probe the extent to which strategies are capable of adaptation and adoption in other countries are cost-effective solutions to the problem of limited resources.

References

Flay, B 1987 Mass media and smoking cessation: a critical review, *American Journal of Public Health* **77**; 153–60

Hastings, G and A Hayward 1990 Social marketing and communication in health promotion, *Health Promotion International* **6** (2); 135–47

Kirp, D L and R Bayer (eds) 1992 *AIDS in the industrialized democracies: passions, politics and policies*, New Brunswick, NJ: Rutgers University Press

Matthews, M, K Wellings and E Kupek 1995 *AIDS/HIV knowledge, attitude and behaviour surveys in the European Community (general population): a report to the European Commission*, Luxembourg: DGV

McCombs, M E and D L Shaw 1972 The agenda setting function of mass media, *Public Opinion Quarterly* **36** (2); 176–87

Palmer, E L 1988 Television's role in communications on AIDS, *Health Education Research* **3** (1); 117–19

Redman, S, E Spencer and R Sanson Fisher 1990 The role of mass media in changing health related behaviour: a critical appraisal of two models, *Health Promotion International* **5** (1); 88–101

Rubery, E 1993 *UK prevention policy*, Medical Research Council AIDS programme workshop, 12–15 September 1993

Wallack, L 1981 Mass media campaigns: the odds against finding behaviour change, *Health Education Quarterly* **8** (3); 209–60

Wellings, K 1992 Selling AIDS prevention, *Critical Public Health* **3** (1); 4–13

2 Setting the agenda

Raising awareness

Very few diseases have appeared quite as precipitously and with as little warning as did the AIDS epidemic. Projections regarding the future spread of the virus, the affected groups and the eventual scale of the problem were at the start inestimable. Since so much was uncertain, the appropriate strategy was difficult to ascertain. The response of some countries was to delay the start of campaigns waiting for greater certainty (Got 1989); others prepared for the worst possible scenario (Berridge 1994), and others treated the problem much like any other public health problem, galvanizing existing resources into action in the fight against a new disease (Kirp and Bayer 1992; Wellings 1994).

The earliest advertisements from governmental agencies appeared in 1986, some five years after the first reported cases of AIDS, although leaflets and some written materials had been produced before this time. In most countries the work of educating specific groups had already begun as NGOs had been advising their own communities and producing educational materials.

The main tasks at the start of campaigns were to raise awareness of the disease, to prevent panic and provide accurate information about the routes by which the virus could be transmitted and the means by which it could be avoided, for example Norway and Switzerland (2.1–4). A preoccupation from the outset was to find an appropriate level of information, so that a campaign could be easily followed up and information digested. A number of contentious issues presented themselves initially, in particular, how to present epidemiological and medical uncertainties surrounding the epidemic. Risk-reduction messages did feature in the advertisements, i.e. to restrict numbers of sexual partners and to use a condom, but the emphasis in these early initiatives was on the importance of acquiring accurate information (hence the endline of the first British mass media campaign: 'AIDS: don't die of ignorance' – **Plates 1–3**), and correcting misinformation.

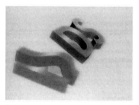

2.1

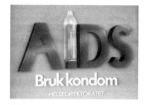

2.2

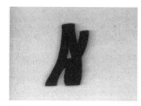

2.3

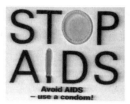

2.4

2.1, 2 Norway, 1986, Directorate of Health, TV. **Voice-over:** *AIDS is a serious transmittable disease. There is no vaccination or treatment for the disease. AIDS is transmitted when blood or sperms from a person with the disease gets in contact with the blood of a healthy person. Avoid sexual intercourse with someone you don't know, and stick to one partner. AIDS is not transmitted just by being close to a person or having social contact, nor through air, water or food.*

A presenter gives the information which is illustrated by means of anthropomorphized letters of

AIDS. Large capital letters spell AIDS on the screen. The male A begins to move and as it does so the I begins to wriggle at the same time as the voice-over provides information on how HIV is transmitted. A female voice says 'no, no', and the I turns red. Both the I and the A disappear from the screen as the words 'stick to one partner' appear under the AIDS heading in the last picture of the film. Already in this early example we see an attempt to portray intercourse, in a manner which will not offend, though there was some controversy when these spots first appeared, over the depiction of sexual intercourse in such an explicit way.

2.3, 4 Switzerland, 1987, Federal Office of Public Health, posters, TV. **Voice-over:** *AIDS is spreading rapidly in Switzerland, and not only among homosexuals and drug addicts. AIDS endangers every man or woman who has more than one sexual partner. Why? Because the virus is transmitted during sexual intercourse, without the partner's knowledge. And there can be a delay of some years between contamination and the outbreak of the disease. You must protect yourself against AIDS. You can protect yourself against AIDS, simply by using a condom. Condoms prevent the transmission and propagation of AIDS. Protect yourself against*

AIDS. Always use a condom. This Swiss TV spot featured blue letters on a pink background. Large capital letters spell AIDS on the screen. The A and I begin wriggling up to one another, smooching until the I is in between the A. A large red letter S comes between them and STOP (in red) separates the A and I with the O as a condom, which at the end opens and slips down over the I in AIDS. The whole sequence is set against a background of soothing vaguely romantic music.

Correcting misinformation

A further important task was to counter the myths disseminated through the media and other informal channels. This task had to be carried out against a background of misinformation and myth generated to some extent by the scientific uncertainty surrounding the epidemic, but most of all by the media. Early media treatment of AIDS issues presented major difficulties for AIDS public education in some countries. The quality of unpaid-for reporting of AIDS issues, particularly by the print media, was initially poor in many countries. Overestimation of the dangers of transmission via social contact began to have serious social and public health consequences – the threat to blood supplies, emergency services, and even health care **(2.5)**. Misinformation relating to casual transmission therefore needed to be tackled with some urgency.

A major consequence of this for the public education campaigns was that a good deal of investment was needed to counter the myths relating to casual

Table 2.1 First AIDS public education campaigns

	Date and agency	Aims	Media	Main message/ endline	Target groups	Tone and style
Austria	February 1987 Ministry of Health	Provide basic and general information about modes of transmission and methods of prevention	TV, brochures, press, seminars	AIDS concerns everybody	General population	Factual
Belgium – Flemish	September 1987 Flemish Community Ministry of Health	Inform public about AIDS/HIV, routes of transmission, etc.	National leaflet drop	Various	General population	Informational, slightly frightening
Belgium – French	1988 French Community Ministry of Health	Raise awareness; inform public about AIDS	TV, leaflet	Open your eyes if you don't want AIDS to close them – AIDS can affect anyone	General population	Serious, sombre
Denmark	1985 National Board of Health	Raise awareness	National leaflet drop	Various	General population	Factual
Finland	1985 National Board of Health	Provide basic information	National leaflet drop		General population, health care staff	
France	1987 CFES[1]	Raise awareness	TV, radio, Minitel, leaflets, posters, press, cinema	AIDS won't happen to me (*il ne passera...*)	General population	Plain, informational
Germany	1985 BZgA[2]	Raise awareness	Letter to all households	Various	General population, special groups	Informational
Greece	1985 NCA and MHWSS[3]	Raise awareness	Leaflet drop	Various	General population, armed forces	Informational
Iceland	1985 General Directorate of Health	Raise awareness	Leaflet drop	Various	General population	Informational
Ireland	1986 HEB[4]	Raise awareness	TV, posters	Casual sex spreads AIDS; Sharing needles spreads AIDS	General population, target groups	Low key, informational
Italy	1988–89 Ministry of Health	Raise awareness, dispel fears	TV, posters, press, brochures	AIDS, if you know it you can avoid it	General population, health professionals	Stark
Luxembourg	1987 Division of Preventive and Social Medicine	Raise awareness	Leaflet drop	AIDS. What everyone should know	General population, young people	Informational
Netherlands	1987 National Committee on AIDS Control	Increase knowledge about transmission and prevention	TV, press, brochures, billboards	Please inform yourselves. Stop AIDS	General population	Serious

Norway	1985 Directorate of Health	Raise awareness	Video, TV	Focus on condoms	General population	Informational, serious
Portugal	1987 CNLCS[5]	Raise awareness; provide basic information	Leaflet, TV, debate	What AIDS is, transmission facts and prevention strategies	General population	Informational
Spain	1985 Ministry of Health	Provide information to those at risk	Leaflets, booklets	Various	General population	Direct, factual
Sweden	1986 AIDS Delegation	Raise awareness	Press, posters	Take action before it's too late	General population	Alarming
Switzerland	1986 FOPH/SAF[6]	Provide and clarify basic facts about AIDS	Leaflet	Stop AIDS	General population	Informational
UK	1986 Department of Health (TBWA agency)	Provide facts about AIDS and risk reduction	Press, posters	AIDS: don't die of ignorance	General population	Informational

[1]Comité Français d'Éducation pour la Santé [2]Federal Centre for Health Education [3]National Committee on AIDS and the Ministry of Health, Welfare and Social Security [4]Health Education Board [5]National Commission for the Fight Against AIDS [6]Federal Office of Public Health/Swiss AIDS Foundation

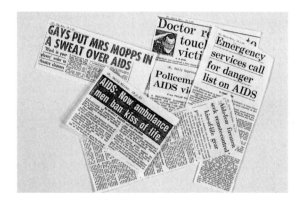

2.5 British newspapers showed fear and panic over the casual transmission of HIV

transmission. Information needed to be provided on the routes by which the virus was transmitted and the means by which it might be prevented, but people also had to be informed of ways in which the virus could not be transmitted. The UK 'No catch' advertisements (**2.6, 7**) represent one attempt to inform the public of the non-contagious nature of the disease. The play on words in the slogan 'No catch' combines a message to the public that this is reliable information and also that the virus cannot be caught in this way. The Swiss 'Keine AIDS-Gefahr' advertisements provide a further illustration of this approach, showing insects and kisses as not presenting risk of HIV transmission (**2.8, 9**), as do the Danish advertisements depicting the safety of public places such as supermarkets and bars (**2.10, 11**).

The twin tasks of alerting the public to the danger of this newly emergent disease at the same time as quelling the rising panic sufficiently to allow

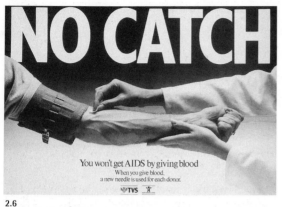

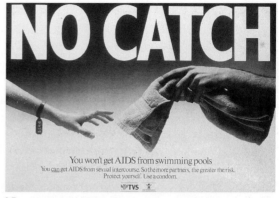

2.6

2.7

2.6, 7 UK, 1987, Health Education Authority/TV South, posters.

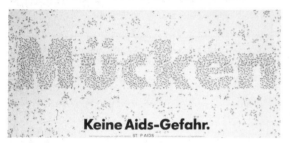

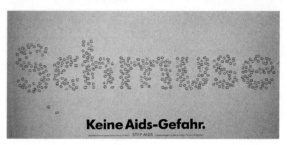

Switzerland, 1989, Federal Office of Public Health, posters.

2.8 *Mosquitos. No danger of AIDS*

2.9 *Necking. No danger of AIDS*

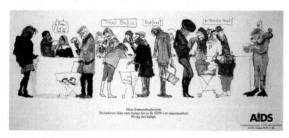

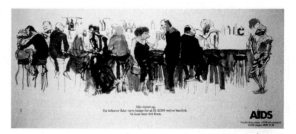

Denmark, 1987, AIDS Secretariat/National Board of Health, posters.

2.10 *Forget the frogman's wetsuit. You don't need to be frightened of getting AIDS in a supermarket, so be cool.*

2.11 *Open up your armour. You don't have to be frightened of getting AIDS in a bar so come on out*

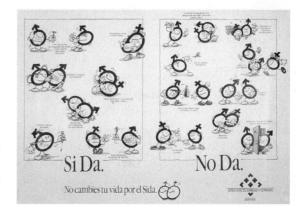

2.12 Spain, 1989, Ministry of Health, posters.
Don't change your life because of AIDS

The Spanish '*SiDa NoDa*' campaign

The Spanish '*SiDa NoDa*' campaign also incorporated information about what were and were not routes of transmission. Cartoon characters were used to enable possibly offensive behaviours to be depicted more easily, and a play on words was used to help answer the basic question 'Do you know what does and does not give you AIDS?' – '*SiDa*' means 'yes it gives', and is also the acronym in Spanish for AIDS.

The first image introduces two male symbols; one of them is injecting drugs into his arm and the other one is apprehensive. The figure injecting drugs has AIDS written inside his circumference and is about to share the needle with the worried-looking figure. The voice-over says 'This way' showing the image and, pausing, 'You can get it. You can get AIDS'.

The same technique is used throughout a whole series of actions depicted by the round cartoon figures. In each case the play on words is used, with '*SiDa*' representing both AIDS and having the meaning 'can give', along with the antithesis '*NoDa*' – 'Can't give'. For each activity illustrated, whether or not the virus can be transmitted in this way is stated clearly:

- female symbol and male symbol sharing a drink from the same glass – '*NoDa*'
- two male symbols having anal sex – '*SiDa*'
- one male symbol puts on a condom, the male symbol has AIDS written inside the circle, and he resumes anal sex with the other male symbol – '*NoDa*'
- female symbol and male symbol kiss on the mouth – '*NoDa*'

The next spot again asks the question: 'Do you know what gives AIDS and what doesn't give AIDS?' This spot depicts the following activities:

- two male figures, one of them with AIDS written inside its body, is about to share the needle he just used with the other character, who looks afraid – '*SiDa*'
- a male symbol with AIDS cuts his face while shaving and offers to lend his razor to another male character

who clearly needs a shave – '*SiDa*'
- a female symbol waiting to use the toilet – '*NoDa*'
- two male symbols wearing sunglasses and looking cool (one has AIDS) sharing a bottle – '*NoDa*'.

The third in the series again begins with the message: 'Do you know what gives AIDS and what doesn't give AIDS?'

- two symbols, male and female, having intercourse, the male symbol has AIDS – '*SiDa*'. On hearing this, the male character puts on a condom, and they resume intercourse – '*NoDa*'
- a male symbol with AIDS brushing its teeth, and about to share his toothbrush with a female symbol – '*SiDa*' – and she refuses to take the toothbrush
- a mosquito which has just bitten a male symbol with AIDS is flying around a second male symbol standing next to the first one, trying to bite him – '*NoDa*'
- a male symbol with AIDS, and a female symbol meeting, shaking hands – '*NoDa*'

Fourth in the series – again, 'Do you know what gives AIDS and what doesn't give AIDS?'

- two male symbols, one with AIDS and wearing a T-shirt which the second wants to borrow – '*NoDa*'
- a male and a female symbol, the male symbol has AIDS and is brushing his teeth and is about to hand the toothbrush to the female figure – '*SiDa*'. As she hears this she refuses the toothbrush
- two symbols, one male, one female, playing in a swimming pool, ducking each other and spitting water at each other – '*NoDa*'
- a male symbol with AIDS cuts himself shaving and is about to hand over the razor to another male symbol, uninfected – '*SiDa*' – he refuses to take the razor
- three childlike symbols, two male, one female, playing together, leapfrogging – '*NoDa*'. Happily playing, they move into the distance.

The message appearing on the screen after all these advertisements was: 'Don't change your life because of AIDS' – The Ministry of Health.

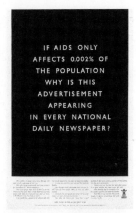

2.13

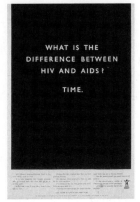

2.14

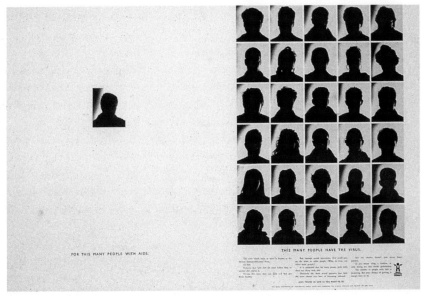

FOR THIS MANY PEOPLE WITH AIDS.

THIS MANY PEOPLE HAVE THE VIRUS.

2.15

2.13 UK, winter campaign December 1988–March 1989, Health Education Authority, BMP DDB Needham agency, press.

The number of people with AIDS, although still quite small, is growing all the time. Not only among homosexuals and drug misusers but throughout the whole community. Over 1,000 people have died of AIDS in the UK. Almost another 1,000 have it now. However, for every person with AIDS it is estimated that there are thirty with HIV, the virus that leads to AIDS. It is possible for a person to be infected with HIV for several years before any signs or symptoms develop. During this time they may look and feel perfectly healthy. But, through sexual intercourse they can pass on the virus to other people (who in turn can affect others). Obviously the more people you sleep with the more chance you have of becoming infected. But safer sex doesn't just mean fewer partners. It also means using a condom, or even having sex that avoids penetration. There is no cure for HIV (as with other viruses it is quite possible that there never will be). AIDS therefore has the potential to be the greatest epidemic the world has known. And while it may still only affect a few people its spread is now something that concerns us all. AIDS. You're as safe as you want to be.

The text of this ad was only slightly modified in other versions, for example **2.14, 15**.

2.14 UK, winter campaign December 1988–March 1989, HEA, BMP DDB Needham agency, press.
This advertisement, presented as a riddle, was only pre-tested with the target group of those as yet uninfected. Immediately prior to the development of this advertisement, the Department of Health and Social Security and the Welsh Office published a report (1988) showing for the first time that HIV infection would lead eventually to AIDS, which in all cases to date had proved fatal. This advertisement unintentionally generated anxiety among those already affected. The HEA responded quickly and promptly withdrew it. This underlines the importance of pre-testing advertisements for unintended consequences, outside of the target audience.

2.15 UK, winter campaign December 1988–March 1989, HEA, BMP DDB Needham agency, press.

normal social life to continue, were to some extent mutually incompatible, particularly where the public education announcements themselves used alarm to motivate.

The Spanish campaign (2.12) included some routes of transmission which represented theoretical rather than practical risks, i.e. although the possibility of infection via this route could not be ruled out, no actual case of infection had occurred by this means. These included shaving, and also – more controversially – sharing a toothbrush, a behaviour which most authorities would dismiss as carrying a very remote risk. That this had an effect on the Spanish public is reflected in the surveys of knowledge, attitudes and behaviour, which show that a third of Spanish people believe HIV can be transmitted via saliva (Ministerio de Sanidad y Consumo 1993).

The scale of the problem

Early campaign components also emphasized the potential scale of the problem. One of the problems in alerting the public to the risk was the credibility gap between the possible worst-case scenario and the lack of visibility of people affected. Long-term predictions had to be made with wide parameters built into them. Because of the long incubation period of the virus and the time lapse between infection and eventual manifestation of the symptoms characterizing the syndrome, the number of people with AIDS was only a fraction of the number of those infected with the virus. A further problem stemmed from the scientific uncertainties surrounding the eventual scale and shape of the epidemic. Many questions were as yet unanswered and possibly unanswerable – how far would the epidemic spread beyond the known risk groups and would it become endemic in the general population?

A major problem relating to AIDS public education was the long incubation period of the virus. Urgent action was immediately required if the epidemic were to be stemmed yet the consequences would not be visible for a number of years. Many of these early treatments incorporated a concept of time lag (2.13–15).

Past campaign components have tended to emphasize the importance of looking beyond actual AIDS cases in order to gain an accurate impression of the scale of the problem, as for example, in the UK DHSS 'Don't die of ignorance' campaign. The fear-provoking aspects of the UK advertisements are dealt with in Chapter 6 but it can be noted here that the use of the image of the iceberg in the UK DHSS 'Don't die of ignorance' campaign served to alert the public to the fact that here was a bigger problem than was currently and immediately visible, which in time would emerge.

References

Berridge, V 1994 *AIDS in the UK: the making of policy 1981–1994*, Oxford: Oxford University Press

Department of Health and Welsh Office 1988 *Short-term prediction of HIV infection and AIDS in England and Wales*, Report of a Working Group (Chair Sir D Cox), London: HMSO

Got, C 1989 Sida: l'ordannance atypique du professeur Got, *Liberation* 10 January 1989

Kirp, D L and R Bayer (eds) 1992 *AIDS in the industrialized democracies: passions, politics and policies*, New Brunswick, NJ: Rutgers University Press

Ministerio de Sanidad y Consumo 1993 *Estudio cuantitivo. Segundo barometro sanitario epigrafe 'Conocimiento y actitudes sociales ante el SIDA'*, Madrid, Spain

Wellings, K 1994 Assessing AIDS preventive strategies: general population, *Social and Preventive Medicine* **39** (Supplement 1); S14–S46

3 Targeting interventions

Two strategies

As in other areas of health education, two possible strategic options were available in AIDS education: to address specific groups selectively or the whole population universally. Metaphors of a 'sniper' and an 'aerosol' approach are useful to describe the distinction between the two – on the one hand quite specifically tailored interventions directed at particular groups; on the other, a blanket strategy directed to all.

Selective targeting of particular groups – most typically carried out at community level – involves identifying specific settings, in which those at whom the educational intervention is aimed may best be reached. The choice of group for targeted approaches has been partly guided by the epidemiology of HIV, and thus directed towards those who, because of particular behaviours, were at greatest risk of infection: men who had sex with men, sex workers, injecting drug users, etc. Targeting has also been guided by communicational precepts – by the informational and educational needs of particular audiences and settings, for example young people in school, ethnic minorities, those in the workforce.

Targeting the general population using broad-spectrum methods of communication most commonly involves the mass media. The broad-spectrum approach nets widely; a distinction can be drawn between seeing the general population as an *audience group* and seeing it as a *risk group*. Where it is viewed as an audience group, the general population can be treated as a broad, undifferentiated heterogeneous group which contains people at differing degrees of risk – covert gay men, those in ethnic minority groups, prostitutes, injecting drug users and their heterosexual partners, travellers, etc. – who are all consumers of the mass media.

The targeted approach has clear advantages in terms of cost-effectiveness and efficacy but presents practical difficulties, particularly since many behaviours implicated in HIV transmission are stigmatized and so may often be covert and concealed. The broad-spectrum approach may lack specificity and sensitivity but has the advantage of reaching those who are potentially at risk but who do not identify as such.

Effective AIDS prevention then needs to combine these two complementary strategies. The two strategies needed to be adopted in parallel. The targeted approach allows tailored information to be disseminated to specific groups, while the broad-spectrum approach reaches those who do not identify themselves as members of a risk group but whose behaviour puts them at risk. In the case of AIDS education there were especially strong arguments for also targeting the population as a whole, as a heterogeneous but undifferentiated mass.

Reasons for the general population approach in AIDS public education

Sexual relationships tend to be temporally dynamic

In practice people do not assemble immutably in fixed epidemiological transmission categories. They move in and out of 'risk' categories through different stages of life, as their situations change. New populations enter the pool of those needing information and motivation as young people mature and become sexually active. Currently monogamous couples may be at low risk, but their status will change should the relationship break down and they find themselves again at the stage of changing partners. In highly mobile societies, risk status also changes with location. Young people in Gloucestershire, in the Basque or in Jutland may be at relatively low risk at home, but on vacation the risk may increase. Old audiences are replaced by new ones as people move from one life-stage or setting to another.

Sexual orientation is relatively unstable

People may constantly discover and rediscover their sexual orientation. Data from surveys of sexual lifestyles show clearly the heterogeneity of behaviour in respect of sexual orientation. The British sexual behaviour survey (Wellings *et al.* 1994) shows, for example, that 90 per cent of men who have ever had sex with a man have also had sex with a woman, and 60 per cent of those men who have had sex with a man in the last five years have also had sex with a woman during this period. Such findings caution against thinking in terms of watertight categories of heterosexual and homosexual.

People may not identify with target groups

Where behaviours are socially stigmatized, people may be reluctant to identify as members of particular groups and so cannot be targeted directly and specifically, but only within the general population as a whole. Additionally, the sexual partners of those practising high risk behaviours might be unwittingly at risk, or else may not identify with health educational messages directed at their partner's behaviour if it is not shared by them.

Transmission routes vary

HIV may be acquired as a consequence of one risk behaviour, but passed on as a result of another. An injecting drug user who has become infected as a result of sharing contaminated needles may infect his or her sexual partner; and by the same token a bisexual man who has acquired the virus from a male sexual partner may pass it to a woman with whom he has sex. There is therefore little to be gained from addressing particular behaviours exclusively.

Information needs vary

Although it may not be necessary for everyone to change their behaviour, there may be a need for everyone to acquire knowledge of, and an appropriate attitude towards, sexual health. Mobilizing the whole population allows open and free discussion which will benefit minorities.

The campaigns

Everyone is at risk

As illustrated in Chapter 2, a universal concern for AIDS public education at the outset was the need to assert and reiterate the risk to everyone, irrespective of risk group. The message that everyone is potentially at risk was incorporated in campaign components addressed to the general population. Aided by endlines like 'AIDS concerns everyone', campaigns across Europe aimed to address the general population. Yet initial AIDS public education campaigns showed considerable crossnational variation in the use of broad-spectrum approaches. In some countries, from the beginning there was a feeling that mass media campaigns do not reach high risk groups, and that the most effective focus for the work was in those settings and among those groups in which the virus was most likely to be transmitted.

At least as important as the epidemiological situation of AIDS/HIV prevalence in determining which target group should be addressed within the campaigns was the moral, social and political climate in each country. In some countries, in Denmark for example, efforts have been made to focus on the general population with no distinction between heterosexuals and homosexuals. AIDS education in Germany also primarily (although not exclusively) addressed the general public on the assumption that people do not identify themselves as members of distinct risk groups. Responsibility for target groups was divided so that the Federal Centre for Health Education (BZgA) – the statutory body with responsibility for health education and AIDS public education – concentrated on the general public, while those at increased risk were chiefly the focus of the NGO, Deutsche AIDS-Hilfe. Where specific target groups have been addressed by the BZgA they have been chosen according to particular communicational needs rather than because they are possibly at increased risk.

In countries in which homosexuality and other minority behaviours are heavily stigmatized, the decision to mount general population campaigns was guided by the need to destigmatize the disease, to normalize it and to minimize the extent to which it was seen as affecting only certain small, minority, deviant groups. A constant theme running throughout AIDS public education in the UK, for example, has been the need continuously to assert and reiterate the risk to everyone, irrespective of risk group membership. This has partly been necessary to counter the refutations of the existence of heterosexual spread in the tabloid press and their constant obsession with seeing AIDS as associated with deviant practices. Ideally, the message that everyone is potentially at risk should have been implicit in campaign components addressed to the general population, and behaviour rather than risk group emphasized.

The issue of targeting has been contentious in many countries. In the UK, the issue of heterosexual spread has been so much a part of heated and controversial debate that health education agencies had little option but to address the issue directly. This was especially apparent in the Health Education Authority (HEA) advertisements, notably the press campaign early in 1989 (3.1) and the 'experts' campaign in 1990 which were used expressly to make the point that everyone was at risk. The advertisements were criticized across a broad front. The right-wing press, which still saw AIDS in terms of retribution, accused the HEA on each occasion of singling out the wrong audience – 'the wrong message for a wrong target' (3.2). These newspapers have large circulations and their impact undoubtedly undermined the message of the HEA. Evaluation of the campaigns needed to take more account of this.

All too often, the press portrayed the heterosexual and the general population as one and the same. This had two important consequences: it encouraged the

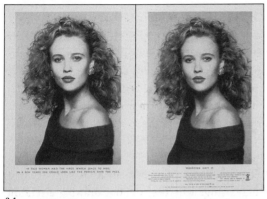

3.1

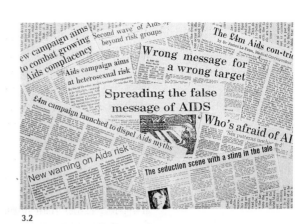

3.2

3.1 UK, winter 1988–89, HEA, BMP DDB Needham agency, press.
Featuring women in advertisements was designed to avoid stereotyping AIDS as a gay disease. This led to criticism from women themselves, and from people infected, who saw the long period of good health as something to celebrate rather than worry about.

3.2 UK, 1988.
Newspaper coverage of campaigns was sometimes critical, and created confusion for the public.

criticism that AIDS public education was being aimed at the wrong target by those who saw AIDS as retribution, as a punishment for deviance; it also allowed a sterile debate to develop as to whether the general population was really at risk – with constant reference to the AIDS statistics in support of the view that there really was no risk to heterosexuals.

The rationale for the 'experts' campaign has to be seen against a background of continuing uncertainty over the future direction of the epidemic. The impetus for this came from heightened controversy over whether or not HIV was efficiently transmitted heterosexually. Throughout 1989, debate was taking place within the scientific community over how far and how fast HIV would spread into the general population. A series of unhelpful articles appeared in the press. From the start of the UK campaigns there was pressure from lobbying and pressure groups with diverse viewpoints. The UK HEA was criticized from time to time for not representing affected groups adequately and for underestimating the threat to the whole population. On the other hand, lobbying groups on the moral Right argued that the HEA was wrongly targeting the 'innocent' and safe heterosexual population, encouraging promiscuity and pandering to the gay lobby.

The Swedish information campaign also initially set out to draw attention to the risk to the general public, aided by endlines like 'AIDS concerns everyone'. One reason for this strategy was that if advertisements deliberately targeted high risk groups, the general population might not identify with the message; but it was also recognized that avoiding targeting groups such as gay men and drug users would help protect them from stigmatization. These groups were able to carry out their own public education more proficiently.

In other countries, it has been possible to target specific groups within the broad-spectrum approach. In the Netherlands for example, where discrimination on the grounds of sexual orientation is actually legislated against, drug users, homosexuals and sex workers were targeted without fear of discrimination and victim blaming. Early Dutch interventions were mainly directed towards high risk groups. There the groups most at risk of HIV infection were served by a solid and extensive infrastructure; statutory and non-statutory organizations already existed with specialist knowledge and a long experience in addressing them. The main targets of interventions from 1983 to 1987 were people whose behaviours placed them at increased risk of infection: men who have sex with men, sex work-ers, those who inject drugs, young people (particularly those with more than one sexual partner), etc. In fact, the decision to introduce a general population cam-paign in 1987 was taken later than in other countries and was made partly on the grounds of crossnational pressure as the Dutch people began to see on their tele-visions the efforts made in other countries to inform and educate the general population in other parts of Europe, in the UK, for example.

Dutch information and prevention policy has been characterized by a twin-track approach. Activities are targeted at people with a high risk of infection using different methods and media. The general population campaign was implemented alongside, rather than in place of, existing activities, without drawing attention from them.

The Norwegian Directorate of Health has openly targeted drug users, homosexuals and prostitutes. The stated rationale was that if they could reduce the size of populations whose behaviour put them at risk, this would indirectly protect the rest of the population. In Norway, from the beginning, those involved in HIV prevention felt the most effective focus for their work was in those settings and among those groups in which the virus was most likely to be transmitted. Initial attempts were therefore not principally targeted at the general population. Criticisms of those who felt more money should be channelled into public educa-tion addressed to the general population were answered by pointing out that high risk behaviours were *within* the general population, which was therefore indirectly being protected. The Directorate of Health, it was stressed, existed for everyone, not only for those already enjoying a healthy lifestyle, but primarily for those with-out such privilege. Again, risk groups were targeted within broad-spectrum approaches with little fear of controversy (3.3).

In France, where the emphasis was on risk behaviours rather than groups, and where campaigns addressed to the general population have stressed that prac-tices rather than people carry risk, the charge was levelled by some that risk groups have been neglected. Pressure to include interventions aimed at men with homo-sexual contacts came from both left- and right-wing pressure groups. In France,

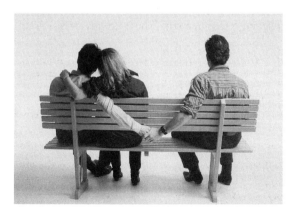

3.3 Norway, 1984–85, Oslo
Board of Health, posters.
*Men who have sex with men
should check their health
regularly*
In some countries there was
early recognition that
behaviours were not discrete
and homogeneous, but diverse
and heterogeneous.

official campaigners responded to this pressure; an advisory expert group for communications with male homo- and bisexuals was established at the Agence Française de Lutte Contre le SIDA (AFLS) at the end of 1989. The 1989 summer campaign (repeated in 1990) 'Condoms wish you a happy holiday' featured gay men, as did the 1990 'Histories of love' TV spot, and the 1991 'Why wait any longer' campaign, which included two spots with gay men talking about safer sex. It was not explicitly stated that they were homosexual, yet anecdotal evidence was that this new orientation was picked up by gay men but not by heterosexuals.

Criticisms have also been levelled at the national Italian AIDS public education campaigns, concerning failure to target specific groups. The first three campaigns (1988–89, 1990–91, 1991–92) were almost entirely directed at the general public despite the fact that those most affected in Italy were injecting drug users. Critics maintained that the campaign messages, 'don't use drugs' and 'don't share needles', were directed towards those who may have had no interest in doing so. Many felt that drug users should have received information from the early campaigns, rather than from drug dependency clinics.

Specific efforts were made in one component of the 1990–91 Italian campaign to demonstrate that the routes by which HIV was transmitted were not discrete, but diverse and interconnected – one person being infected via one route but passing on the virus via another. A TV spot featured an infected drug-injecting man sharing syringes with another man, who then had sexual contact with a woman who subsequently has sex with a man; each in turn infects the other – a continuous pink line connotes contagion (**Plates 4–12**). It received over 3,000 TV showings. The endline – 'If you know about it, you can avoid it; if you know about it, it won't kill you' – was, however, criticized on the grounds that it was discriminatory: it could be misinterpreted as 'If you know him, you can avoid him', since the pronoun for a man and the indefinite object is the same in Italian.

The balance between targeting and broad-spectrum approaches has varied with the nature of the epidemic. In some countries the targeting strategy reflected the dominant risk transmission category. In Spain and Switzerland for example, injecting drug users (IDUs) received attention in the mass media because of the prominence of this risk group in the HIV statistics. Targeting high risk behaviours, particularly IDUs and homosexual men is acknowledged as difficult in Spain, yet attempts have been made to do so by including these in campaign components (see Chapter 2, '*SiDa NoDa*').

Risk groups to risk behaviours

In many countries a perceivable shift in targeting strategy has occurred since the earliest campaigns. The emphasis has gradually moved from risk groups to risk behaviours. The risk group model was predicated on the belief that particular subgroups of people had to be identified as at higher risk. The alternate view, that particular behaviours put people at increased risk, depends far less on the need to target particular people directly and far more on pointing out to everyone how to

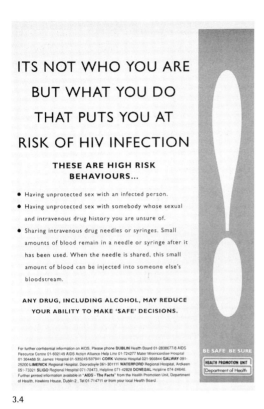

ITS NOT WHO YOU ARE
BUT WHAT YOU DO
THAT PUTS YOU AT
RISK OF HIV INFECTION

**THESE ARE HIGH RISK
BEHAVIOURS...**

- Having unprotected sex with an infected person.
- Having unprotected sex with somebody whose sexual and intravenous drug history you are unsure of.
- Sharing intravenous drug needles or syringes. Small amounts of blood remain in a needle or syringe after it has been used. When the needle is shared, this small amount of blood can be injected into someone else's bloodstream.

**ANY DRUG, INCLUDING ALCOHOL, MAY REDUCE
YOUR ABILITY TO MAKE 'SAFE' DECISIONS.**

For further confidential information on AIDS, Please phone DUBLIN Health Board 01-2838677/8 AIDS Resource Centre 01-602149 AIDS Action Alliance Help Line 01-724277 Mater Misericordiae Hospital 01-304488 St. James' Hospital 01-535245/537941 CORK Victoria Hospital 021-966844 GALWAY 091-25200 LIMERICK Regional Hospital, Dooradoyle 061-301111 WATERFORD Regional Hospital, Ardkeen 051-73321 SLIGO Regional Hospital 071-70473, Helpline 071-42828 DONEGAL Helpline 074-24646. Further printed information available in "AIDS - The Facts" from the Health Promotion Unit, Department of Health, Hawkins House, Dublin 2. Tel 01-714711 or from your local Health Board

BE SAFE BE SURE

HEALTH PROMOTION UNIT
Department of Health

3.4

**IGÅR DELADE
HAN SPRUTA MED
TRE KOMPISAR**

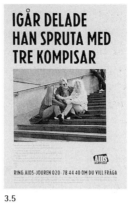

RING AIDS-JOUREN 020-78 44 40 OM DU VILL FRÅGA

3.5

**FÖR ETT ÅR SEDAN
VAR HAN
PÅ GAY-KLUBB
I KÖPENHAMN**

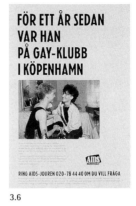

RING AIDS-JOUREN 020-78 44 40 OM DU VILL FRÅGA

3.6

**DU FÅR ALLA
HANS
ERFARENHETER**

RING AIDS-JOUREN 020-78 44 40 OM DU VILL FRÅGA

3.7

**VILL DU VETA HUR
EN HIV-SMITTAD KAN SE UT!
VARSÅGOD OCH TITTA:**

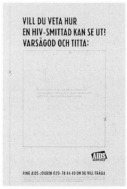

RING AIDS-JOUREN 020-78 44 40 OM DU VILL FRÅGA

3.8

3.4 Ireland, 1991, Health Promotion Unit, Department of Health, posters.

Sweden, March 1987, AIDS Delegation, Ted Bates agency, posters.

3.5 *Yesterday he shared needles with three friends*
3.6 *A year ago he went to a gay club in Copenhagen*
3.7 *You get all his experiences*
3.8 *Do you want to know what someone with HIV looks like, here have a look*

avoid risk to themselves personally. Sometimes this message was explicitly and expressly transmitted as in the 1991 Irish public lavatory advertising campaign (**3.4**). A poster, placed in public toilets in Ireland, makes it clear that what you do, rather than who you are, is important in determining risk. The contrast between the risk group and the risk behaviour approach is clearly illustrated in a comparison between some early advertisements from the Swedish campaign (**3.5–8**) with later examples from the Norwegian campaign (**3.12–15**). A set of posters produced for the Swedish campaign in 1987 aimed to encourage people to recognize risky situations, gay bars, foreign locations. Colour pictures feature couples in everyday encounters, their body and eye contact showing them to be clearly attracted and absorbed by one another. The fourth advertisement (**3.8**) has an empty square in place of the image, which the reader is told to cut out and position at the bathroom mirror, in order to see what an HIV-infected person could look like.

While it is true that the focus of the text is on behaviours, the images suggest otherwise. A chilling contrast is created between the stark message of the text and the warmth of the pictures, confirming the message that a threat can lurk under the surface of everyday life, and the danger is linked with other individuals, groups or settings, rather than on any aspect of personal behaviour within the actor's control. The recommended risk-avoidance strategy is avoidance – avoidance of particular kinds of people and places. The message is to take an HIV test

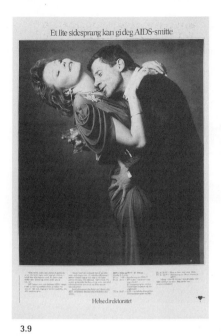

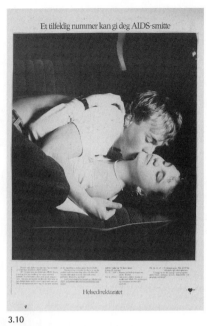

Norway, Directorate of Health, posters, transport posters, press.

3.9 *A little sidestep can give you AIDS*
(February 1987)

3.10 *A one-night stand can give you AIDS*
(February 1987)

3.11 *Happiness and care. Safer sex*
(1990–91)

3.9

3.10

3.11

or phone the AIDS hotline. No other risk-reduction strategy is mentioned.

In Norway there was early recognition that behaviours were continuous not discrete, as is apparent in **3.3**. In the more recent summer campaigns (1988–91), the emphasis has been not on identifying and avoiding *other* people who might present a risk to self, but on taking appropriate action in relation to one's own personal behaviour to avoid risk – compare **3.9** and **10** with **3.11**. Other later posters

Norway, 1988 and 1991,
Directorate of Health, posters,
transport posters, press.

3.12 *Of course you'll fall in
love this summer! Take AIDS
seriously!*

3.13 *Of course you'll fall in
love this summer! Take AIDS
seriously!*

3.14 *Never share needles! If
you're taking drugs it's safer to
give up. Take AIDS seriously!*

3.15 *Summer holiday! Travel
where you want, it's what you
do that matters. Take AIDS
seriously!*

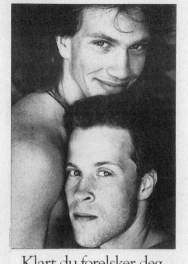

3.12

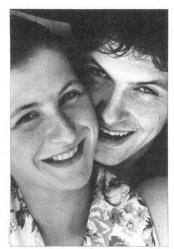

3.13

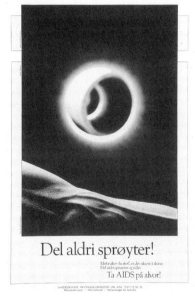

3.14

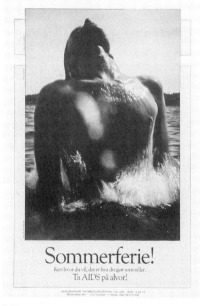

3.15

depict a homosexual couple, a heterosexual couple, a drug user and a vacation
traveller, with the same message for each (**3.12–15**).

The most recent advertisements show a definite shift towards the importance of generic risk-reduction advice using the same message and treatment for
all, again with the emphasis on behaviour instead of target group. The Swiss 'Stop
AIDS' campaign, for example (**3.16–20**), used the same message in portrayals of

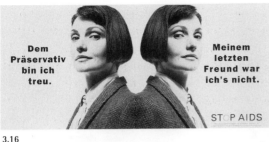

3.16

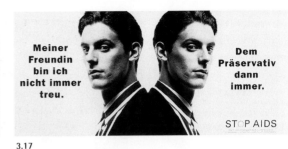

3.17

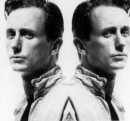

3.18

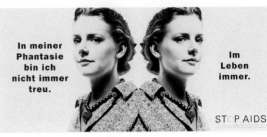

3.19

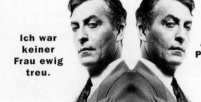

3.20

Switzerland, summer 1993, FOPH/SAF, cR Advertising agency, posters.

3.16 *To the condom I'm faithful.*

To my last friend I wasn't

3.17 *To my friend I am not always faithful.*

To the condom always

3.18 *To the condom I am faithful.*

To my friend I was unfaithful

3.19 *In my fantasies I am not always faithful. In life always*

3.20 *I was never lastingly faithful to a woman.*

But I am to a condom

The rationale for the change of emphasis from risk groups to risk behaviours has been:

- a recognition that behaviour is a more important focus than groups
- evidence that groups are not discrete in their behaviour
- the difficulties of identification inherent in risk group approach.

several different couples. The trend is now to see the general population not as an undifferentiated mass, but as containing different targets who can each be dealt with in one intervention in which they are addressed with only slightly different messages.

The Dutch 1993 'Three steps to heaven' campaign (see Chapter 8) addressed gay men and ethnic minorities as part of a campaign aimed at the general population as a whole. The campaign comprised a three-part TV and cinema spot – the first 'step' holding hands, the second kissing, the third sex. The second 'step' featured gay men. Gay men were regarded as a target audience *within* the general population. The campaign aimed to get through to those who would not be reached by targeted efforts and also to reduce further stigmatization and discrimination. For the same reasons, two of the couples featured in the posters were non-white. There was no opposition to this from the Ministry of Health, Welfare and Culture (MHWC), who accepted the National Committee on AIDS Control sub-committee of Education and Prevention's (NCACEP) and the STD Foundation's (STDF) advocacy of integration of homosexuality into mass media campaigns, since gay men remain the most important risk group. Ultimately the NCACEP and the STDF control the campaigns. Although the MHWC are consulted, the lead of the NCACEP and STDF is accepted and respected.

References

Wellings, K, J Field, A M Johnson and J Wadsworth 1994 *Sexual behaviour in Britain. The national survey of sexual attitudes and lifestyles*, London: Penguin Books

4 Getting the message

The messages disseminated in AIDS public education have been largely determined by the distinctive nature of AIDS and HIV. AIDS is a communicable disease whose viral agent, HIV, is transmitted through limited and highly specific routes. The fact that the spread of HIV is linked with well-defined human behaviours has enhanced opportunities for prevention; had this been an air- or waterborne virus the consequences would certainly have been far more grave.

A further distinctive feature of this virus is that it is almost exclusively transmitted through *social* encounters, either through sexual relations or as a result of sharing needles with injecting drug users. Unlike preventive strategies for chronic diseases, which tend to be targeted mainly at the individual level, AIDS preventive strategies have to take account of the dyad of, on the one hand, infected persons needing advice on how to avoid infecting others, and on the other uninfected persons needing advice on how to avoid infection. Messages have also had to take account of the diversity of transmission routes – through heterosexual sex, homosexual sex and injecting drug use.

Modification of the behaviours which determine HIV transmission has formed the basis of risk-reduction advice to the general public. In relation to the sexual transmission of HIV, two messages have predominated in public education campaigns: condom use and restriction of numbers of sexual partners, preferably to one mutually exclusive relationship. Other messages, including being careful about the choice of partners, practising safer-sex techniques and abstinence, have featured less commonly in campaigns. Advice to avoid penetrative sex has not been fully developed in any of the countries, despite being a predominant message in the literature intended for gay men. In some countries, the symptom-free nature of HIV has been emphasized, and hence the difficulty of knowing who is infected, with the consequent need for protective measures to be taken at all times (**4.1, 2**). Very few countries, Spain and Switzerland being notable exceptions largely because of the high prevalence of HIV among drug users in those countries, have attempted to introduce the message to avoid needle sharing into campaigns addressed to the general public. The advice to take an HIV test has also featured somewhat rarely, although with increasing regularity over time as the circumstances relating to testing have changed.

4.1 Sweden, 1990, AIDS
Delegation, BRO agency,
posters.

HIV can't be seen
Doesn't show
New faces
Sweet music plays
But who is most likely to be a
carrier?
So don't take the risk
Protect yourself

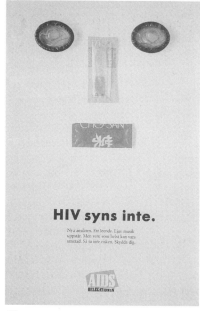

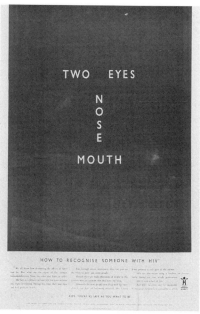

4.1

4.2

4.2 UK, winter 1988–89, Health Education Authority, BMP DDB Needham agency, magazines.
How to recognise someone with HIV. We all know how devastating the effects of AIDS can be. But
what are the signs of the Human Immunodeficiency Virus, the virus that leads to AIDS? The fact is, a
person can have HIV for years without any signs developing. During this time they may look and feel
perfectly healthy. But through sexual intercourse, they can pass on the virus to more and more people.
Already there are many thousands of people in this country who are unaware that they have the virus.
Obviously the more people you sleep with the more chance you have of becoming infected. But having
fewer partners is only part of the answer. Safer sex also means using a condom, or alternatively,
having sex that avoids penetration. HIV is now a fact of life. And while infection may be impossible to
recognise, fortunately it is possible to avoid. AIDS. You're as safe as you want to be

Condom use or fewer partners?

Risk-reduction advice for the general public has mainly featured messages to use
a condom and restrict numbers of sexual partners. The selective emphasis on each
of these two main messages has varied between countries. On scientific grounds,
the condom message makes better preventive sense; there is epidemiological evidence that it is not primarily the number of sexual partners that creates risk of
infection, but rather the exchange of body fluids by direct routes. Therefore a
monogamous relationship with a partner already infected with HIV will not lessen
the risk of infection. Moreover, health educational messages most likely to meet
with compliance are those which provide practical advice on preventive action
(Blaxter 1989).

Yet although the condom message is likely to meet with greater compliance
than messages promoting abstinence and monogamy, it has led to political resistance in some countries; few have escaped controversy over the condom message.

Influences on the choice of primary risk-reduction message

Closeness to government
Mass media campaigns by definition have a high profile; the visibility of AIDS/HIV campaigns roused fears of public disapproval which prevented decisions being made on purely scientific grounds. Much depended on how closely the agency responsible for the campaigns was affiliated to the government. Where control of the public education programme was, initially, taken directly by the government, there has been a greater emphasis on the moral than the pragmatic message. By contrast, where the campaigns were initially removed from government control, the relevant ministry could distance itself from more controversial advertisements, and condoms could be promoted more freely.

Scale and nature of the epidemic
The degree of willingness to espouse the condom message was also determined by the scale of HIV and AIDS prevalence. The moral message could be subordinated to the more pragmatic concern where the need was felt to be urgent – hence the positive promotion of condom use in countries where opposition might have been anticipated, but where high rates of infection led to such qualms being quashed and resistance challenged. High prevalence rates warranted radical solutions, and this accounts for acceptance of the condom message in Switzerland and France.

The nature of the agency
Who had responsibility for executing the campaigns had important implications for the manner in which the campaigns were conducted, and the messages transmitted. Where responsibility for the interventions lay with professional public health agencies, who had firm convictions based on sound health educational principles and were confident enough to dictate the conditions to the commercial agencies contracted to execute advertisements, promotional activities, etc., the campaigns were more likely to choose realizable messages.

The social and historical background
This also influenced the content of messages. Traditional obstacles to the uptake of preventive messages had to be overcome. Where there was resistance to condom use, for example, campaigns needed to address this directly.

Degree of consensus/conflict
An important factor determining choice of messages was whether the environment was characterized by consensus or conflict. Too many factions with competing claims on the content of risk-reduction messages resulted in compromise, which led to mixed and confusing messages.

The message to be monogamous has the advantage of being compatible with traditional values while the pragmatic message to use a condom might be seen as undermining them, appearing to encourage casual sex. Whether the 'moral' message to practise monogamy and/or restrict numbers of partners, or the 'pragmatic' message to use a condom was promoted was determined largely by what was politically feasible rather than what was desirable in public health terms.

Even in countries with a liberal reputation, such as the Netherlands and Sweden, there has been some opposition to reliance on promoting the condom as a means of protection. The difference lay in the strength with which objections were expressed and the degree to which they influenced the programme. 'In many countries ... the moral agenda was more prominent than it was in others, and the conviction of those responsible that condoms should be promoted was weaker' (Kraft and Rise 1988). Some countries – France and Switzerland, for example – resolutely promoted condoms and dealt robustly with opposition. Some like the Netherlands took a more circumspect view that people needed to be able to make a personal choice from a range of messages. In Spain, promotion of condom use has been an important component of nearly every mass media campaign. At the beginning of the AIDS epidemic, this provoked moral and political debate but has since become accepted. In others – Belgium, for example – the choice was framed by fear of possible political reaction if too heavy a reliance was placed on the condom message, thereby seemingly condoning promiscuity.

France

The dominant message of primary prevention in the French campaign – that condoms should be part of everyday practice – was tailored specifically to the national situation, one in which there was widespread resistance to the use of condoms. The heavy reliance on condoms in the French campaign partly reflects the obstacles to be overcome in promoting condom use as a means of prevention.

Traditionally, attitudes towards abortion and contraception in France have been hostile and restrictive. This has partly been attributable to strict adherence to the ruling of the Vatican on these issues. In addition, because of the dramatic loss of life after the Franco-Prussian, then the First World War, a harsh law was enforced in 1920 making both contraception and abortion illegal. Police were empowered to enter pharmacies and confiscate all contraceptive devices except condoms, which were exempt because of the protection they provided against STDs.

Before the AIDS public education campaign, condoms had a poor image, could not be advertised on TV (until March 1987), and were little used; fewer than 10 per cent of the population in France used condoms before the AIDS epidemic. They were associated with illicit sex and prostitution, and seen as outmoded, socially embarrassing and as an interruption to lovemaking (BVA 1988). In addition they were expensive and difficult to obtain.

The first task was therefore seen as removing the obstacles to condom use and promoting their everyday use. A condom promotion campaign was launched in March 1989 by the Comité Français d'Education pour la Santé (CFES), together with the Agence Française de Lutte Contre le SIDA (AFLS), with the aim of improving the image of the condom and normalizing its usage. A commercial company was especially contracted to design a campaign in which condoms were promoted in an explicit and open way (**4.3**). Disassociation of

4.3 France, 1989, Agence Française de Lutte Contre le SIDA, Belier agency, TV, press. *Condoms protect against everything, everything except love*

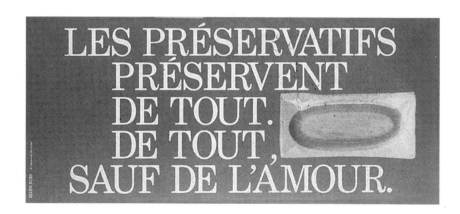

AIDS from the recommended action for risk reduction has been a distinctive feature of the French campaigns, and a radical departure from the strategy adopted in any other European country. Two campaigns have been developed along separate lines: one encourages solidarity and sympathy with AIDS sufferers, the other promotes condoms. Nowhere in the condom campaign is AIDS mentioned (solidarity campaigns are dealt with in Chapter 5). The separation of the two has enabled condoms to be promoted positively, thus avoiding being stigmatized by association with a fatal and sexually transmitted disease.

The attitude of the Catholic church in France towards representation of issues relating to sexuality or condoms has been ambivalent. Although those in the upper echelons of the established church have taken a predictably hard line on issues relating to public morality, ecclesiastical views at local level have been more moderate. When the first condom campaign was launched, the established church stressed the need for recourse to values of family life and fidelity as the only acceptable solution. The clear statement from the government supporting the condom message did much to defuse and dissipate opposition and persuaded the church to adopt a more liberal stance. Introducing the National Plan Against AIDS in 1989, the Minister of Solidarity, Health and Social Protection, Claude Evin, made clear reference to the central role of the condom in the campaign strategy: 'the only vaccine, the only mode of prevention is the condom' (*Le Monde* 18 April 1989) **(4.4)**.

Government endorsement of the campaigns did much to legitimize them. But this endorsement itself was made possible and indeed necessitated by the severity of the problem in France. The high prevalence of AIDS in France has been in large part responsible for overriding concerns about offending moral sensitivities.

4.4 France, 1988, *Le Monde.*
The Catholic authorities
condemn the use of condoms
France, 1989, *Le Monde.*
To prevent AIDS there's only
the condom or mutual fidelity

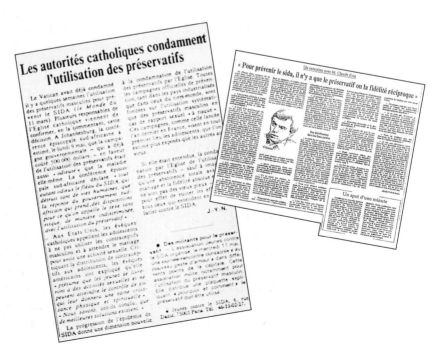

Switzerland

The Swiss 'Stop AIDS' campaign has similarly depended on a strong emphasis on condom use. Switzerland is also characterized by higher prevalence rates than in the rest of Europe, *the* highest in fact until 1990. The Swiss campaign is described more fully in Chapter 8, but has been distinctive for its use of the condom as a common symbol throughout. The circular rim of the condom (variously depicted as a moon over Swiss cities, the sun on holiday, the O of 'OK' and 'Tonight') and a slogan, 'Stop AIDS' (in which a condom forms the O) have unified the campaign to create a strong visual and verbal image (**4.5 and Plates 21–7**).

A unique feature of the Swiss campaigns has been the way in which messages are introduced cumulatively in each wave of advertising, adding to, rather than replacing, earlier messages. Each campaign wave has built on and reinforced the previous one. The first and the enduring message to be associated with the campaign against AIDS was the condom message. The primary message 'Condoms protect' was incorporated into slogans of the type: 'Everybody's speaking about AIDS so let's talk about condoms'; 'Make war on AIDS, make love with condoms', and so on. While the first wave (1986) of the 'Stop AIDS' campaign concentrated on the basic condom message, the second (1987) broadened attention to injecting drug use and the need for fidelity. In the third phase of the campaign (1987–88), messages relating to the ways in which HIV is not transmitted were added to the three permanent basic messages, and subsequently the solidarity message was included. Messages promoting condom use have continued to be a consistent feature of the Swiss campaign (Keller *et al.* 1994).

From the start the Swiss campaigns were marked by a considerable degree of consensus. Switzerland has no federal health ministry; issues relating to public health fall under the auspices of the Ministry of the Interior. A special group was created by the Ministry of the Interior and was given autonomous control over AIDS education campaigns, with little interference from the Ministry. The Federal Office of Public Health (FOPH), staffed by public health professionals, is responsible for the AIDS campaigns and there is no necessity on the part of FOPH to consult the Ministry, only to inform.

Acceptance of the Swiss 'Stop AIDS' campaign has been generally good and there has been very little opposition from either public, press, or church (Gromyko 1993). Catholic and Protestant authorities alike gave their official approval willingly. The subject of AIDS has been greatly aired in the Swiss media, and journalists and editors have generally been largely supportive of the Swiss campaign. Especially valuable collaboration was achieved with the TV and broadcasting media. In the principal edition of television news following the launch of the 'Stop AIDS' campaign, the presenter began his announcement on the subject of the press conference by taking a condom from his pocket, unrolling it on to his finger and declaring: 'Ladies and gentlemen, this little thing can save human life.' Politicians may not always have agreed with the manner in which campaigns were conducted, but they deferred to the professional judgement of those whose responsibility it was to execute them.

4.5 Switzerland, 1987, Federal Office of Public Health, cR Advertising agency, posters.

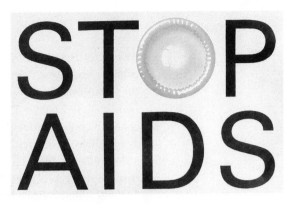

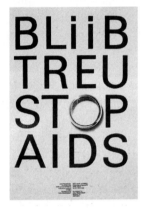

4.6 Switzerland, 1987, Federal Office of Public Health, cR Advertising agency, posters.
Stay faithful, Stop AIDS

Part of the credit for this harmonious state of affairs is attributable to efforts made by the FOPH to represent and take account of all interests. From the start of the campaign, representatives of the three main churches in Switzerland have met twice a year with the creative team, which has itself incorporated NGOs, media groups and representatives from local level. Prevention is to a large extent the responsibility of each canton, and policy varies greatly from one canton to another.

Yet even in Switzerland where the condom message has been the mainstay of the campaign, there have been campaigns stressing the need for fidelity. Misgivings about an exclusive reliance on the condom message prompted the introduction of a message which stressed fidelity. In June 1987, the second wave of the campaign featured two additional messages, 'Faithfulness protects' and 'Take care not to exchange syringes.' In the advertisement relating to fidelity, a wedding ring replaced the condom in the O of 'Stop AIDS' (**4.6**). This part of the campaign attracted a good deal of attention. While it found favour with those who objected to the exclusive emphasis on condoms, many others argued that it was not the role of the FOPH to issue imperatives and prescribe for moral lifestyles.

Subsequently, a new message was introduced combining the strategies of condom use and fidelity, designed to restrict its relevance to those who were already in an exclusive, monogamous relationship, and offering an explicit choice of preventive action: 'Stay faithful *or* use a condom.' This was incorporated into a poster and TV spot which featured the by now familiar condom shape as a wedding ring, and the message 'Faithfulness protects' was replaced by the slogan 'Stay faithful.' This may have succeeded in reaching a compromise, but by that time the controversy over the message had reached such a pitch as to have completely deflected attention from other important messages disseminated simultaneously, e.g. not to inject drugs. The modification was, in addition, neither well received nor well understood and although this information may have achieved some success in political terms, having lent some semblance of respectability to the campaign, the problem was that people paid closer attention to it than they did to other equally important messages (F Dubois-Arber, personal communication 1990). By the early 1990s, the approach to condom use and fidelity was clearly more pragmatic. Posters produced in 1993 took for granted the existence of non-exclusive sexual relationships (see **3.16–20**).

Sweden

Sweden provides an example of a country in which responsibility for the campaigns was closer to the government, in which there were numerous vested interest groups and in which the prevalence of AIDS placed it lower on the public agenda. Although Sweden has the reputation of being a country relatively free from sexual repression the official response to sexual issues has been marked by some apparent contradictions (Henriksson 1988). Some of these contradictions are apparent in an early TV spot (March 1987) in which a couple begin to make love, touching hands, caressing bodies to the sound of hearts beating in the background. The advertisement bears the logo of the AIDS Delegation. In each frame of the spot one partner in each couple moves on to a new partner and the text identifies each by name (**4.7**). The advertisement seems to bear all the hallmarks of the Swedish sexual stereotype: freedom in expressing scenes of lovemaking, naked bodies and sexual pleasure. Yet there is some ambiguity between the text and the visual imagery. Although the overt and explicit risk-reduction message in the endline is to use a condom, the covert and implicit message emerging from the images of partner change is to reduce numbers of partners. The voice-over further confuses by presenting several messages.

The state's National Audit Bureau or Riksrevisionsverket (RRV) was commissioned by the state AIDS Delegation to carry out an independent evaluation of its public education campaign. The result was an unusually open criticism by one government body of another. The RRV observed that the values conveyed by mass information did not correspond with those in the AIDS Delegation's objectives. The AIDS Delegation was charged with conveying a traditionally moralistic attitude to sex, recommending monogamy and sexual restraint: 'The underlying tone of the campaign is somewhat puritanical, with an abundance of warnings and negative statements about casual sex and sex abroad but very little positive information about safe sex. The tone is sometimes didactic' (RRV 1988). In the opinion

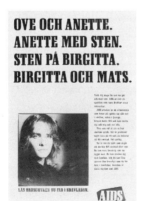

**OVE OCH ANETTE.
ANETTE MED STEN.
STEN PÅ BIRGITTA.
BIRGITTA OCH MATS.**

LÄS BROSCHYREN DU FÅR I BREVLÅDAN.

4.7 Sweden, March 1987, AIDS Delegation, Ted Bates agency, posters, TV, cinema.
Ove and Anette.
Anette with Sten.
Sten on top of Birgitta.
Birgitta and Mats.
Voice-over: *Think carefully what you do and with whom. AIDS is not a disease which only affects certain people. AIDS is caused by a virus which is threatening to spread further in the world, even in Sweden. The virus is called HIV and can be transmitted to you and me and every one of us. Thank goodness we know how the disease is transmitted; there is practically only one way of catching it. During intercourse. And now it's you who decides if you want to catch HIV or not. You can be careful who you sleep with. You can protect yourself with condoms and you can read the leaflet you will get through the letterbox. Knowledge is the protection against AIDS. Use a condom*

of the RRV, the campaigns contained confusing information and complicated messages; practical risk-avoidance advice would have been more effective.

Most of the messages in the campaign set out to increase knowledge about how the virus spreads, yet they were, on the whole, of a very general nature or offered indirect advice about where knowledge could be obtained, e.g. 'Ring AIDS-Jouren!', 'Be tested for HIV! Read the brochure!' Warnings and negative recommendations dominated the advice, the most common ones being against 'casual sex' (one-night stands, infidelity, prostitution, promiscuity, etc.): 'Promiscuity causes AIDS'; 'You can be more easily infected abroad'; 'Beware of drug users'; 'Beware of having sex with gay and bisexual men'; 'Take an HIV test because you are probably not infected. The test will reassure you.' Advertisements targeting young holidaymakers, for example, did not provide safer-sex advice, but instead recommended 'If you have been abroad and been to bed with someone that you really can't trust, you should go and get the test.' Condom use was a subsidiary message at this stage and was not actively promoted until 1990. In contrast to earlier campaigns, in 1993 the Federal Health Institute together with the Swedish Federation for Sex Education and the Swedish Federation for Gay and Lesbian Rights ran a campaign which not only aimed to encourage condom use but also provided information about their correct use and the choice of water-based lubricants.

United Kingdom

In the UK too, the earliest campaigns originated in the government, and the original government message was to 'stay with one faithful partner, and if this is not possible use a condom', emphasizing sexual exclusivity as the first option, with condom use as a failsafe. There too, diverse interests competed for claims on the content of advertisements, including health educators in the field anxious to see a realistic and theoretically sound message, and a particularly vociferous moral lobby which, in an adverse climate, succeeded in making ministers nervous about overexplicit messages. There were those, for example, on the moral Right who strongly protested against the condom as a message, claiming that it encouraged and condoned casual sex. The moral nature of the objection was often disguised

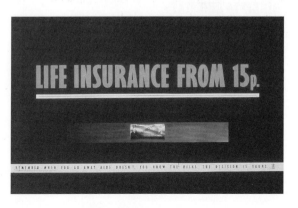

4.8 UK, summer 1988, Health Education Authority, BMP DDB Needham agency, posters. *Life insurance from 15p. Remember when you go away AIDS doesn't. You know the risks. The decision is yours*

4.9 UK, March–June 1988, Health Education Authority, TBWA agency, posters.

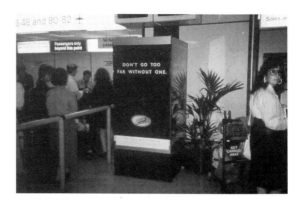

as concern for the reliability and efficacy of condoms as a means of protecting against HIV transmission.

The conflict between the views of different bodies and sections of society at times prevented clear messages of positive emerging. The simpler statements of some later advertisements won awards and helped to legitimize this approach (**4.8, 9**).

The Netherlands

The Dutch campaign has been characterized by an emphasis on freedom of choice backed up by good information. Human rights and liberties play a dominant part in Dutch society, and the starting point of messages relating to the Dutch campaign was that people should take responsibility for themselves. The approach has been pragmatic rather than moralistic, aiming for what is feasible and achievable, in the belief that the most effective approach will be one which stimulates people to adapt their lifestyle, rather than requiring them to change it drastically. In this sense, it takes reality as a starting point, asking people to use a condom if they are not monogamous, to clean or avoid sharing needles if they inject drugs. Campaigns have attempted to create a positive social environment for AIDS and STD prevention and to adopt a supportive rather than a repressive approach to sexuality.

The Dutch campaign aimed to pre-empt any criticism that promoting condom use increases sexual promiscuity. Restricting the campaigns to the promotion of condom use might have antagonized some people and would, consequently, have reduced the effectiveness of the various campaigns. Safer sex in general was promoted, not simply condom use. Roughly half of the messages in the Netherlands were about condom use, the other half about ways of having safer sex. This included postponing sexual intercourse, restricting sexual contact to a mutually monogamous relationship, and practising only non-penetrative sexual techniques.

Yet again, despite the permissive climate and the efforts made to defuse any opposition, the condom message has come under attack from a number of factions. The first condom campaign, by the STD Foundation, was contentious. Some church groups opposed the condom message as the predominant one on the grounds that it might be seen to be encouraging casual sex, while homosexual groups also objected to a reliance on the condom message, believing that hetero-sexuals should be encouraged, like gay men, to explore other ways of having safer sex and to avoid an exclusive focus on penetrative sex.

Have condom campaigns had any effect?

Against this background, it is interesting to note the degree to which the choice of messages officially transmitted might appear to have influenced the public's per-ception of risk-reduction strategies – whether the Swiss public, for example, were more or less likely than the British or Swedish to cite condom usage as the primary risk-reduction strategy.

An attempt has been made in Figures 4.1 and 4.2 to compare responses in terms of condom use and numbers of partners in those countries for which data are available.

The data on sexual relationships do not lend themselves readily to direct comparisons, but they do give some indication of the scale of changes over time in different countries. As Figure 4.1 shows, more or less irrespective of the country, there is little change in reports of sexual partnerships. By contrast, figures for con-dom use (Figure 4.2) show some remarkable achievements over the period of most intensive campaigning, 1986–89. The most noticeable change in sexual behaviour is an increase in condom use among those at risk. Claims of increased condom use are more dramatic than those with respect to restrictions in numbers of partners. Furthermore, while it is clear (as far as we can tell from the data) that higher rates of condom use seem to have been achieved in some countries than in others, this is not the case for reductions in numbers of partners, exclusivity in relationships, reductions in the prevalence of casual sex, etc.

The limited evidence available seems to suggest that little success has been achieved in persuading people to limit the numbers of partners or to restrict them to one. There is evidence, at least from claimed behaviour, that the risk-reduction strategy taken up by larger numbers was that of condom use and, further, that those countries in which this message was stated unequivocally and with authority, and where the confusion of mixed messages was avoided, seem to have been more successful than countries in which this was not the case.

Furthermore, some interesting patterns emerge from graphical representa-tion of these data. It seems as if those countries in which AIDS public education has maintained a constant presence and a continuous flow, e.g. Switzerland, are characterized by a smoother and more consistent profile for condom usage than do those in which campaigns have been characterized more by peaks and troughs of campaign activity, e.g. the UK. Despite the fragility and limitations of the data and the frustrations of dealing with results from differently designed and conducted surveys, it is difficult to avoid the conclusion that those campaigns which set out single-mindedly to increase condom use, and in which those responsible for pub-lic education were most resolute in countering resistance, seem to have made greater progress in achieving their goals than have countries in which there was a greater degree of hesitancy over the condom message.

Figure 4.1 Respondents reporting multiple partners in recent time period

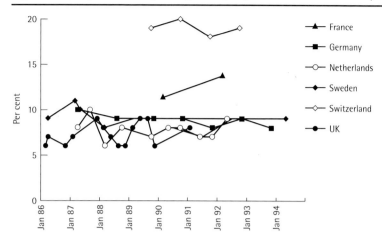

France *In the past twelve months, how many different sexual partners have you had? (write down the number)*

per cent writing down more than one partner in last twelve months

n = 916 (1990), n = 1,927 (1992) (18–69 years)

Germany *During the course of a year it is quite possible that one has more than one partner, and many people sometimes have a casual fling which then becomes intimate. In the last twelve months, have you had more than one partner with whom you were intimate, I mean, with whom you had sexual intercourse?*

per cent answering 'yes'

n = 2,295 (16–65 years)

The Netherlands *In the past six months, have you had sex with a steady partner only or also with other people?*

per cent answering 'with steady partner and other(s)' or 'casual partners only'

n = 1,015 (15–45 years)

Sweden *Have you had more than one sexual partner during the last six months?*

per cent answering 'yes'

n = 2,369 (16–44 years)

Switzerland *Have you changed steady partners once or met a new partner in the course of the year?*

per cent answering 'yes'

n = 2,602 (17–45 years)

UK *In the last twelve months, how many men/women have you had sexual intercourse with? Please include every man/woman you have had sexual intercourse with in the last twelve months, even if only once.*

per cent reporting two or more partners of opposite sex in last year

n = 1,963 per quarter (16 years and over)

(Source: Matthews *et al.* 1995)

Figure 4.2 Condom use for respondents reporting multiple partners

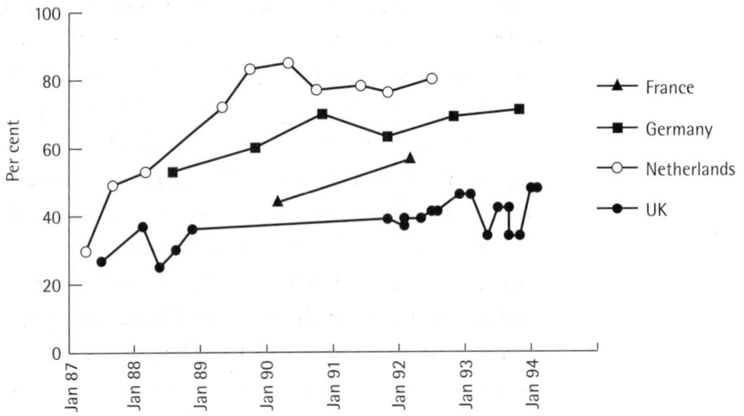

France *In the last twelve months have you used condoms?*
per cent of multipartners answering 'yes'
n = 105 (1990), n = 279 (1992) (18–69 years having more than one sexual partner in last twelve months)

Germany *In the recent past, how often have you used a condom when having sexual intercourse?*
per cent of multipartners answering 'always', 'often' or 'occasionally'
n = approx. 165 (16–65 years with more than one sexual partner in last twelve months)

The Netherlands *How often have you used condoms in the last six months?*
per cent of multipartners answering 'always', 'almost always', 'sometimes' or 'rarely'
n = approx. 75 (15–45 years non-monogamous in last six months)

UK *Was a condom used at all?* [last sexual experience]
per cent of multipartners answering 'yes'
n = approx. 130 per quarter (16 years and over with two or more sexual partners in last twelve months)

(Source: Matthews *et al.* 1995)

References

Blaxter, M 1989 *AIDS behavioural research,* paper prepared for the Economic and Social Research Council, UK (unpublished)

BVA 1988 *Le SIDA connaissances et attitudes. Premiers resultats,* appendix of press pack, Paris: Ministère de la Solidarité, Santé et Protection Sociale and Comité Français d'Education pour la Santé

Gromyko, A 1993 Evaluation of the Swiss national programme on AIDS prevention and control, *Social and Preventive Medicine* 38 (2); 96–104

Henriksson, B 1988 *Social democracy or societal control – a critical analysis of Swedish AIDS policy*, Stockholm, Sweden: Glacio Bokforlag

Keller, A, F Wasserfallen, F Dubois-Arber 1994 *Seven years of promotion of condom use in the framework of the national Stop AIDS campaign: experiences and results in Switzerland*, paper presented at 'AIDS in Europe – the behavioural aspect'. European conference on methods and results of psycho-social AIDS research, 26–29 September 1994, Berlin, Germany

Kraft, P and J Rise 1988 AIDS – sources of information and public opinion in Norway 1986, *NIPH Annals* **11** (1); 19–28

Matthews, M, K Wellings and E Kupek 1995 *AIDS/HIV knowledge, attitude and behaviour surveys in the European Community (general population): a report to the European Commission*, Luxembourg: DGV

Riksrevisionsverket (RRV) 1988 *Informationskampanjen om HIV/AIDS – samhällsinfomration som styrmedel* [The information campaign about HIV/AIDS – national information as a means of direction], Stockholm, Sweden: Regeringsuppdrag

5 Influencing the social climate: solidarity campaigns

In addition to *primary prevention* aimed at reducing the prevalence of new HIV infection, an important feature of AIDS prevention has been the formulation of messages relating to *secondary prevention*, aimed at enabling those with the virus to avoid infecting others and to postpone serious illness (Shernoff and Palacios-Jimenez 1986). In the case of AIDS/HIV, a communicable disease, the boundary between these two is blurred since advice needs to be given both to those already infected on how to avoid passing on the virus, and to those uninfected on how to protect themselves.

Mobilizing support for those who are ill has been a characteristic feature of AIDS prevention. In the case of most other infectious diseases the need for such a task does not arise. But the behaviours associated with HIV infection are often stigmatized and the affected groups marginalized in society.

In this context a key challenge has been to fight the prejudice which threatened the success of preventive and therapeutic activities. In many countries, AIDS has been virtually synonymous with the term 'gay plague' in the public imagination; the retributive way in which the disease has been seen by some has suggested that this was a disease which was visited on deserving minorities (Wellings 1988; Pollak 1992).

There is evidence that proximity encourages greater empathy (Moatti *et al.* 1990). In high prevalence countries, knowing someone who is ill is likely to prompt empathetic responses. But in countries where AIDS prevalence is too low for the likelihood of knowing someone affected to be high, the media can play an important role in putting a human face on the disease.

Rationale

The presence and severity of discrimination against various groups in society is a major 'risk factor' for HIV transmission (Mann 1993). In addition to humanitarian concerns, there are other issues which threaten the success of preventive efforts. First, where a disease is associated with retribution and victim blaming, there is a danger of public resistance to funds being spent on it. Second, where prejudice and intolerance exist there is a tendency for groups to be driven underground, making prevention and treatment more difficult. Unlike chronic diseases – which require preventive efforts only by the person not yet affected – AIDS is a communicable disease; preventive action needs to be taken both by those not yet affected and by those already affected. Research shows high levels of intolerance towards those affected.

Figure 5.1 'I would not like to have people with AIDS as neighbours'

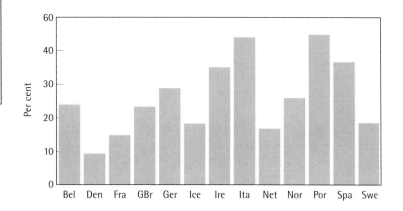

(Source: Barker *et al.* 1990)

The campaigns

In several countries campaigns have been conducted with the aim of changing the social climate in order to facilitate prevention work, and to create a sympathetic environment for the care of the sick. Campaigns designed to increase empathy with, and support for, people with HIV have been carried out in Norway, Spain, Italy, Switzerland, Sweden, France, the Netherlands, Germany, Portugal and in Iceland (see **5.1–7** for some examples). The approach taken has, to some extent, reflected the national situation. In those countries in which prevalence rates are high enough for the problem to be visible, it has been possible to appeal to the need for universal concern because of the proximity of the problem. For example in France, the endline for the 1989 and 1990 TV spots was 'AIDS: any one of us can come up against it.' In some countries irrational concerns about contagion have been addressed directly, as for example in the Netherlands (**5.8–11**). Some have attempted to put a human face on suffering, inviting identification: one of the endlines for a Norwegian AIDS Association (an NGO) poster was 'The loneliness is what kills me' (**5.12–15**). Direct pleas from those affected for affection and attention have characterized other campaigns, for example in Germany (**5.16–20**).

5.1 Italy, 1990–91, Ministry of Health/Commissione Nazionale per la Lotta Contro l'AIDS, Armando Testa agency, magazines.
Encouraging solidarity was a major feature of all Italian campaigns. The second, running from 1990–91, like the first aimed to be anti-discriminatory. Campaign materials included magazine advertisements featuring a group of well-heeled people at work with the caption 'One of these people is seropositive. Their colleagues can rest easy.' The theme was continued into the third campaign in 1991–92, which featured the crowd scene **(5.2)**.

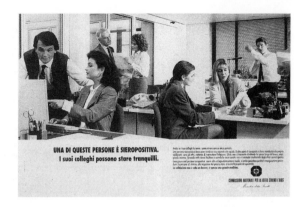

UNA DI QUESTE PERSONE È SIEROPOSITIVA.
I suoi colleghi possono stare tranquilli.

5.2 Italy, 1991–92, Ministry of Health/Commissione Nazionale per la Lotta Contro l'AIDS, Young & Rubicam agency, magazines, TV.
This is one of the most striking Italian solidarity advertisements, featuring a crowd of people with linked arms walking forwards, united under the slogan 'AIDS. The wish to stop it is contagious.'

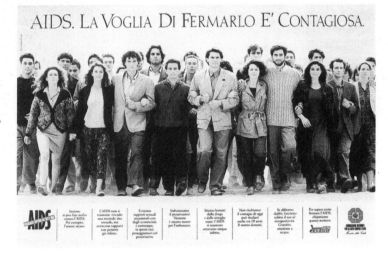

AIDS. LA VOGLIA DI FERMARLO E' CONTAGIOSA.

5.3 Portugal, 1993, Abraço, posters, leaflets.
Make the first move
AIDS is not transmitted by friendship
The Portuguese NGO Abraço took a more didactic approach in this poster, providing guidelines on how to treat those affected.

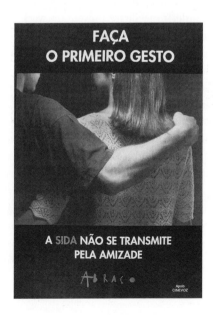

FAÇA
O PRIMEIRO GESTO

A SIDA NÃO SE TRANSMITE
PELA AMIZADE

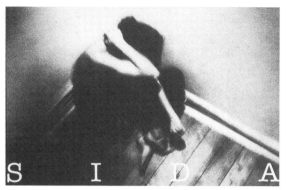

5.4

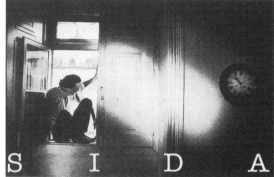

5.5

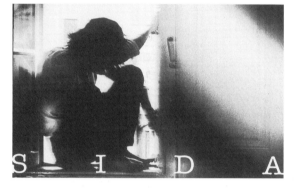

5.6

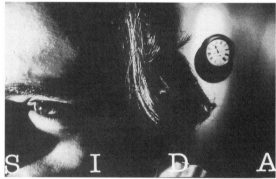

5.7

5.4–7 Portugal, 1993, Comissão Nacional Luta Contra a SIDA, Ministério de Saúde, posters, press, postcards, radio.

These examples from the Portuguese solidarity campaign show the negative effects of discrimination, in terms of

loneliness and isolation, on sufferers. The caption on the reverse side of this postcard reads '*Solidarity...why not?*'

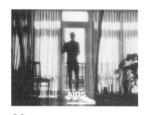

5.8

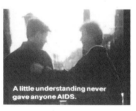

5.9

5.10

5.11

5.8–11 The Netherlands, 1990–92, NCAC, TV.

A little understanding

A young man gets up from his bed, looks at his alarm clock, goes up to the window and stares outside. Next he sits in a chair and starts reading a newspaper. After a while he

puts it down, puts on his clothes and goes out on the street. Two neighbours watching him as he walks downstairs look worried and frightened and go inside as soon as they see him. As he walks out on the street, another man comes up to him and puts

his hand on his shoulder, giving him a sympathetic look.

Voice-over: *AIDS. You can't do much against it. But we can reassure sufferers they are not alone. A little understanding never gave anyone AIDS*

This Dutch example adopts an

alternative approach, showing the effect of both rejection and acceptance. Here advice to extend warmth and companionship to those affected is combined with information that HIV is not contracted through everyday contact.

Jeg er hiv-smittet.

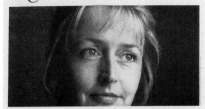

Gi meg en klem.

Dette er historien om Hanne.

Hanne er 26 år, hun er ugift, har fast jobb og tjener omtrent det samme som folk flest.

Ikke er hun sprøytenarkoman og ikke er hun prostituert. Har hatt verken flere eller færre seksualpartnere enn andre. Kunne ha vært hvem som helst.

Men Hanne har hiv. Ble smittet for et år siden. Deler skjebne med 2–3.000 andre her i landet.

Det er ikke mange som vet "det". Bare de aller nærmeste vennene. Og kjæresten.

Vet ikke om hun tør å fortelle det til flere heller. Redd for hvordan de vil reagere. Redd for å bli alene, miste venner, familie. Det er så mange som er redde for hiv og aids fordi de ikke vet nok. De tror mye og har hørt enda mer.

Hadde hudkontakt vært smittsomt, hadde mange rundt Hanne vært smittet for lengst.

Men Hanne er fremdeles Hanne. Med de samme behov, tanker og følelser som før.

Er det så vanskelig å skjønne?

Er det?

Omsorg smitter ikke.

5.12

Er det slik vi vil løse aids-problemet?

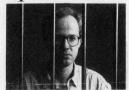

I mange land merker hiv-positive og aids-pasienter en økende grad av diskri- minering.

I ett tilfelle brant hjemmet til tre barn ned. Naboene hadde tent på fordi barna var hiv-positive.

En domstol i USA har nektet en seks år gammel jente adgang til skolen dersom hun ikke plasseres i eget bur, to ganger to og en halv meter.

I Norge har en professor foreslått å tato- vere alle hiv-positive i lysken.

"La oss få dem vekk!" Vi kjenner stem- mene. Mytene innhenter oss.

Det er ikke sant. At en hiv-smittet kollega

eller venn er en trussel mot din helse.

Det er ikke sant. At det er farlig å gi en hiv-smittet en klem.

Sannheten er at din mangel på kunnskap og vilje til forståelse, påfører med- mennesker en smerte som nesten ikke er til å bære.

Men heldigvis finnes det også lyspunkter. Norsk Høyesterett har nylig fastslått at hiv-smitte ikke er oppsigelsesgrunn i arbeidslivet. Det er likevel svært få av de 2–3.000 hiv-positive i Norge som tør stå frem av frykt for å miste jobb, venner og familie.

Hvordan ville du reagere hvis en av dem var en venn, kollega, bror eller søster?

Omsorg smitter ikke.

5.13

Det er ensomheten som dreper meg.

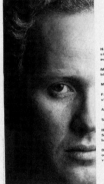

Han hadde fått vite det for et par år siden. Hiv-positiv. Angsten hadde nesten ødelagt ham.

Men han behøvde jo ikke bli syk. Ikke alle ble det.

Medisiner. De arbeidet med nye medisiner.

Familie. Venner. Livredde. Han var stemplet.

Alene.

Så forferdelig alene.

Han trengte noen. En å snakke med. Snakke ordentlig. Noe å holde i. En varm hånd.

Det var det viktigste. At noen brydde seg om ham. Tenkte på ham. At han slapp å være alene med alle tankene.

Omsorg smitter ikke.

5.14

Dette barnet hadde aids. Men det døde av mangel på hudkontakt.

Italia. September 1984.

Hiv-smittede barn. Noen hadde fått blod- overføring, andre var smittet i mors liv.

Antonio ble lagt på isolat. Akkorat som alle de andre. Avstengt fra alt og alle. Sykehuspersonalet var livredde.

Hva smittet? Tårer? Urin? Hudkontakt? Man visste ikke sikkert. Man tok ingen sjanser.

Masker. Hansker. Store hvite frakker. Barnehud mot steril plast.

Overlatt til seg selv. Uten å skjønne

hvorfor ingen tok på ham. Hvorfor ingen ga ham en klem, strøk ham over håret, holdt ham inntil seg.

I 1984 visste man ikke så mye. Så han døde. Alene. Akkorat som alle de andre. Antagelig altfor tidlig.

Norge. Høsten 1988. 37 barn og unge er smittet av hiv-viruset.

"Jeg er ikke syk," sa en av dem. "Men i kroppen min finnes et virus som sover. Medisinene skal få viruset til å sove enda bedre. Kanskje sovner det for alltid."

Kanskje.

Omsorg smitter ikke.

5.15

Norway, 1988, Norwegian AIDS Association, posters.

5.12 *I'm infected with HIV. Give me a hug*

5.13 *Is this the way we want to solve the AIDS problem?*

5.14 *The loneliness is what kills me*

5.15 *This child had AIDS. But it died from lack of physical contact*

One of the earliest attempts to promote solidarity was made by the Norwegian AIDS Association. The text of the advertisements draws attention to the problems facing those with HIV and AIDS, for example loneliness and deprivation of physical contact.

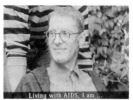

5.16

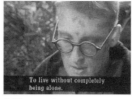

To live without completely
being alone.

5.17

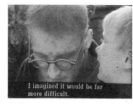

I imagined it would be far
more difficult.

5.18

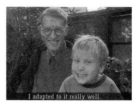

I adapted to it really well.

5.19

5.16–19 Germany, 1992, BZgA,
TV, cinema.

Neighbourhood help

'Hi, sweetheart.'

'There'

'Ready'

'Yes'

'Living with AIDS, I am...so to
say, connected to it, come what
may and...For me it was

*important when I suddenly
became seriously ill...to find a
way back to everyday life. That
somebody is there. Simply to
talk to. To live without
completely being alone. I must
keep in touch with people. I
imagined it would be far more
difficult. I adapted to it really
well.'*

If you have any questions
about AIDS, please call us.
The personal telephone
conversation will name
advisory centres in your area.
Don't give AIDS a chance

The testimonial approach was
also successfully used in this
German campaign to put a

human face on suffering and to
show how compassion could
help sufferers live with AIDS.
Solidarity was encouraged by
showing the need for
acceptance in the community
and authenticity was assured by
avoiding the use of actors.

5.20 Germany, 1990–92, BZgA,
posters, TV.
Sick people belong to us

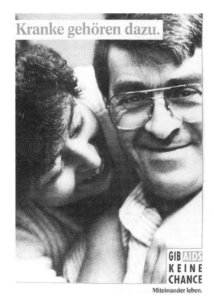

Kranke gehören dazu.

GIB AIDS
KEINE
CHANCE
Miteinander leben.

Preventing stigmatization

In addition to countering the effects of social stigmatization and discrimination, those responsible for carrying out public education have had to take care to ensure that the preventive interventions themselves were not discriminatory. Where a discriminatory tone did creep into the intervention it was generally the result of inadequate pre-testing of the campaign component.

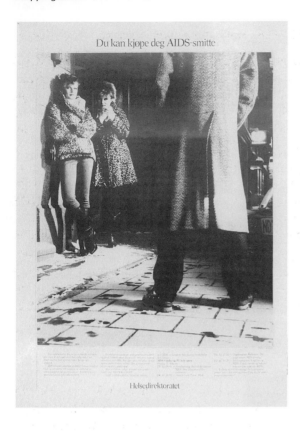

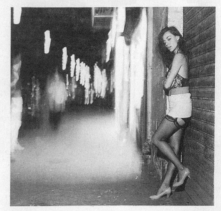

5.21 Norway, 1990–91, Directorate of Health, posters (abandoned).
You can buy yourself AIDS infection

5.22 Sweden, autumn 1987, AIDS Delegation, Ted Bates agency,
posters, press, magazines.
Today she has had sex with fourteen men – without a condom

    Some subgroups of the population have presented particular difficulties in terms of avoiding stigmatization. A comparison of the representation of prostitutes in the Swedish and Norwegian campaigns illustrates this. It is now accepted that prostitutes do not present as large a risk to others as they face themselves in their trade generally, often as a result of their regular partner's drug-using habit which they are working to fund (Day and Ward 1990). Although Norway and Sweden are renowned for enlightened attitudes to sexuality, in both countries the agencies responsible for the advertisements produced images of prostitutes as predatory and dangerous **(5.21, 22)**.

    The Norwegian Directorate of Health, having a high degree of autonomy over the campaigns, managed to block distribution of the posters, albeit belatedly, and replace them with others that were more in keeping with the epidemiological evidence. In Sweden, by contrast, the advertisements – which gave the impression that prostitutes were a potent reservoir of infection – were disseminated without interference from the state AIDS Delegation, the government agency responsible for coordinating the campaigns.

The French testimonial campaign 1989–93: a case study in promoting solidarity

France is one of the few countries where a political party has tried to exploit AIDS and the fear of becoming infected in order to reach its objectives. The extreme right National Front has blamed both non-European immigrants and indigenous ethnic minority groups for the spread of HIV infection, as a means of attempting to stop immigration. 'SIDA-toriums' have been advocated, where those with AIDS could be incarcerated; people with AIDS have been dubbed '*Sidaique*' – a pun on *Judaique*. The free distribution of AZT in hospitals has resulted in an influx of people from abroad seeking medication, with further potential for inflaming prejudice. One in five French people favoured isolation of AIDS patients in 1987 (Moatti *et al.* 1988).

As a result, clear anti-discriminatory measures have been implemented in France. Explicit official reference to any possible connection with African communities has been avoided. In December 1987, it was ruled that seropositivity could not be used as the basis for refusal to authorize residence in France for aliens. Legislation has been introduced prohibiting all kinds of AIDS/HIV-related discrimination.

Formative evaluation

The Comité Français d'Education pour la Santé (CFES) commissioned the BVA Institute to carry out a survey (BVA 1988) with a national sample of 1,000 people aged 18 to 49 in order to target AIDS information more precisely and, together with the results of qualitative research, help shape the communication strategy. The BVA survey demonstrated that the French were relatively tolerant towards people with AIDS/HIV. However, although as many as 94 per cent said they would work with a person with AIDS, a smaller proportion (though still a large majority – 84 per cent) said they would eat with one, but only 64 per cent would leave their children with someone with AIDS.

As the number of people affected has increased over time, it has proved possible to use the stories of those directly affected to transmit the need for empathy. The testimonial approach was used in the French campaign to encourage solidarity, tolerance and caring by showing the response of real individuals (or that of friends or family members affected) to direct experience of illness. Authenticity was assured by avoiding the use of actors. Finding people who were willing to expose themselves in this way (especially women) sometimes proved difficult. There was no mention in any of the films of how the virus was contracted so that viewers were less likely to distance themselves from the situation. The French AIDS information campaigns have separated primary and secondary preventive messages by presenting the solidarity message independently from messages promoting condoms (**5.23–5**).

The testimonial campaign on TV was followed a year later by a poster campaign in which common doubts and concerns of those affected were articulated and reassurance sought. For example, a photograph of the face of a small boy was

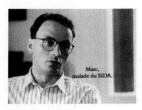

5.23

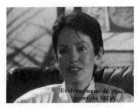

5.24

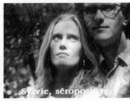

5.25

France, June and November 1989, June 1990, AFLS, TV.
5.23 *Marc, ill with AIDS*
5.24 *Evelyne, whose brother Pascal died of AIDS*
5.25 *Sylvie, HIV positive*

June 1989 Epernay, Marne
Marc, ill with AIDS: *I never imagined I would be seropositive at the age of 26. We were going out, we didn't think about being careful, we were having fun, we just wanted to have fun. Every month since 1986 I've been seeing a doctor and he helps me a lot, especially because he's young. It helps when you have someone in front of you who understands, who helps you to keep up morale when you need it. It's really important to help someone who has AIDS; you can save his life by sustaining his morale.*

Voice-over: *For the prevention of the illness, and the understanding of those who are ill, we fight against AIDS. AIDS: any one of us can come up against it.*

November 1989
Juvisy-sur-Orge
Evelyne: *Pascal was my brother. When I learned that Pascal had AIDS I refused to believe it, I thought that it could happen to other people but not to Pascal. The day after, I went to the hospital, and I told him that I knew. He gave me a glazed look and I could tell he was afraid of my reaction. I took him in my arms and he understood that we were going to help him and that we were going to fight with him against the illness which we did up to the very end. There are so many things we can't express.*

Voice-over: *For the prevention of the illness, and the understanding of those who are ill, we fight against AIDS. AIDS: any one of us can come up against it.*

June 1990
Sylvie, seropositive: *In 1986 I learnt I was seropositive status. I thought that was it, I thought I was going to die, I was going to die, I would die tomorrow. Now I've been under treatment for over a year and I am now feeling much better. At first I didn't want to talk about it – I was too scared about what people would say about me.*

Husband: *We went through difficult moments and what saved us was being able to talk about it with people who understood. For example, – who helped us a lot, and who didn't overdramatize things.*

Woman: *And there is also Georgette, I can call her any time of the day or night if I am not feeling well, she is always present in the difficult moments to help me.*

Older woman: *That's what friendship is. And why shouldn't I kiss her because she has AIDS. You have to love people the way they are, with or without their illness, it doesn't change anything.*

Husband: *It is true that the illness, we don't think about it the way we used to, and that is something very recent, it comes with time, and thanks to all the people who are here around us.*

Voice-over: *Today in France, thousands of people are seropositive, or ill from AIDS, we can help them to live.*

For the prevention of the illness, and the understanding of those who are ill, you help fight against AIDS. AIDS: any one of us can come up against it.

captioned 'If I am seropositive, will you play with me? Say yes'; other posters featured captions such as 'If I am seropositive will you stay? Say yes' (photograph of man) and 'If I am seropositive, will we still meet at the canteen? Say yes' (photograph of a schoolgirl's face). Similar themes featured in the 1993 solidarity poster campaign **(5.26, 27)**.

France, 1993, AFLS, posters.

5.26 *You wouldn't like to stay alone when things aren't working out. Why should someone who's seropositive be any different from you?*

5.27 *You expect your friends to listen to you. Why should someone who's seropositive be any different from you?*

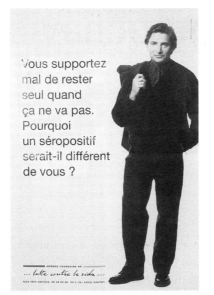

Vous supportez mal de rester seul quand ça ne va pas. Pourquoi un séropositif serait-il différent de vous ?

5.26

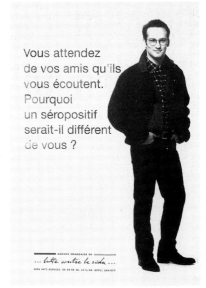

Vous attendez de vos amis qu'ils vous écoutent. Pourquoi un séropositif serait-il différent de vous ?

5.27

References

Barker, D, L Halman and A Vloet 1990 *European values study 1981–1990 summary report*, London: European Values Group

BVA 1988 *Le SIDA connaissances et attitudes. Premiers resultats, appendix of press pack*, Paris: Ministère de la Solidarité, Santé et Protection Sociale and Comité Français d'Education pour la Santé

Day, S and H Ward 1990 The Praed Street Project: a cohort of prostitute women in London. In M Plant (ed.) *AIDS, drugs and prostitution*, London: Routledge, pp. 61–75

Mann, J 1993 *AIDS policy in evolution: learning from experience,* report of the 1993 Conference of European Community Parliamentarians on HIV/AIDS, April 1993, British All-Party Parliamentary Group on AIDS, London

Moatti, J P, L Manesse, C Le Gales, J P Pagès, F Fagani 1988 Social perception of AIDS in the general public: a French study, *Health Policy* **9**; 1–8

Moatti, J P, W Dab, M Pollak, P Quesnel, A Anes, N Beltzer, C Ménard and C Serrand 1990 Les attitudes et comportements des Français face au SIDA, *La Recherche* **223** (July–August); 888–95

Shernoff, M and L Palacios-Jimenez 1986 Three levels of prevention, *Focus: A Review of AIDS Research* **2** (1); 3

Pollak, M 1992 *AIDS: a problem for sociological research*, London: Sage Publications, pp. 24–35

Wellings, K 1988 Perceptions of risk – media treatment of AIDS. In P Aggleton and H Homans (eds) *Social aspects of AIDS*, London: The Falmer Press, pp. 83–105

6 Motivating behaviour change

Using emotions to motivate

The persuasive impact of communication is determined by emotional as well as cognitive responses (Dubé *et al.* 1993a,b). The two most commonly used emotions in AIDS campaigns have been fear and humour.

Using fear to motivate

Early prevention campaigns which relied on fear to motivate behaviour change emphasized the mortal consequences of AIDS, underlining the cataclysmic scale of the disaster and the dire threat to humanity. The imagery used to convey this was clearly death related rather than life enhancing. The juxtaposition of images of death with those of sexuality was particularly dramatic, since it combined two major taboos in western society.

The European campaign most associated with the use of fear was the 'Don't die of ignorance' campaign in the UK, which ran from autumn 1986 to spring 1987. The TV advertisements used in this campaign used images of death, such as lilies and tombstones, and juxtaposed them with subliminal images of sexuality – erupting volcanoes and nails being hammered (into coffins). Such visual imagery left the viewer in no doubt that the epidemic had the potential to be a momentous problem – the iceberg as yet only partially visible but about to emerge, the volcano about to erupt. In both cases the physical and natural worlds were used as metaphors for the social world, suggesting disruption to the social order mirrored and paralleled in the natural disasters (**6.1, 2** and **Plates 1–3**). No subsequent campaigns in the UK have used fear in this way.

Although the UK examples have been widely cited, and criticized (Sherr 1987; Lund and Uldall Jepson 1992) as the prime illustrative examples of this genre, they were not unique in Europe. Early campaigns in other countries were also characterized by some reliance on the use of fear. In the Dutch campaigns, the symbolism was less dramatic but the idea of death was conveyed by the sudden death of a promiscuous bee in the 1987 TV advertisement (and the leaflet associated with this which was delivered to every household), and in the progressive snuffing out of candles in the 1989 TV advertisement (**6.3–6**).

Many countries in Europe stated before the start of the campaigns their

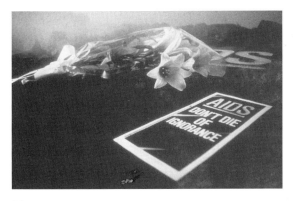

6.1

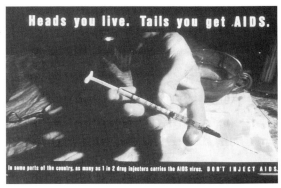

6.2

6.1 UK, autumn 1986–spring 1987, DoH, TBWA agency, posters, TV.

6.3, 4 The Netherlands, spring 1987, National Committee on AIDS Control, posters, press, brochures, TV.
There is a disease which spreads though sex, so if you don't always have sex with the same partner, you are at risk. It is an incurable disease, and its name is AIDS. This brochure tells you how you can prevent/avoid AIDS. Stop AIDS

6.2 UK, 1986, DoH, TBWA agency, posters.
The use of fear in UK advertisements can be contrasted with the more life-enhancing approach used in examples **6.7** and **6.8** from Portugal and France.

6.5, 6 The Netherlands, 1989, NCAC, TV.

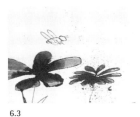

6.3

6.4

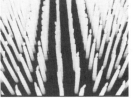

6.5

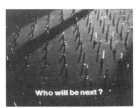

6.6

6.7 Portugal, 1992, Abraço (NGO), McCann Erikson/JM agency, posters.
Saves lives
In Portuguese 'salva vidas' is the name given to a lifebuoy.

6.8 France, 1988, CFES, posters.
AIDS. For the love of life...

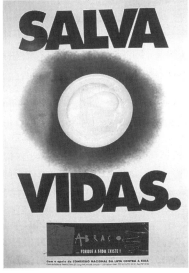

6.7

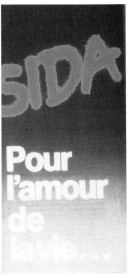

6.8

antipathy to the use of fear. In Switzerland, France and Norway, for example, it was stated explicitly as part of early campaign philosophy that fear would form no part of the strategy (see also **6.7, 8**). This was particularly characteristic of those countries in which responsibility for the interventions lay with professional public health agencies who had strong, firm convictions based on sound health educational principles, and were confident enough to dictate the conditions to the commercial agencies contracted to design advertisements.

Much hinged on whether there was consensus in the creative team. In Switzerland and in Norway, teams of experts from relevant disciplines and areas of experience could agree on what the interventions should aim to achieve. Differences of opinion between the ministries and public health professionals did occur, but the latter always had the ultimate right of sanction. In less harmonious teams, health educators found it difficult to accept the philosophy of those from a public relations or advertising background, and vice versa. The resultant compromise was revealed in advertisements containing confusing and mixed messages.

Rationale for the use of fear

In the face of a need to prevent a deadly disease, public education approaches using dire threats and warnings have intuitive appeal. A typical strategy in market research is to ask consumers what sort of approach they themselves think should be adopted in order to motivate the public. A plea for advertisements with a strong emotional charge, generating high levels of fear and anxiety, is commonplace. Formative research carried out to guide strategy for the early UK Health Education Authority AIDS campaigns found consumers to be firm in their views on the need for such an approach; in focus-group discussions and personal interviews consumers regularly called for illustration of sick people in hospital beds as the necessary images to alert people to the dangers of infection (J Hitchins, personal communication 1990). One of the most vexed questions around the pre-testing issue is what credence should be given to the views of consumers themselves on the style and tone of advertisements.

With regard to the shock-horror approach, the consumer's view is more in line with the old medical model of health education, which relied heavily on the generation of high levels of fear, than the more recent 'lifestyles approach' which aims to be more positive and less punitive. The charge might be levelled that it is paternalistic to claim that the health educator is privy to some wisdom about the motivations of individuals which they themselves do not possess, but it seems reasonable to assume that empirically based studies of human motivation may generate more reliable insights than the top-of-head responses of consumers. Consumers may be enticed by the intuitive appeal of fear-provoking images, but are often ignorant of the actual effects achieved by such approaches.

Overstating the case, as in the early heavily fear-dominated campaigns in the UK and in Australia, for example, has resulted in interventions which are difficult to follow up, and also confusing for the public when the most pessimistic predictions are clearly not observable.

Figure 6.1 HIV antibody tests in England and Wales January 1985–June 1988

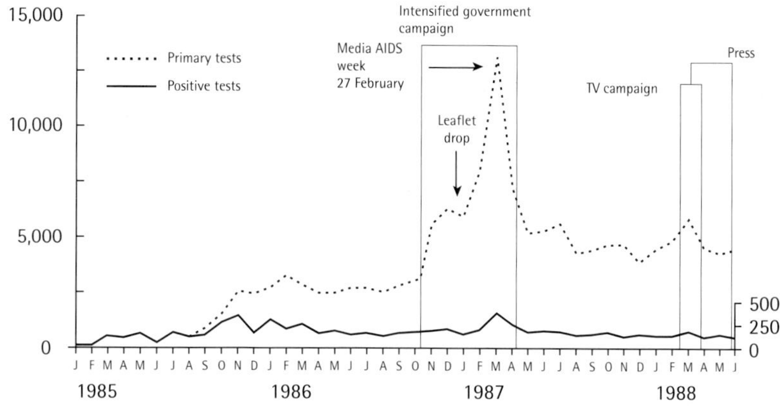

(Source: Communicable Disease Surveillance Centre)

Figure 6.1, which charts HIV-testing figures for England and Wales, illustrates clearly the peaks of public concern which coincided with periods of maximum AIDS public education activity.

HIV-testing data provide a proxy measure of levels of public concern possibly resulting from public education interventions. Attendances at clinics for testing increased by more than 300 per cent over the period of the initial government health education campaign, the increase being higher among the 'worried well' than among those who were infected.

Any intervention attempted after the initial panic about AIDS would have experienced difficulties of raising public concern to its previously high level, whatever the approach used. Initial public response to the AIDS epidemic verged on the hysterical, and this was by no means attributable solely to public education efforts; hysteria was fuelled by the press and professionals alike.

In countries in which AIDS public education campaigning began later, the agencies responsible were able to take advantage of the experience gained from the use of fear in earlier campaigns in other countries, with the result that the explicit message *not* to be afraid was incorporated into many campaigns. In general NGOs were quicker to note the need to avoid the use of fear-provoking campaigns. As early as 1987, Austrian cinema advertisements by AIDS-Hilfe were saying 'Being frightened can be a sensible thing sometimes, especially when the number of people infected with AIDS is on the rise, and therefore also a general risk of infection. But enjoyment is better than being afraid, especially when it comes to sex…'

In Italy, where campaigns began in 1988, slogans of the Ministry of Health campaigns emphasized the avoidable nature of the disease and the need to avoid fear: 'AIDS: if you know about it, you can avoid it; if you know about it, it won't kill you' was to become a much-repeated slogan in the campaigns. Slogans in other advertisements read: 'AIDS. A phone-call against fear' and 'AIDS. Overcome fear.'

One of the canons of health education philosophy is that high levels of fear may well be counterproductive, leading to denial and dissociation from the message. However, it must be noted that the evidence relating to the use of emotion to motivate behaviour change is sparse and equivocal (Lund and Uldall Jepsen 1992). There have been few controlled studies or evaluations of the effect of the use of fear. Relevant material either derives mainly from USA and thus reflects different social and cultural relationships, or else is related to the use of fear in other areas of health behaviour – alcoholism and road safety, for example (Robertson 1974; Fritzen and Mazer 1975; Steele and Southwick 1981; Nelson and Moffit 1988) – and although helpful, we should clearly be cautious in generalizing the conclusions of these studies to the field of sexual health. An evaluation of syphilis campaigns conducted early this century which sought to arouse fear in the troops showed that although such strategies changed general impressions of STDs they had little effect on knowledge and behaviour (Lashley and Watson 1921). American fear-appeal campaigns intending to prevent syphilis, gonorrhoea and other venereal diseases during the Second World War similarly had limited effects (Brandt 1987).

Evidence on whether *some* level of fear is necessary to influence behaviour is equivocal (Janis and Feshbach 1953; Leventhal *et al.* 1967; Rhodes and Wolitski 1990; Lund and Uldall Jepsen 1992). The consensus of research (from other areas of health promotion and AIDS prevention) seems to be that the use of fear, if it has the desired effect of motivating behaviour change, only does so conditionally (Leventhal *et al.* 1967; Ben-Sira 1981; Kleinot and Rogers 1982; Becker and Joseph 1988; Job 1988). For example: the level of fear generated should be sufficiently high to motivate individuals to take action, but not so high as to paralyse them into inaction or to cause them to deny their susceptibility (Janis and Feshbach 1953; Bishop 1974; Ben-Sira 1981); and the threat should be perceived to be real and accompanied by clear practical guidelines on what action to take to avoid the risk (Becker and Joseph 1988; Job 1988). Effectiveness depends on the size and nature of the threat, the probability that it will occur if no action is taken and the perceived effectiveness of the measures taken to prevent the danger (Leventhal *et al.* 1967; Kleinot and Rogers 1982). Programmes relying on fear will be unsuccessful where the fear is associated with a low probability event and – as in the case of AIDS – where there is a substantial time-lag between risk-associated behaviour and adverse outcomes (Des Jarlais and Hunt 1988).

The use of fear may be effective in motivating behaviour change where:

- the threat is seen to be real
- the level of fear is appropriate
- advice on avoidance action is provided
- preventive action is seen as effective.
      (Job 1988)

Several of these criteria were met at the time of the UK 'Don't die of ignorance' campaign. Survey evidence showed perceived personal susceptibility to be high, as was knowledge of the efficacy of condoms. More problematic was the perception of the threat as real. At the time the 'Don't die of ignorance' campaign was run, only 466 cases of AIDS had been reported by December 1986 (according to the European Centre for the Epidemiological Monitoring of AIDS) in a country with a population of 55 million, which presented real difficulties in terms of proximity and visibility. Moreover, these campaigns provided few realizable pointers to action other than to read the leaflet when it arrived. At the time there were possibly apocryphal, but nevertheless telling, stories of schoolchildren asking their parents, 'What is ignorance? I don't want to die from it.'

The interventions described above have primarily used fear of the physical consequences of risk behaviour, i.e. death and disease, to motivate behaviour change. Since death is a remote and far-off concept for many young people, the more immediate and emotionally salient fear may be that of offending group norms, of social ostracization. Less attention has been paid to the potential of using fear of social disapproval and rejection. A promise of social acceptance may be a better means of convincing than using the fear of death, and may be especially influential among young people (Clark 1988). (For further discussion of using 'costs' and 'benefits' to motivate, see the final part of this chapter.)

Using humour to motivate

Opinions on the capacity of humour to motivate are varied. Some think humour diminishes the ability to understand and hence act upon the message, others that humour increases the acceptance of the message. McGuire (1984), for example, warns against the use of humour because of its potential to distract from and decrease acceptance of the message. However, in health promotion, evidence of the effects of humour is virtually non-existent, despite an increasing interest in using humour in this context (Lund and Uldall Jepsen 1992).

Comparing the two approaches, fear-inducing interventions have often been perceived as more effective in terms of awareness raising (Janis and Fesbach 1953; Leventhal *et al.* 1967; Rhodes and Wolitski 1990), although with problems of follow-up; provoking humour is seen to be easier to maintain, but less effective in raising awareness. Yet high levels of awareness (Matthews *et al.* 1995) were also achieved in countries in which campaigns have been typified more by a humorous approach, as in Switzerland and Norway, for example. The earliest campaigns run by the UK Department of Health were unprecedentedly effective in raising the profile of AIDS (DHSS and Welsh Office 1987), but they also produced waves of anxiety which militated against a steady and constant awareness of the disease.

Few studies have compared the effectiveness of fear and humour. Canadian research (Baggaley 1988) has shown humorous AIDS spots to be judged more positively than others; because of the use of humour, individuals with risk behaviours were especially likely to look favourably on such approaches. A rare piece of investigative work showed three versions of a condom pamphlet (one containing neutral information, one using fear and another using humour) to a sample of young people. Responses to the pamphlet using humour were more positive and more supportive than responses to either fear appeal or neutral versions, which did not differ greatly (Dubé *et al.* 1993a). Respondents who had been exposed to a fear-appeal communication had a lower rate of recognition, as well as a more negative attitude towards the communication and toward condom use. Neither perceived risk nor behavioural intention between the two groups differed significantly (Dubé *et al.* 1993b).

Major progress has been made in deflecting opposition to the frank presentation of pragmatic messages through the use of humour, permitting the use of material which might otherwise have brought the charge of overexplicitness. The use of cartoon characters depicting safe and unsafe sex helped ease the passage of more explicit campaign components in Spain, a Catholic country, in which difficulties might have been expected (see Chapter 2).

Research is beginning to show that the public react more favourably to communications using humour than they do to those using fear (Poelman *et al.* 1992; Servant 1992; Dubé *et al.* 1993a,b). Such findings have contributed to a gradual shift of tone in AIDS public education in Europe to lighter, more amusing campaigns and to a life-enhancing rather than a death-orientated approach.

By contrast with interventions which evoke fear – where punishment is intended to motivate behaviour – those using humour offer a reward since laughter is positive reinforcement. Humour has the further advantage of allowing us to raise issues which would otherwise not be allowed expression (Lund and Uldall Jepsen 1992). An alternative view is that humour has the potential to increase the recipients' attention. It has been stressed that AIDS is a disease surrounded by taboos – death and sex. Humour, by using fictional characters and thereby distancing the audience from reality, offers the possibility of breaking down taboos. As in the case of fear, the effectiveness of the use of humour will depend to some extent on the trustworthiness and credibility of the source or agent transmitting the message, and on the receptivity of the recipient. Campaigns using humour have been found to have less effect on religious and conservative population groups than on freethinking liberal audiences (Lund and Uldall Jepsen 1992).

The Danish 'Think twice' campaign 1988: a case study in the use of humour

Despite the lack of empirical evidence on relative effectiveness, the Danish AIDS Secretariat within the National Board of Health decided to avoid a fear-based approach in their campaigns in favour of humour. The 1988 Danish public education campaigns involved a series of humorous TV spots, including adaptations of Hans Christian Andersen's famous fairy stories. The adaptation of these classic tales was given an up-to-date twist, using a condom in the moral of the story. Other spots featured famous media personalities in various non-risky settings (a swimming pool, an office, a public toilet) to correct misinformation (described in Chapter 2). Others used the quiz genre, a cartoon and a parody of Shakespeare's *Hamlet*.

The princess and the pea (6.9–14)

A theatre curtain is raised to show a castle. It is stormy and cold, and thunder is heard outside. A king stands next to the fireplace, warming his hands. He takes his glass of wine which is on the mantelpiece and puts on his crown. In the mirror on the mantelpiece, we see a queen and a prince playing chess. The narrator begins: 'One night it was horrible weather, it was thundering and lightening', the scene cuts to outside, where a young woman with a shawl over her head runs to the front door and pulls the bell. The queen opens the door with a candle in her hand and tells the visitor, 'The rain and the evil weather has made you look horrible.' The young woman replies, 'But I am really a princess.' The queen lets the young girl into the castle and the narrator tells us that the queen is unsure whether it is a true princess or someone who wants free lodging. As she closes the door the queen says knowingly to the camera, 'We'll soon find out.' Inside we see her making a bed with some twenty mattresses on top of each other, standing on a ladder and tucking in the sheets.

The queen then tells the young girl her bed is ready, and points to where she can change. The princess curtsies to the queen. The prince peeps inside the door and watches her undress. As she puts on her nightdress he sneaks into the room.

6.9–14 Denmark, 1989–90, Danish Board of Health, TV.

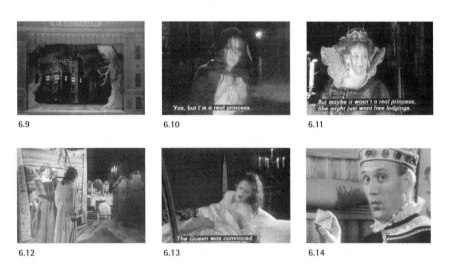

6.9

6.10

6.11

6.12

6.13

6.14

The queen blows out the candles, but as the prince creeps up the ladder after the young girl, the queen grabs hold of his arm and warns him 'Think about it.' We then see the queen slip something between two mattresses. The young woman tosses and turns in bed, clearly uncomfortable and crying out in pain, and the prince looks at his mother questioningly. The narrator tells us 'Now the queen was convinced.' The young girl sits up in bed and suddenly looks at the camera, smiling and then whistles the AIDS tune which features throughout this campaign. The queen cries delightedly 'It *is* a true princess!' The prince then puts his hand between the two mattresses and pulls out a packet of condoms. He looks at his mother, smiles and he too whistles the AIDS tune, and rushes eagerly up the ladder. The narrator then says 'The prince thought about it for ever and ever.'

Numbskull Jack (6.15–24)

As two doormen open the door to the castle, a man falls clumsily inside. He walks towards the king and the princess on their thrones. 'Umm … ahh …', he begins, but the princess interrupts him, saying 'Won't work, go away.' Three valets act in unison, writing down everything that is said with quills. The man

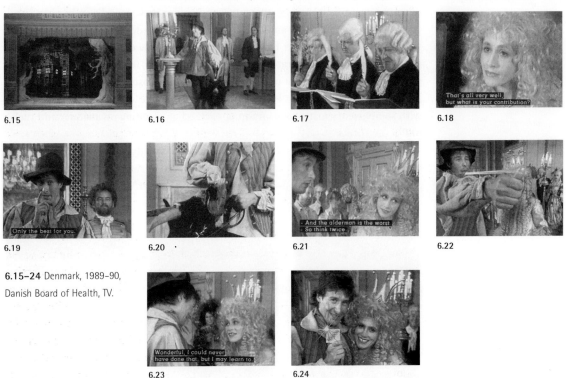

6.15

6.16

6.17

6.18

6.19

6.20

6.21

6.22

6.15–24 Denmark, 1989–90, Danish Board of Health, TV.

6.23

6.24

begins to cry. The doorman with a gold stick in his hand thumps it into the ground and says 'next one' and the trumpets sound again. The next suitor enters, and the next, and much the same action ensues. As the fourth suitor approaches we hear the sound of a goat, and a young man wearing a peasant hat stumbles over the doorstep. Instead of writing, the valets are now waving their feathers in front of their noses as the young man obviously smells. He looks at the princess, touches his hat and then says, as the previous suitors did, 'It's roasting hot in here', and again the princess smilingly replies 'That is because I am roasting cockerels today.' The young man replies 'That's good, maybe I can have a bit too, I'm really, really hungry.' The princess then leans forward and asks him what he will bring to the dinner. The young man reaches into his pocket and brings out a fluorescent orange packet of condoms and whistles the AIDS tune, together with the goat. The princess smiles at him 'I like you, you can speak for yourself.' She looks towards the valets and says 'But do you realize that everything we say is being written down and gets printed in the monthly newspaper?' She walks towards one of the valets and says, 'and the alderman is the worst one'. The alderman angrily points at the young man, saying 'Think about it.' The young man replies, 'But that is exactly what I am doing', smiles at the princess and flicks a condom towards the alderman. The condom lands on the alderman's finger to the amusement of the court. 'That was well done, I couldn't have done that, but I will probably learn how some day', says the princess to the young man. The king has woken up and is smiling. The two then kiss and look towards the camera, and the young man whistles the AIDS tune showing the packet of condoms.

Evaluation of the Danish 'Think twice' campaign

In autumn 1990, the Communication Research Institute at Roskilde University was commissioned by the AIDS Secretariat to carry out an evaluation of the 1988 campaign, one aspect of which was an enquiry into the use of horror and humour in health education.

The humorous TV spots for the 'Think twice' campaign, with the endline 'Think about it – use a condom' were tested in 1988 with two sets of focus groups, one comprising key AIDS policy personnel, the other young people aged 16 to 26.

Recall was highest for the Hans Christian Andersen fairytales. However, these were interpreted as largely entertainment by the policy personnel, who felt they failed to transmit the intended message. The sketch featuring the swimming pool was judged most successful in transmitting information and also for representing homosexuality on screen in a non-sensational manner. The *Hamlet* parody, in which the main character (a member of a famous Danish comic trio) quotes the words 'To be' followed by a skull, continuing with an echo sound effect 'or not to be' was less well received. The main character completes the quotation with 'That is the question' and 'but not to me', as he (whistling) presents a pack of condoms. In particular, the AIDS personnel saw the juxtaposition of humour and death as unfortunate and inappropriate, and neither amusing nor stimulating.

The petrol station spot (see Chapter 7) drew such comments as: 'it was quite funny'; 'it's good to show that it's natural to buy condoms'; and 'it does turn things upside-down'. Humour was judged as an appropriate tool to encourage condom purchase.

Reactions were sought to fear-invoking AIDS information campaigns used in other countries. The evaluators showed the focus groups the Australian 'Grim reaper', in which a scythe is shown cutting its way through the human race. Reactions were that this was antithetical to the Danish spirit: 'this is so unDanish'; such approaches 'do more harm than good' and couldn't be taken seriously; that the horror component made them unintentionally comical. The Danish AIDS personnel also objected to the hidden tone of guilt and morality: 'it makes the sick look like murderers and criminals'; 'it reminds me of cold-war propaganda'; 'it is unbelievable rubbish'. These comments perhaps underline the importance of taking account of social context in planning campaigns. (Source: Lund and Uldall Jepsen 1992)

Using role models to motivate

Little is known about the effectiveness of using role models in mass media, but in the field of health promotion and education it is suggested that learners are most likely to learn by following the example of those they respect and admire; educators have to try and ensure that their students wish to identify with the role models and learn positive behaviour and attitudes from them (Weare 1992). Peer education programmes are much used in health promotion. The use of group members, or opinion leaders within a community, as sources of information can be an effective strategy for changing attitudes (Downie *et al.* 1990; Kelly *et al.* 1992). Obviously peer education is not possible in the mass media but role model campaigns can be seen to provide 'peer education by proxy'; those seeking to promote healthy behaviour through the mass media can use role models – either famous or 'ordinary' – with whom the target audience can identify.

Several possible approaches to using role models in AIDS education mass media campaigns can be identified. Examples may be made of those who have acted unwisely, showing the public how not to behave (see Chapter 7, 'excuses' campaigns). These are rather negative approaches. Alternatively, good behaviour can be held up as an example of behaviour to be emulated. Advertisements which celebrate young people behaving in such a way as to stay healthy, describing why they wear condoms rather than why they neglect to do so seems to hold more promise in terms of empowering young people. The latter option has the obvious advantage of being positive but the models must clearly be chosen with care. Government officials are not the obvious choice in the area of sexual health if the aim is to persuade young people to identify with the advice and its source.

From time to time in the AIDS epidemic, opportunities have arisen to present such a role model through the experience of a famous person with HIV. In November 1991, for example, the charismatic sportsman Magic Johnson held a press conference to announce that he was HIV positive and would be retiring from basketball. Magic Johnson was seen by most as the archetypal fit and active heterosexual. Several researchers opportunistically monitored the effect of this. Surveys of knowledge, attitude and behaviour change among young people in school following the publicity revealed that Magic Johnson's appearance increased perceived personal vulnerability (Whalen *et al.* 1994) and reinforced knowledge and increased saliency, albeit temporarily (Sigelman *et al.* 1993). Other studies in STD clinics in Maryland (MMWR 1993) and in Philadelphia (Langer *et al.* 1992) showed that following the announcement patients were more likely to express an intention to take an HIV test and to change their behaviour.

The simulation of such a scenario clearly lacks the authenticity and therefore the impact of real people. Campaigns using popular figures – whether media celebrities, prominent actors or folk heroes – to motivate necessary action have been mounted in several European countries, in Ireland, Greece, Sweden and Belgium. Although not strictly comparable, the use of figures known to be a specific authority on a particular issue might also be included here though there are obvious differences.

The 1993 Greek AIDS public education campaign for World AIDS Day made ample use of heroes or role models. Though the association may be neither deliberate nor conscious it seems unsurprising that this approach should be adopted by a nation in whose history the gods have played such a major role. The TV spots featured nationally famous personalities – a singer, a basketball player, an actress and actor – who all urge solidarity with those infected and encourage condom use.

The Irish 'Straight talking about sex and AIDS' campaign 1993–94: a case study in the use of role models

The 1993–94 Irish Health Promotion Unit's TV and radio spots used role models – TV presenters, a mother whose son had AIDS, a journalist, the National Union of Students president – to promote condom use; these personalities sat close to the camera and talked directly and candidly to the audience about con-

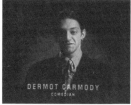 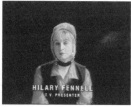 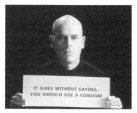

6.25

Ireland, May 1993–94, DoH Health Promotion Unit, BMB&B agency, TV.
Dermot Carmody: *Irish people are funny. I mean, we're different, as in ordinary Irish people don't get AIDS or HIV, not at all, that's reserved for drug abusers, homosexuals, people who sleep with prostitutes. So you see, ordinary Irish people don't get HIV or AIDS. Therefore it follows that ordinary Irish people don't need to wear a condom if they're having sex. Now that's a joke*

6.26

Hilary Fennell: *When a guy's trying to impress a girl, he sometimes pays her a little compliment but, if he were to whisper in her ear 'I think you're stupid and I don't give a damn about you', she wouldn't be very impressed at all, now, would she? Well, that's exactly what he is saying if he expects you to have sex without a condom. Because if he asks you, he might have asked others, so you can't be sure he's safe. Here's some sound advice: never sleep with a man who's prepared to kill you*

6.27

The diceman (a mime artist) holds up a sign. The spot ends with a black screen and the text 'Protect yourself with a condom'.

dom use (6.25–7). Although there was some criticism of this campaign for not warning people of the dangers of sex, the pressure for moral messages has dropped considerably (see Chapter 8).

Evaluation of the Irish role model campaign

A survey was carried out by Irish Marketing Surveys on behalf of the Department of Health among the Irish population into their attitudes to AIDS, based on a nationally representative sample of 1,507 people aged 15 and over. Younger age groups were weighted. Interviews were face to face. Fieldwork was conducted from 18 to 30 March 1994.

Of particular interest in the context of the use of role models were responses relating to sources of information. Television was seen as the most appropriate medium for public education and three-quarters of all respondents claimed to have been aware of the Irish advertising campaign on AIDS at around the time of research (mid- to late March 1994). The performance of this campaign was ranked as good, ahead in terms of awareness of advertising on road safety though behind advertising on smoking.

The message of the campaign was clearly recalled, with approximately two in every three people claiming awareness of either television or radio advertising saying that the main message was to use a condom. Recall of the characters who appeared was not as good, though television performed better than radio in this respect. Pat O'Mahony (a TV show presenter) was recalled by over one-quarter of those aware of TV advertising, while 12 per cent remembered the character who played the mother of the person with AIDS. Among those aware of radio advertising this ranking was reversed; 15 per cent of listeners remembered the mother while 9 per cent associated Pat O'Mahony with the campaign. This tends to suggest that the use of celebrities depends for its effectiveness on their being recognized by their physical appearance. (Source: Irish Health Promotion Unit 1994)

Using 'empowerment' to motivate

Although the use of the mass media may not be the first or the obvious choice of channel through which to encourage self-empowerment, several campaigns have tackled the issue with some success. One approach chosen by campaigns in Switzerland and the UK has been to use evidence of change in behaviour in apparent response to the AIDS epidemic to encourage and stimulate continued efforts. This is illustrated in the UK Health Education Authority cinema advertisement featuring Mrs Dawson, a worker in a condom factory who applauded the good sense of young people in using more condoms and 'keeping her busy' (8.66–9); in the Swiss ad the message '*continuez*' overprints a graphical illustration of increasing condom use (**Plate 47**).

Empowerment models of health education view the ability to make an informed choice as crucial. In this model, knowledge is valued as a necessary condition for informed choice, but must be combined with values such as consideration for others and self-esteem (Kemm 1991).

The Spanish 'Póntelo, pónselo' campaign 1990–91: a case study in the use of empowerment

The rationale for the Spanish '*Póntelo, pónselo*' campaign was prompted by the recognition that both STDs and unwanted pregnancy among young people were on the increase. Both had been a problem during the 1970s in Spain, and had then begun to decrease, but during the latter 1980s there was a resurgence in incidence. Pregnancies in 15- to 19-year-olds reached approximately 23,000 per year by 1985, and have since risen to 30,000 per annum. An estimated 1,000 young people under the age of sexual consent have an abortion each year in Spain (*El Independiente*, 25 October 1990). One contributory factor may have been the greater freedom in Spanish society after Franco, with inadequate provision of sex education to equip young people to deal with it. The evidence in Spain is that young people tend to take problems and questions relating to sexuality to sex shops, despite the provision of special health services for young people (J L Bimbela, personal communication 1994).

The '*Póntelo, pónselo*' advertisements were aimed at young people aged 15–24 and used the school setting to reach them. The TV spot features a group of high school students in a gym. An older man (a teacher) walks into the dressing room and sees a condom on a towel. He looks angry as the young people get into a group at the prompt of his whistle. The young people become quiet and look worried. The teacher shows the group the condom that he has found – the condom can be seen plainly in a clear wrapper – saying 'I found this in the dressing room. Whose is it?' The group look at each other in embarrassment and start giggling. The teacher looks more angry and serious, and the group becomes more serious too. He then becomes impatient and repeats his question: 'I said, Whose is this?'

The camera focuses on one of the young men in the group who nervously stands up, saying 'Mine'. The teacher looks disapproving but at that point, another young man stands up and says 'Mine', followed by a girl, each with their arms crossed, somewhat defiantly. Little by little almost everybody in the group stands up and says 'Mine', owning up to being the owner of the condom. The spot ends with a white screen in the centre of which appears a yellow condom, accompanied by the voice-over: 'The condom is the most effective way of preventing unwanted pregnancy and sexually transmitted diseases.' The next message on the screen reads: 'Put it on, put in on him.' (6.28–33). The logos of the Ministry of Health and Consumer Affairs, the Ministry of Social Affairs, the Institute for Women and the Institute for Young People then appear on the screen.

Accompanying posters placed in the subway and on street boards carried the same slogan 'Put it on, put it on him' over the same yellow circular condom. Above the condom, the words 'unwanted pregnancies, gonorrhoea, AIDS, fungal infection, hepatitis B, vaginitis, trichomoniasis, genital herpes, syphilis,

6.28–33 Spain, 1990–91, MOHCA, MSA, Institute for Women, Institute for Young People, TV, radio, subway posters, phone boxes, bus stations, billboards, leaflets, T-shirts, stickers, badges.

The '*Póntelo, pónselo*' campaign aimed to empower young people to use condoms to protect themselves against HIV. The TV spot shows a group of young people defending their need to practise safer sex. The controversy surrounding this campaign was as well recalled as the campaign components themselves.

The spot finishes with a white screen in the centre of which appears a yellow condom, accompanied by the voice-over: 'The condom is the most effective way of preventing unwanted pregnancy and sexually transmitted diseases.' The next textual message says: 'Put it on, put it on him.'

The advertisements were aimed at young people aged 15–24, using the school setting in the TV spot to reach them.

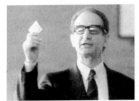

6.28

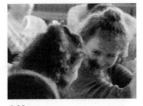

6.29

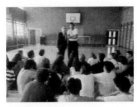

6.30

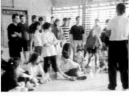

6.31

6.32

Póntelo. Pónselo.

6.33

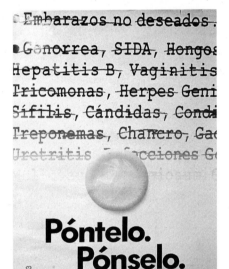

6.34 Spain, 1990–91, Ministry of Health and Consumer Affairs, posters, TV, radio. 'Put it on. Put it on him.' The reference to other sexually transmitted diseases in the Spanish '*Póntelo, pónselo*' campaign broadens the scope beyond the prevention of AIDS/HIV.

candida' and other STDs start to fade out and have been crossed through **(6.34)**. In addition radio spots adapted the lyrics of well-known songs, aired on national radio and a few private channels: 'Nothing embarrasses me. Putting it on can be funny… carry it with you in your pocket and ask for it in the chemist's shop'; 'I use a condom for pleasure'; 'You're doing it very well' (i.e. using/putting on the condom); a 'condom rap' featured a man and woman singing/rapping: she wants him to use a condom, when he resists, she gives him reasons why they should, and he finally accepts her putting it on him.

Evaluation of the Spanish 'Póntelo, pónselo' campaign

Research was carried out for the Ministry of Health and Consumer Affairs in July 1991 to evaluate this campaign. A pre- and post-test was carried out with a sample of 783 people aged 15–24 years and 479 aged 25–54 years.

The campaign was recalled by 81 per cent of the total sample, and by a higher proportion (88 per cent) of young people. Unprompted recall showed the impact of the TV spot to have been greatest, posters in bus stations and phone boxes were the next most commonly recalled, and the least well recalled was radio. Newspaper coverage also refers only to the TV spot, the radio spots seem to have gone largely unnoticed. The impact of the slogan '*Póntelo, pónselo*' was very strong, the term almost became a catchphrase; other campaigns by other groups with different aims paraphrased the slogan to suit their own ends.

The research showed that 38 per cent linked the campaign with the Ministry of Health and Consumer Affairs. In terms of the messages received (spontaneous response) 38 per cent said the message was about preventing unwanted pregnancy, 40 per cent said prevention of STDs. Fewer than 10 per cent liked nothing about the campaign. Four out of ten (39 per cent) said they found nothing offensive at all in the messages, although they thought that the teacher looked overly angry. People thought that the campaign had changed opinions about condoms. One of the most important consequences was that people now felt more comfortable about discussing condoms and STDs at home, at school and at work, etc.; the campaign seemed to have made a major contribution to breaking down barriers. Fewer than 5 per cent saw the message as encouraging immoral behaviour. Around one in ten (10.3 per cent) doubted the effectiveness of the campaign.

According to the survey, 79 per cent of men and women interviewed felt condoms were the method of contraception to use. 30 per cent felt comfortable using condoms and 16 per cent felt them to be an effective and safe method of contraception; 18 per cent found them easily accessible. 33 per cent reported using them to avoid pregnancy, and 13 per cent against STDs. Analysis showed recall of the campaigns to be higher among more habitual users of condoms.

This campaign provoked unprecedented national debate which continued for several months. Posters, especially, were everywhere. More people remembered the debate surrounding the campaign than the campaign itself. Only 71 per cent of those who recalled the campaign were aware of and had seen the actual advertisements. (Source: Ministerio de Sanidad y Consumo/Cuanter 1991)

An important feature of the evaluation of any campaign must be to monitor response at the level of the social context as well as at the individual level, given, for example, that some chemists still conscientiously object to selling condoms. As the summary of the campaign evaluation shows, an unintended but extraordinarily effective consequence of this campaign (in terms of raising awareness) was the huge amount of controversy it generated. The Spanish media provided full coverage of the debate over whether young people should be persuaded to use condoms, and so aired important issues which would not normally

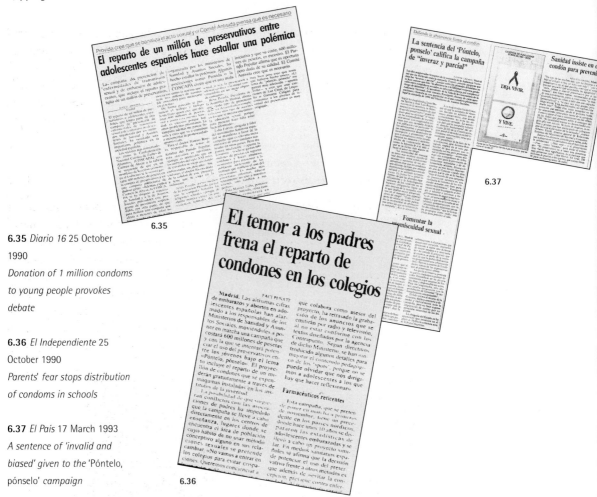

6.35 *Diario 16* 25 October 1990
Donation of 1 million condoms to young people provokes debate

6.36 *El Independiente* 25 October 1990
Parents' fear stops distribution of condoms in schools

6.37 *El País* 17 March 1993
A sentence of 'invalid and biased' given to the 'Póntelo, pónselo' campaign

have been brought into the open. Some examples of the newspaper coverage are given in **6.35–7**.

The *Diario 16* and *El Independiente* articles illustrate the opposition to the planned distribution of free condoms in schools which caused such controversy. The pro-life organization Provida and the National Catholic Conference of Parents of Pupils (CONCAPA) were among the NGOs who protested; both had support although this was not widespread. The planned distribution of condoms in schools was stopped when CONCAPA complained. The Institute of Youth, linked to the Ministry of Social Affairs but at some distance from government, did distribute condoms but not directly in schools. To justify the campaign the Ministry certainly encouraged political debate around related issues.

As shown in the cutting from *El País* (17 March 1993), the furore rumbled on as late as 1993, 'a sentence of "invalid and biased" was given to the "*Póntelo, pónselo*" campaign'. Two magistrates declared the campaign invalid and biased on the grounds that the messages in the campaign did not give abstinence and fidelity as the no-risk option, and the campaign promoted sexual promiscuity. This article coincided with the new government campaign 'Live and let live.' Answering the charge that the campaign promoted condoms, the administration answered that its aim was not to promote a model of sexual behaviour. All national newspapers covered the story. The tone of the coverage – i.e. whether critical or supportive, supporting the church or the administration – depended on whether the editorial perspective was right- or left-wing. The view of the right-wing church was not the view of the general public and indeed, the conservative Popular Party ratified the use of condoms.

Using 'costs' and 'benefits' to motivate

Social marketing is predicated on the fact that there can always be a 'reward' or 'benefit' – or an 'expected positive utility' to use the term from health economics – resulting from a particular exchange. Positive utilities are more difficult to think of for condom use or sexual exclusivity. The only reward the purveyors of the 'goods', or preventive strategies, have to offer is the absence of a disease which the target audience is so far free from, and sees very long odds on contracting. At the same time, the price asked is high: the surrender of sexual freedom, potential loss of spontaneity and pleasure in sex, possible embarrassment and loss of face, etc. All the preventive messages carry negative utilities, since they all require us to give up

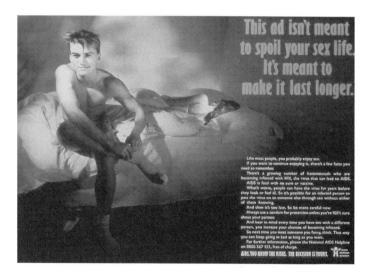

6.38 UK, summer 1988, HEA, magazines, posters.
This ad isn't meant to spoil your sex life. It's meant to make it last longer.
AIDS. You know the risks.
The decision is yours
This example from the UK highlights a possible benefit of safer sex for the individual.

or modify a behaviour we have chosen for its personal benefits. Although advertising agencies have made good creative use of the need to transmit positive messages about sex, for example 'This ad isn't meant to spoil your sex life. It's meant to make it last longer' (**6.38**), perhaps the good news is still overshadowed by the bad.

An approach used in some countries was to emphasize the high cost of the risk behaviour and/or the low cost of the risk-reduction strategy. The German advertisement stresses the high cost of casual sex abroad, while the examples from Switzerland and the UK stress the low cost of condom use (**6.39–42**).

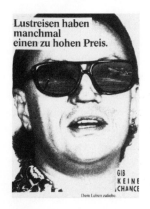

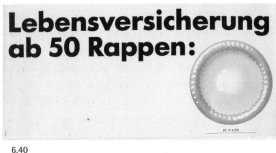

6.40

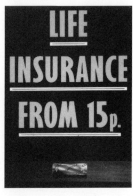

6.42

6.39 Germany, 1990–92, BZgA, posters, TV.
Wanderlust sometimes has too high a price

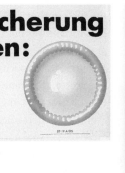

6.41

Switzerland, 1989, FOPH/SAF, posters.
6.40 *Life insurance policies from 50 cents*
6.41 *Much protection for little cost*

6.42 UK, summer 1988, HEA, BMP DDB Needham agency, posters.
*Life insurance from 15p
Remember when you go away AIDS doesn't. You know the risks. The decision is yours*

References

Baggaley, J P 1988 Perceived effectiveness of International AIDS Campaigns, *Health Education Research* **3** (1); 7–17

Becker, M H and J G Joseph 1988 AIDS and behavioural change to reduce risk: a review, *American Journal of Public Health* **78**; 394–410

Ben-Sira, Z 1981 Latent fear-arousing potential of fear-moderating and fear-neutral health promoting information, *Social Science and Medicine* **15** (E); 105–12

Bishop, R L 1974 Anxiety and readership of health information, *Journalism Quarterly* **51** (1); 40–6

Brandt, A M 1987 *No magic bullet: a social history of venereal disease in the United States since 1880*, New York: Oxford University Press

Clark, E 1988 *The want makers*, London: Coronet Books

Des Jarlais, D C and D E Hunt 1988 AIDS and intravenous drug use, AIDS Bulletin, National Institute of Justice, US Department of Justice

DHSS (Department of Health and Social Security) and the Welsh Office 1987 *AIDS. Monitoring response to the public education campaign February*

1986–February 1987, London: HMSO

Downie, R S, C Fyfe and A Tannahill 1990 *Health promotion. Models and values*, Oxford: Oxford University Press

Dubé, L, G Reaidi and C Descombes 1993a *Comparing affective and cognitive responses to informational vs emotional messages on AIDS prevention: a field study among Canadian young adults*, PO-C22-3160, IXth International Conference on AIDS/IVth STD World Congress, Berlin, 6–11 June 1993

Dubé, L, G Reaidi and C Descombes 1993b *A field study on communication effectiveness in promoting condom use for AIDS prevention: fear may not be a good approach*, PO-C22-3161, IXth International Conference on AIDS/IVth STD World Congress, Berlin, 6–11 June 1993

Fritzen, R D and G E Mazer 1975 The effects of fear appeal and communication upon attitudes toward alcohol consumption, *Journal of Drug Education* **5** (2); 171–81

Irish Health Promotion Unit 1994 *AIDS awareness survey July 1994*, Dublin: IHPU

Janis, I L and S Feshbach 1953 Effects of fear-arousing communications, *Journal of Abnormal and Social Psychology* **48**; 78–92

Job, R F S 1988 Effective and ineffective use of fear in health promotion campaigns, *American Journal of Public Health* **78** (2); 163–7

Kelly, J A, J S St Lawrence, Y Stevenson, A C Hauth, S C Kalichan, Y E Diaz, T L Brasfield, J J Koob and M G Morgan 1992 Community AIDS/HIV risk reduction: the effects of endorsements by popular people in three cities, *American Journal of Public Health* **82** (11); 1483–9

Kemm, J 1991 Health education and the problem of knowledge, *Health Promotion International* **6** (4); 291–6

Kleinot, M C and R W Rogers 1982 Identifying effective components of alcohol misuse prevention programs, *Journal of Studies on Alcohol* **43** (7); 802–11

Langer, L M, R S Zimmerman, E F Hendershot and M Singh 1992 Effect of Magic Johnson's HIV status on HIV-related attitudes and behaviours of an STD clinic population, *AIDS Education and Prevention* **4** (4); 295–307

Lashley, K S and J B Watson 1921 *A psychological study of motion pictures in relation to venereal disease campaigns*, Washington DC: US Interdepartmental Social Hygiene Board

Leventhal, H, J C Watts and F Paguno 1967 Effects of fear and instructions on how to cope with danger, *Journal of Personality and Social Psychology* **6** (3); 313–21

Lund, A B and M Uldall Jepsen 1992 Skræk og humour som virkemilder i adfædspåvirende sundhedsoplysning, Arbejdspapir nr. 7, Roskilde Universitetscenter [Humour and horror in health education, an analysis of Danish and foreign experiences with different information strategies], Paper 7: Communication Research Institute, Roskilde University

Matthews, M, K Wellings and E Kupek 1995 *AIDS/HIV knowledge, attitude and behaviour surveys (general population) in the European Community*, report for the European Commision (DGV), London: LSHTM

McGuire, W J 1984 Public communication as a strategy for inducing health promoting behaviour change, *Preventive Medicine* **13**; 229–319

Ministerio de Sanidad y Consumo/Cuanter 1991 *Evaluacion de la campaña sobre el uso del preservativo (Póntelo, pónselo). Informe de resultados*, Madrid

MMWR (Morbidity and Mortality Weekly Report) 1993 Sexual risk behaviours of STD clinic patients before and after Earvin 'Magic' Johnson's HIV infection announcement, *Morbidity and Mortality Weekly Report* **42** (3); 45–8

Nelson, G D and P B Moffit 1988 Safety belt promotion: theory and practice, *Accident Analysis and Prevention* **20**; 27–38

Poelman, J, J Reinders, H Schaalman, M Paalman 1992 *A comic strip about AIDS*, POD02 3471, VIIIth International Conference on AIDS/IIIrd STD World Congress, Amsterdam, 19–24 July 1992

Rhodes, F and R J Wolitski 1990 Perceived effectiveness of fear appeals in AIDS education: relationship to ethnicity, gender, age and group membership, *AIDS Education and Prevention* **2** (1); 1–11

Robertson, L S, A B Kelley, B O'Neill, C W Wixom, R S Eiswirth and W J Haddon 1974 A controlled study of the effect of television messages on safety belt use, *American Journal of Public Health* **84** (11); 1070–80

Servant, A M 1992 *Love object...condoms with humour*, POD 5150, VIIIth International Conference on AIDS/IIIrd STD World Congress, Amsterdam, 19–24 July 1992

Sherr, L 1987 An evaluation of the UK government health education campaign on AIDS, *Psychology and Health* **1**; 61–72

Sigelman, C K, A B Miller and E B Derenowski 1993 Do you believe in magic? The impact of Magic Johnson on adolescents' AIDS knowledge and attitudes, *AIDS Education Preview* **5** (2); 153–61

Steele, C M and L Southwick 1981 Effects of fear and causal attribution about alcoholism on drinking and related attitudes among heavy and moderate social drinkers, *Cognitive Therapy and Research* **5** (4); 339–50

Weare, K 1992 The contribution of education to health promotion. In R Burton and G Macdonald (eds) *Health promotion. Disciplines and diversity*, London: Routledge

Whalen, C K, B Henker, R O'Neil, J Hollingshead, A Holman and B Moore 1994 Preadolescents' perceptions of AIDS before and after Earvin Magic Johnson's announcement, *Journal of Pediatric Psychology* **1**; 3–26

7 Eroding barriers to preventive action

By 1987, knowledge of HIV transmission routes was already high in most western European countries as was awareness of the means of protection, but there was little evidence of behaviour being modified accordingly and there was only weak evidence of increases in the practice of safer sex. People knew well enough that condoms protected against HIV but still failed to use them (Becker and Joseph 1988; Kraft and Rise 1988; Schmidt *et al.* 1989; Tikkanen and Koskela 1992).

There were a number of possible reasons for this. Throughout most of Europe by the 1980s, a 'post-pill' generation had grown up accustomed to the convenience and efficacy of oral contraception, for whom condoms were simply unfamiliar. Even among older people condoms had fallen into disuse. Efforts to encourage usage in the context of the AIDS/HIV epidemic were further thwarted by the condom's poor image and by the significant barriers to its use. Research revealed considerable resistance to and distaste for condoms: they were seen as difficult to use, old-fashioned, objects of fun, unromantic and unspontaneous (Dubois-Arber *et al.* 1993; BZgA 1994; Dorozynski 1994).

Theoretical framework

Models of health behaviour acknowledge the importance of overcoming barriers to preventive action. The health belief model (Rosenstock 1974a,b) refers to perceived barriers of performing preventive behaviours, including estimates of physical, psychological, financial, and other costs incurred in performing the behaviour. The theory of reasoned action (Fishbein and Ajzen 1975; Ajzen and Fishbein 1980; Ajzen 1988) also identifies factors which can act as barriers to taking up preventive action, perhaps most importantly the extent to which the behaviour is under volitional control (Ajzen 1988; Sheppard *et al.* 1988; Terry *et al.* 1993). An important next step in AIDS prevention then is to address some of the barriers to behaviour change.

Motivational barriers: the 'excuses' campaigns

Resistance to chang-
ing behaviour, despite
high knowledge levels,
highlighted the need
to address the barriers
to preventive action.
Research showed that
many, particularly
young people:

- give excuses for not
  using condoms
- feel embarrassed
  when buying
  condoms in public
- find it difficult to
  raise the subject with
  a partner
- may not know how
  to use a condom
  properly.

Research (de Vries 1990) showed that people rationalized their reluctance to use condoms either by understating the seriousness of the HIV epidemic (some believed a vaccine would be found, for example, while others believed it to be just another of life's risks) or by exempting themselves from risk (by not sleeping with foreigners, not being homosexual, etc.). Others claimed they employed alternative risk-reduction strategies, for example, being careful about the choice of a partner by paying attention to appearance or cleanliness and previous sexual history, or using the pill.

A strategy adopted in several campaigns across Europe was to address some of these false reasons or excuses which acted as barriers to behaviour change, and to invalidate them. Condom 'excuses' campaigns have been run in the Netherlands, the UK, France and Switzerland, with the aim of exposing the (irrational) excuses people provide for not using condoms.

Models of information processing suggest the presence of cognitive and emotional biases in information processing which prevent good decision making. Tversky and Kahnemann (1974) suggest that in situations where there exists doubt and uncertainty, people use a variety of heuristics or 'short-cuts' to handle the information they are presented with. These mental techniques generally serve us well in making sense of complex and contradictory information, but in some circumstances they can lead to bias and error in our perceptions of the world, leading us to under- or overestimate the probability of certain events occurring.

United Kingdom 1988

The UK excuses campaign launched in 1988 featured single individuals reflecting on their failure to take preventive action. The tone of these advertisements was somewhat victim blaming. The advertisements make an example of someone who acts unwisely. The first line of the advertisement suggests that the reader is also capable of such imprudent action, and then provides information intending to impress on the reader the need for condom use.

The advertising agency responsible for the advertisements (TBWA) was the same as had been commissioned for the 'Don't die of ignorance' campaign (see Chapter 2). Although the message had changed, the tone and style of the advertisements was reminiscent of the earlier sombre tone, featuring dramatic and funereal colours of red, dark blue and black (**Plates 13 and 14**).

The excuses represented reflect the national situation. In Britain, periods of relative inactivity following bursts of energetic media campaigns had fostered the view that AIDS had gone away, so that it was necessary to remind the public of the ever-present threat. In addition, as in many other countries, including the Netherlands and Switzerland, the equation by the free media coverage of the disease with high risk groups, in particular gay men, provided those whose behaviour was exclusively heterosexual with a ready-made excuse for exempting themselves from the need to use a condom.

The rationale for the French campaign was informed in part by research commissioned by the Comité Français d'Education pour la Santé (CFES) and carried out by the survey agency BVA (BVA 1988). This research showed a high level of knowledge of modes of transmission of HIV – 83 per cent of the French population knew that condoms provide protection – and major gains in condom use in the recent past (in 1987 11 per cent of young people of 18 and over in the Paris region claimed to have used condoms in the last twelve months, a figure which rose to 18 per cent in 1989). But despite these positive changes, more than half the sample – some 53 per cent of those who were potentially at risk, according to the survey – did not use condoms, suggesting a need to examine more closely the reasons for non-use.

Obstacles to condom use in France again very much reflected specific features of the national context relating to the use of '*le capote Anglais*' (for further discussion of this see Chapter 4). This traditional resistance emerged in research. 70 per cent of respondents held the view that condoms killed romanticism; 63 per cent said they were artificial and reduced sensitivity. The use of the condom in the context of HIV prevention served to reinforce some of these positions. If a partner were to use a condom, the fear would be that they had something to hide. 34 per cent of the sample said they would link the suggestion of condom use with doubt about the partner (BVA 1988). The separation of AIDS information campaigns from those which promote condoms, and the dissociation of the two messages, was a strategy deliberately adopted to enable condoms to be positively promoted to avoid negative associations with a fatal and sexually transmitted disease.

The excuses campaign executed by CFES and the advertising agency Belier Conseil in 1988 carried the slogan 'Nowadays, condoms protect you from everything, even ridicule' and aimed to address the silence surrounding condoms, placing emphasis on open discussion. Eight-second TV spots expressed the suspicions about condoms and then invalidated them. The formula was to show a couple, who were varied each time in terms of coming from different age groups, but a common feature of each was the fact that it was the male partner who expressed the stereotypical view of the condom (since research had shown greater resistance on the part of men). The excuse was followed by joint laughter. The stereotypical excuses were: 'But it's hell to put on', 'It seems women hate them', 'You can't feel anything'.

The advertisements concluded with the voice-over 'Nowadays, condoms protect you against everything, even ridicule.' This final slogan appeared on the screen alongside a condom in its wrapping (7.1–4).

The design of these French advertisements incorporated several important principles. First, the couple *themselves* invalidate the excuse for not using a condom, rather than a third person in the guise of an expert correcting them. Second, the object of laughter is the *excuse given for not wearing a condom* and not the idea of using one, so shifting the focus of ridicule to non-use rather than use.

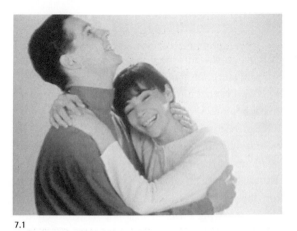

7.1

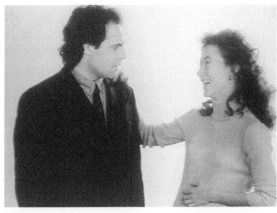

7.2

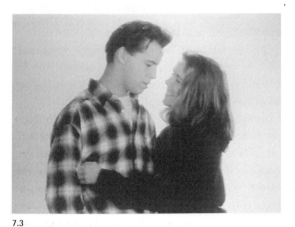

7.3

Aujourd'hui les préservatifs préservent de tout même du ridicule

cfes comité français d'éducation pour la santé

7.4

7.1–4 France, 1988, CFES, Belier Conseil agency, TV.

Third, the couple laugh at themselves, the viewer is invited to laugh with them and not at them. Finally, in each case the focus is on the couple and not the individual, emphasizing that just as sex is a matter for two people, so too is discussion of risk-reduction behaviour. There is thus no suggestion that one person is unilaterally protecting themselves against another riskier person. An evolving feature of the French campaigns was to locate messages firmly within a relationship. The everyday language used, the light laugh, the confidentiality and the relaxed feel to the advertisements was designed to ease worries and create a positive feeling around sexuality.

Research carried out by the Agence Nationale de Recherches sur le SIDA (ANRS) and the Agence Française de Lutte Contre le SIDA (AFLS) (1992) showed a slight shift of opinion in favour of condom use on a number of dimensions, though in the absence of a controlled evaluation, no claims can be made that these outcomes can be attributed to the campaigns.

Table 7.1

Opinions on condoms – per cent who agree or maybe agree that condoms:

	1990	1992
ruin romanticism	68.2	54.9
ruin pleasure	65.8	57.5
are expensive	58.6	62.0
are not needed when in love	52.6	41.4
cast doubts on partner	54.7	40.0
are for young people	34.6	24.7
are complicated to use	34.1	23.1
are not normal	26.4	26.1
are embarrassing to buy	24.0	12.4
are old-fashioned	18.8	11.3

(Source: ANRS and AFLS 1992)

The Netherlands 1989

In the Netherlands, the STD Foundation ran a campaign in 1989 aimed at confronting young people with the excuses they commonly use to avoid having safe sex. The target group was 18- to 25-year-olds, men and women, heterosexual and homosexual. The focus was not solely on condom use but on safer sex in general, reflecting government policy on prevention strategy. A series of photographs were used depicting either a young man, a young woman, or a couple; above each, a sentence described their reason for not using a condom or having safer sex (7.5–8).

The tone was somewhat cynical; the complacency of the young people was attacked in each case by the phrase 'sleep well', which was placed in a bar across the eyes of the models. The models looked ordinary and two represented ethnic minority groups to increase identification by the audience. The photographs appeared on black and white posters at railway stations, on billboards and in discotheques, and in several national newspapers and magazines. They featured in booklets which presented additional information about AIDS prevention. The concept was also broadcast as a radio message and cinema spot. This mixture of communication channels led to free media publicity.

The tone of these advertisements is more ironic than the French advertisements, the sarcastic tone less likely to encourage feelings of sympathy with the individuals, but the tone is not one of victim blaming. The excuse 'I don't need condoms because I take the pill' was omitted after pre-testing to avoid this particular message being misunderstood as a legitimate reason rather than as an excuse (de Vries 1990). All the same, this campaign did result in some confusion, which was revealed in the outcome evaluation. Some of the young people with less formal education interpreted some of these excuses literally, for example, that one *can* stop using condoms after three weeks.

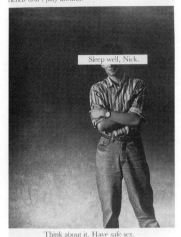

This is Nick. He doesn't need safe sex, because his friends don't play around.

Sleep well, Nick.

Think about it. Have safe sex.

7.5

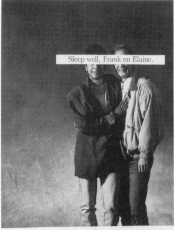

This is Frank and Elaine. They don't have to use condoms because they've known each other 3 weeks already

Sleep well, Frank en Elaine.

Think about it. Have safe sex.

7.6

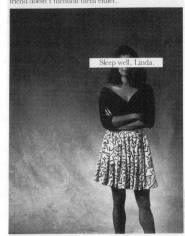

This is Linda. She doesn't need condoms because her friend doesn't mention them either.

Sleep well, Linda.

Think about it. Have safe sex.

7.7

7.5–7 The Netherlands, July 1989, STD Foundation, Reclamebureau PMSvW/Y&R agency, posters, brochure, cinema.

At the foot of each ad appeared the general message: 'Love is blind. And deaf. And especially dumb. That's probably why there are these excuses for unsafe sex at the start of a new relationship. On top of that it's not romantic. And not cool enough. And also it feels a bit silly to talk about it. But it's still stupid. Because you are playing with your life.'

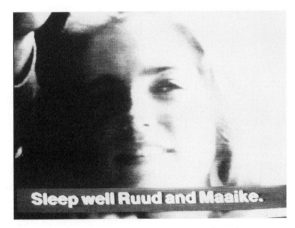

Sleep well Ruud and Maaike.

7.8 Cinema spot

Switzerland 1990

Research also showed the widespread use of excuses to justify not using condoms among Swiss youth. Most (80 per cent) of respondents felt that the AIDS problem concerned them, but for those who didn't, reasons given included excuses such as 'I have talked about it at length with my friend' and 'I am not a drug addict and I don't change partners' (Hausser *et al.* 1991).

The Swiss agencies saw their task as one of persuading people to confront reality by exposing myths without embarrassing or ridiculing people. The implicit message was that everyone is personally responsible, since infection occurs wherever the opportunity arises. Research had shown that many saw AIDS as someone else's problem (Schmidt *et al.* 1989; Hausser *et al.* 1991). A

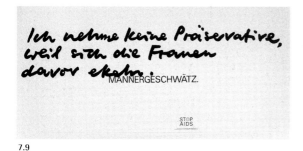

7.9

Je n'ai pas besoin de préservatifs.
Je prends la pilule. LA PILULE NE PROTÈGE
PAS DU SIDA.

ST⊙P
SIDA

7.10

Ich nehme keine Präservative,
weil ich immer wieder
den Test mache. TESTEN SCHÜTZT NICHT VOR AIDS.

ST⊙P
AIDS

7.11

Switzerland, January 1990,
FOPH/SAF, cR Werbeagentur AG
agency, billboards

7.9 *'I don't use condoms
because they put women off'*
That's a man's fear

Booklet text: *Here is a man
speaking on behalf of not one
but all women. Did he ask
them all, every one of them?*

*What makes him think that
condoms put women off?
Statements such as this are no
more than a man's way to
project male fantasies into
what women seemingly want.
Chances are that instead,
women are put off by men
who refuse to do the
responsible thing – use a
condom.*

7.10 *'I don't use condoms
because I take the pill'*
*The pill doesn't protect against
AIDS*

Booklet text: *A common error
among very young women,
probably because they consider
the simultaneous use of the
pill and condoms redundant. It*

*is not up to an AIDS campaign
to examine the pros and cons
of pill versus condoms. Women
– as well as men – must realize
that the pill protects against
conception. It takes a condom
to protect against sexually
transmitted diseases, such as
AIDS.*

7.11 *'I don't use condoms
because I take regular AIDS
tests'*
*The test doesn't protect against
AIDS*

Booklet text: *The HIV antibody*

*test is not a means of
prevention just as a pregnancy
test is no protection against
becoming pregnant. In either
case, if the test result is
positive, the time to practise
prevention is past.*

billboard campaign in winter 1990 featured excuses, misinformation, apologies
and evasions encountered by AIDS counsellors as 'one-liners', (represented in
7.9–11 as excuses and rejoinders). A TV spot and an additional booklet with
fuller text augmented the campaign. Posters featured the most common excuses,
handwritten to convey a personal note, and accompanied by no other image.

This campaign was not evaluated for its specific impact; the Swiss AIDS
prevention strategy as a whole is evaluated each year.

Practical barriers

Barriers to buying condoms

In addition to cognitive barriers, practical obstacles have inhibited the use of condoms. One such was the problem associated with buying condoms. During the course of the AIDS epidemic, condoms have become considerably more accessible. Retail outlets have expanded to include garages, supermarkets, pubs, clubs and cafés in addition to existing outlets such as mail order and pharmacists. They have also come out from under the counter and are now commonly displayed openly in racks.

Nevertheless, there remains some resistance to their purchase, largely stemming from the potential embarrassment which surrounds the product. Buying condoms is an open statement of sexual activity and while this may be a proud boast for some, for others – particularly the young – it is likely to lead to discomfort. Campaigns in several countries addressed precisely this difficulty. Examples are shown here from Germany and Denmark. Both use well-known actors (for a discussion of the principle behind this strategy, see Chapter 6).

In the German TV and cinema spot (**7.12–16**), a well-known actor plays the part of a young man buying condoms in the supermarket. At the cash till, we see the last transaction being completed and the key character takes his turn looking shamefaced and furtive. He does his best to place his condoms on the till discreetly, but the cashier dashes his hopes of doing so by shouting loudly to her colleague 'Tina! How much are the condoms? 3.99?' To underscore the positive message, a fellow shopper, an elderly woman, replies 'No, 2.99 … they're on special offer' and beams approvingly at the young man. The young man also finds his actions win the approval of a pretty female shopper who throws him an admiring glance.

The matter-of-fact attitude of the other shoppers contrasts sharply with the embarrassment of the young man. The message is not only that there is nothing shameful about buying condoms but that, on the contrary, it is socially approved by others.

7.12–16 Germany, 1989–95, BZgA, cinema, TV.

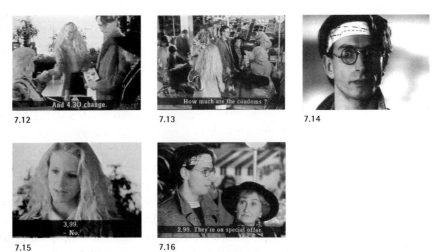

7.12

7.13

7.14

7.15

7.16

7.17–22 Denmark, 1988,
National Board of Health, TV.

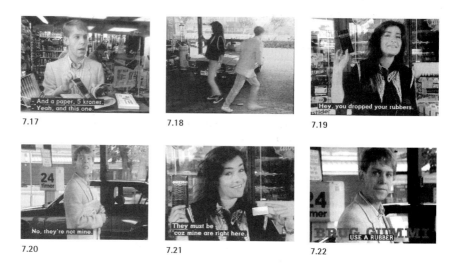

7.17   7.18   7.19

7.20   7.21   7.22

In a similar vein, one of the Danish 1988 'Think twice' campaign spots addresses practical barriers to condom purchase **(7.17–22)**. A young man walks into a garage to pay for his petrol, puts a newspaper on the counter, picks up a pack of condoms from the counter stand and tucks them inside the newspaper, looking behind him to see if anyone is watching. The shop assistant asks 'And a newspaper? Five kroner.' He replies 'Yes, and these', giving her a quick glimpse of the condoms inside the newspaper. He is clearly flustered. He reaches for the money in his pocket, and she says, 'That's 247 in total.' He folds up the newspaper and puts it under his arm, fiddling nervously with his fingers, as he waits for his change. In the next scene he leaves the shop and the pack of condoms begins to slip out of the newspaper. As he walks towards his car, he bumps into a young woman on her way into the shop and the condoms fall on to the floor. Not noticing that he has dropped his condoms, he continues walking. The young woman looks down and, seeing the condoms, picks them up, holds them up in the air and shouts at him, 'Hey, you dropped your rubbers.' He turns round, looks shocked and stutters, 'No, no, that's … no, they're, they're, they're not mine.' She replies, 'They have to be', and grinning, she says '…because I have got mine here.' She takes a pack of condoms from her pocket and holds them up in the other hand. He then checks through his newspaper, and is clearly embarrassed. We hear the AIDS tune whistled, and at the same time, the words 'Use rubber' appear on the screen and the man and woman smile at each other.

In 1989 a sequel to this was developed **(7.23–8)**. It begins in the same way as the previous spot, with a petrol pump being put back on the stand. In the shop, the assistant (this time an older man) says 'That will be 200 kroner, anything else?' The young man (a different one) replies quite openly, 'A pack of rubbers, the black pack.' The queue of people behind are taking no notice at this point. The owner gives him the pack, the young man looks furtively around, leans forward to the shop assistant and whispers 'And a packet of cigarettes with filters.' The owner is taken aback at first but then laughs, and is joined by all the other customers in the shop. The young man throws his money down and runs from the

7.23–28 Denmark, 1989, National Board of Health, TV, cinema.

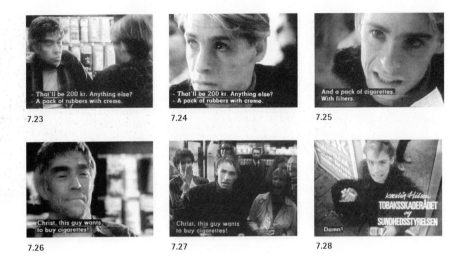

shop (with cigarettes and condoms), looks up at the camera, saying 'Damn.'

These advertisements show the fears people have when buying condoms of exposing themselves to shame and ridicule. These fears are then demonstrated to be unfounded. Contrary to their expectations, fellow shoppers and sales assistants alike turn out to be supportive and approving. The contrast between the obvious embarrassment and discomfort of the shopper is contrasted with the relaxed and matter-of-fact approach of those he comes into contact with. It is interesting to note, however, that all these examples feature men not women, though women give their approval.

Barriers to correct condom use

Low efficacy of condoms is more commonly the result of user failure than method failure (Riley 1989). As a result it is vitally important to provide instruction on the correct use of condoms. There are obvious difficulties in so doing via the media, not least the common prohibition of showing an erect penis in mass communication. Nevertheless these were partly surmounted in the German advertisements featuring the popular cartoon character Rolf (see **8.18–21**) and the Swiss advertisements using the cartoon character Leo.

Communicational barriers

Problems are not only associated with buying condoms, but also with the discussions which are necessary before they are used. Using a condom in a sexual encounter necessitates talking about it in advance and this may be a further impediment to safer sex. The advice to negotiate safer sex with a partner is common in AIDS public education and although well meaning, it has often failed to take into account the fact that sex is often conducted without much discussion. Especially in more casual relationships, couples often say very little. These problems have been addressed in some campaigns, many of which begin by

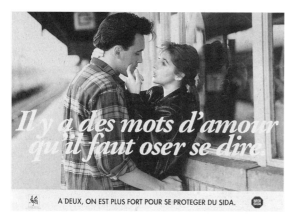

Il y a des mots d'amour qu'il faut oser se dire.

A DEUX, ON EST PLUS FORT POUR SE PROTEGER DU SIDA.

7.29

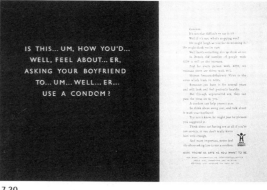

IS THIS... UM, HOW YOU'D...
WELL, FEEL ABOUT... ER,
ASKING YOUR BOYFRIEND
TO... UM... WELL... ER...
USE A CONDOM?

7.30

7.29 Belgium, 1991,
INFORSIDA, posters.
*There are some words of love
you must dare to say.
Together, you have more
strength to protect against
AIDS*

7.30 UK, December 1988–late
1989, HEA, BMP DDB Needham
agency, women's magazines.
*Condom. It's not that difficult
to say is it? Well if it's not,
what's stopping you? He might
laugh at you for mentioning it.
He might think you're easy. Well
here's something else to think
about. In Britain the number of
people with AIDS is still on the
increase. And for every person*

*with AIDS, we estimate there
are thirty with HIV. Human
Immunodeficiency Virus is the
virus which leads to AIDS.
Someone can have it for several
years and still look and feel
perfectly healthy. But through
unprotected sex, they can pass
the virus on to you. A condom
can help to protect you. So
think about using one, and talk
about it with your boyfriend.*

*You never know, he might just
be pleased you suggested it.
Think about not having sex at
all if you're not certain, or if
you don't know him well
enough. And more important,
never feel shy about asking him
to use a condom.
AIDS. You're as safe as you
want to be*

acknowledging the difficulties people experience in talking about sex, with the aim of enabling people to realize that this not a problem peculiar to themselves.

Exactly when to talk about sex is problematic since as soon as condoms are mentioned the assumption has been made that the relationship, whatever its duration, will be sexual. Discussing condom use also raises the whole issue of sexual etiquette since the suggestion by one partner that a condom should be used may be seen by the other as inferring that they were seen to be 'risky'. The fact that raising the subject takes courage is recognized in the Belgian example, which stresses that what is at stake is too serious to allow issues of apprehension or pride to get in the way **(7.29)**.

The first example from the UK **(7.30)** addresses more directly just how difficult talking about safer sex can be. This advertisement appeared in magazines aimed at younger women, and acknowledged in the stuttering and stumbling text that the difficulty of finding the words to talk about sexual matters is a problem shared by everyone.

The second example from the UK **(7.31)** points out the irony that people may feel comfortable enough to be totally intimate, yet may still feel embarrassed at the thought of discussing condom use.

7.31 UK, 1989–90, HEA, BMP
DDB agency, women's
magazines.

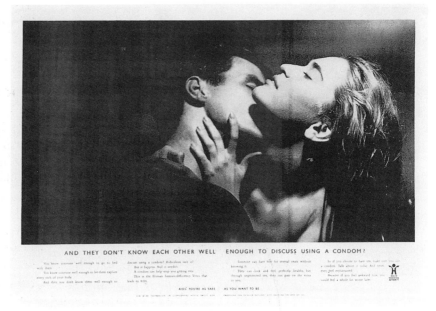

AND THEY DON'T KNOW EACH OTHER WELL   ENOUGH TO DISCUSS USING A CONDOM?

AIDS. YOU'RE AS SAFE   AS YOU WANT TO BE

7.31

A later example from the UK which was also placed in women's magazines aims to prompt people to consider when to raise the subject of condom use – at the beginning of the encounter when the prospect of sex might not yet have arisen and the idea could seem premature, or in the height of passion when reason may no longer prevail. In smaller text, underneath the photographs, the text asks 'When is the easiest moment to say you want to use one? How about while you're still wearing your knickers?' (see **8.16**).

References

Ajzen, I 1988 *Attitudes, personality and behaviour*, Chicago: Dorsey Press

Ajzen, I and M Fishbein 1980 *Understanding attitudes and predicting social behaviour*, Englewood Cliffs, NJ: Prentice Hall

ANRS and AFLS (Agence Nationale de Recherches sur le SIDA and Agence Française de Lutte Contre le SIDA) 1992 *Evaluer la prévention du sida en France: un inventaire des données disponibles*, Paris and Vanves: ANRS and AFLS

Becker, M H and J G Joseph 1988 AIDS and behavioural change to reduce risk: a review, *American Journal of Public Health* **78** (4); 394–410

BVA 1988 *Le SIDA connaissances et attitudes. Premiers resultats*, appendix of press pack, Paris: Ministère de la Solidarité, Santé et Protection Sociale and Comité Français d'Education pour la Santé

BZgA (Bundeszentrale für geshundheitliche Aufklärung) 1994 *AIDS im öffentlichen Bewußtsein der Bundesrepublik 1993*, Cologne: Bundeszentrale für gesundheitliche Aufklärung

Comité Français d'Education pour la Santé and Ministère de la Solidarité, Santé et Protection Sociale 1988 'Aujourd'hui, les préservatifs preservent de tout, même du ridicule', press pack, Paris

de Vries, K 1990 *SOA Stichting procesevaluaties vrij veilig campagne 1989 'De Smoezencamapigne'*, Utrecht: SOA Stichting

Dorozynski, A C 1994 France examines its poor record for using condoms, *British Medical Journal* **308**; 676

Dubois-Arber, F, A Jeannin, G Meystre-Augustoni, F Guet and F Paccaud, 1993 *Evaluation of the AIDS prevention strategy in Switzerland mandated by the Federal Office of Public Health, fourth assessment report 1991–1992*, Lausanne: University Institute of Social and Preventive Medicine

Fishbein, M and I Ajzen 1975 *Belief, attitude, intention and behaviour: an introduction to theory and research*, Reading, Mass.: Addison-Wesley

Hausser, D, E Zimmerman, F Dubois-Arber and F Paccaud 1991 *Evaluation of the AIDS prevention strategy in Switzerland, third assessment report 1989–90*, Lausanne: Institut Universitaire de Médecine Sociale et Préventive

Kraft, P and J Rise 1988 Aids – sources of information and public opinion in Norway 1986, *NIPH Annals* **11** (1); 9–18

Riley, A 1989 The condom, *British Journal of Sexual Medicine* **16** (June); 242–6

Rosenstock, I M 1974a Historical origins of the health belief model, *Health Education Monographs* **2**; 328–35

Rosenstock, I M 1974b The health belief model and preventative health behaviour, *Health Education Monographs* **2**: 354–86

Schmidt, K W, A Krasnik, E Brendstrup, H Zoffmann and S O Larsen 1989 Attitudes towards HIV infection and sexual risk behaviour. A survey among Danish men 16–55 years of age, *Scandinavian Journal of Social Medicine* **17** (4); 281–6

Sheppard, B H, J Hartwick and P R Warshaw 1988 A theory of reasoned action: a meta-analysis of past research with recommendations for modifications and future research, *Journal of Consumer Research* **15**; 325–43

Terry, D J, C Gallois and M McCamish (eds) 1993·*The theory of reasoned action: its application to AIDS-preventive behaviour*, Oxford: Pergamon Press

Tikkanen, J and K Koskela 1992 A five year follow up study of attitudes to HIV infection among Finns, *Health Promotion International* **7** (1); 3–9

Tversky, A and D Kahnemann 1974 Judgment under uncertainty, *Science* **185**; 1124–31

Wellings, K 1988 *Perceptions of risk – media treatment of AIDS*. In P Aggleton and H Holmes (eds) *Social aspects of AIDS*, London: The Falmer Press, pp. 83–105

8 Specific issues in AIDS public education

A number of issues feature more prominently in a discussion of AIDS/HIV public education than in other areas of health promotion. These include the problem of handling sensitive material in the public domain, the difficulty of sustaining interest and maintaining a place for AIDS/HIV on the public agenda, the need to integrate AIDS into allied health problems, and AIDS 'normalization'.

DEALING WITH SENSITIVITIES

A major problem in AIDS public education stems from the sensitivities around open discussion of behaviours associated with the transmission of HIV and its prevention. The routes of HIV transmission and the methods of preventing further spread demand detailed and explicit description of drug use and sexual practices – behaviours which are highly socially regulated and traditionally subject to prohibition and taboo. They are certainly not topics normally aired in public in the context of health education.

Yet many of these issues have now been dealt with for the first time by the mass media; explicit mention of the risks of sexual behaviour in a health promotional context in the past has been limited to contraceptive campaigns designed to prevent pregnancy, and STD campaigns specifically targeted, for example, at travellers and those working in the armed forces.

The problem of social acceptance was exacerbated in the 1980s by the prevailing climate around sexuality. The advent of the AIDS epidemic coincided with a period of retrenchment in moral values. Several countries were seeing repressive measures reintroduced in relation to this area of conduct after the more permissive decade of the 1960s. Sex education was surrounded by renewed controversy in many countries, notably the UK and Belgium. In Germany there was increasing support for retrogressive reform of abortion legislation, and laws relating to drug use were considerably tightened in Italy and Spain. AIDS public education therefore took place against a background of renewed censoriousness in much of Europe.

The problem of causing offence is heightened in the context of interventions targeted at the population as a whole. Public education through the mass media is high profile, and visibility is unavoidable. Furthermore, because of the scale of the exercise and the costs involved, governmental involvement in campaigns is inevitable, which brings further problems in terms of what is possible with regard to sexual explicitness and openness.

Examples of controversy

These difficulties were by no means academic. There are examples from throughout Europe of AIDS public education campaigns which were aborted because of official sensitivities. For example, in the autumn of 1989, a TV condom campaign in the UK aimed at young people – developed and scheduled for launch in October of that year – was abandoned. In fact development research showed the advertisements to be poorly accepted by the target group of young people. The general feeling was that the aim of bringing a light and humorous note to the advertising had not been achieved. But doubts cast over the threat to the general population made the climate a more hostile one in which to mount a campaign solely promoting condoms. Exclusive reliance on the condom message brings criticism of condoning casual sex, and this more radical approach is more likely to be tolerated where it is justified by the perceived scale of the epidemic. The condom advertisements were aborted and replaced by the 'experts' campaign in spring 1990, in which health professionals and scientists talked authoritatively about the UK AIDS epidemic.

Problems of sensitivity have been experienced even in those countries in which the scale of the epidemic warranted radical measures. Even in France, where condom promotion campaigns have run smoothly since 1988, there have been some problems of sensitivity. The Agence Française de Lutte Contre le SIDA (AFLS) planned to run a condom campaign in the Métro to support their TV campaign, but this was halted by the information service attached to the Prime Minister's office and the advisers to the Prime Minister and President. Several explanations were given – that the creative idea worked better in the press, that there were insufficient funds available to cover posters in addition to the other media used. There was, however, speculation in the press and among AIDS associations that the real reason may have been connected with the fact that the Métro spots would be difficult to target specifically and therefore visible to everyone (see country report for France).

Language

Difficulties are often related to the language used. An example is to be found in the third (1991–92) Italian campaign in which a comic book entitled '*Come Ti Frego Il Virus!*' (How to Cheat the Virus!) was produced for young people featuring *Lupo Alberto* (Albert Wolf). HIV was depicted as a black bug to show how the virus could and could not be transmitted. The booklet addressed young people in the kind of argot they themselves used and in a medium – the comic – which they found congenial. Its distribution was impeded by the Ministry of Education. The Ministry of Health (MoH) noted that young people preferred this to other offi-

> The ease with which sex-positive messages can be conveyed depends on:
>
> • the social context in which campaigns are conducted
> • the status of the agency seen to be intervening
> • the severity of the AIDS epidemic.

cial leaflets because it was funny, which also made it popular with teachers. The MoH distributed it on request. Independent distribution was subsequently organized by some NGOs, and by young people themselves through discos and a music magazine. 1,375,559 copies were distributed between 1991–93 by the Centro Informazioni AIDS alone (see Italy country report).

The controversy created by such campaigns has proved a double-edged sword. Where efforts meet with controversy and confrontation between different agencies, the communicational advantages of the intervention have to be weighed against the damage done in terms of undermining the campaign. Public attention tends to focus on the political issues rather than the health educational messages. Alternatively, they may create even more public awareness of the campaign as in the case of the Spanish '*Póntelo, pónselo*' campaign (Chapter 6). Few attempts have been made to evaluate such effects but they certainly rank as unintended outcomes of campaigns.

The social context in which campaigns are conducted

Some countries experienced fewer problems than others in this respect, but few have escaped controversy. Campaign components such as those produced by the Danish Board of Health as early as 1987 (8.1–3) which succeeded in adopting a positive approach towards sexuality, were atypical of the rest of Europe, and the result perhaps of historically more liberal attitudes.

While virtually no European country has escaped some political difficulty in transmitting the condom message, varying degrees of success have been achieved in circumventing the sources of opposition. Some countries have done unexpectedly well in this respect. In Spain for example, a country whose Catholic tradition might have been expected to militate against the frank and explicit presentation of pragmatic messages to use condoms, major progress has been made in deflecting

Denmark, 1987, AIDS Secretariat, Danish National Board of Health, posters, TV.

8.1 *Sex is lovely*

8.2 *Sex is nice*

8.3 *Sex is beautiful*

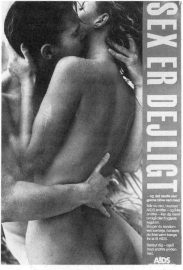

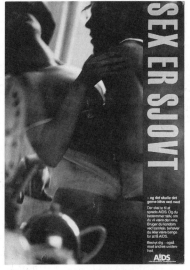

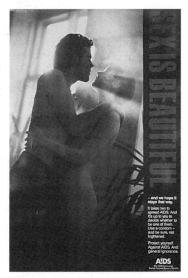

8.1

8.2

8.3

opposition through the use of cartoon characters depicting safe and unsafe sex. In Switzerland, too, the authority of the Roman Catholic Church was used to help fight discrimination against people with AIDS (8.4).

8.4 Switzerland, 1991, FOPH/SAF, cR Basel agency, posters.

Discrimination towards people with AIDS is irreconcilable with the gospel

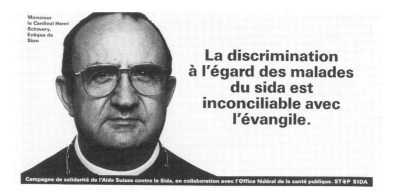

The status of the agency seen to be intervening

Governmental involvement in campaigns creates problems in terms of what is possible with regard to sexual explicitness and openness. The boundaries of acceptability were often quite finely drawn, as in the example of the UK HEA's press campaign of 1988–89, one strand of which aimed to encourage the adoption of safer-sex practices among gay men. This advertisement was produced in two forms. In the first (8.5), which appeared in general readership London listings magazines, the torsos of the two young men were cut off above the nipple and in

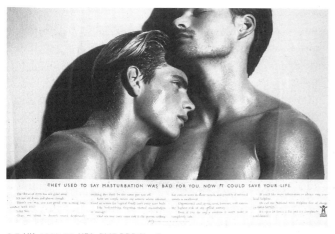

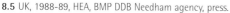

8.5 UK, 1988-89, HEA, BMP DDB Needham agency, press.

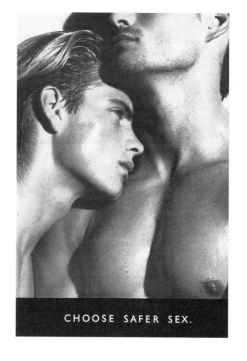

8.6 UK, 1990, HEA, BMP DDB Needham agency, gay press.

the second **(8.6)**, destined for the gay press, the nipple was shown.

The freedom health educators have to promote topics is different from that accorded to commercial advertisers of consumer goods. In general, provided advertisements avoid offending public decency, commercial advertisers have a fairly free rein. In the case of AIDS, interventions are mostly publicly funded and the association with the government and the high visibility of mass media campaigns has led to sensitivities over the content. As a result the treatment of certain issues has been more conservative than health educators would judge ideal.

The use of NGOs

Mass media campaigns are high profile and governmental involvement in campaigns brings further problems with regard to candour and openness, as indicated above. In western European countries, more sensitive work may be handled by NGOs so as to relieve the government of embarrassment and harmful controversy, although not all countries have well-developed networks of NGOs.

An ideal compromise combining the authority conferred by governmental agencies with the grassroots support of the NGO is a coalition of the two. Such an example is to be found in the Swedish 'Love power' campaign **(Plates 16–20)** which was the result of collaboration between the Federal Health Institute (a government agency), the RFSL (the Swedish Federation for Gay and Lesbian Rights) and the RFSU (the Swedish Federation for Sex Education), the latter two of which are NGOs.

The distinctive feature of this Swedish campaign was its use of the flower as a metaphor for sex. Images of arum lilies, tulips and paeonies have a strong aesthetic appeal at the same time as conveying sexual imagery through the striking and powerful resemblance to male and female genital parts. The rubber tree flower is used in the context of the condom message. The campaign used posters, TV and cinema, and postcards with love messages. Condoms were distributed in flower packets. This use of imagery helped ensure fewer objections to explicitness.

Evaluation in autumn 1993 (Levy and Posner-Körösi 1993) showed the campaign to be well received by young people who found the flower language both sensual and attractive and a non-threatening alternative to the fear-provoking treatments of former campaigns. Audience research showed that 80 per cent of young people noticed the campaign compared with the target of 60 per cent, and 97 per cent of those who saw it felt positively about it. Staff in youth centres reported young people spontaneously talking about the messages on cards. 'Love power' also won critical acclaim for the 45-second film *Come together*, and its multi-media campaign (Hiv-Aktuellt 1993).

The severity of the AIDS epidemic

In general, the greater the perceived seriousness of the epidemic, the greater the acceptance of radical solutions and explicit approaches. This may well help to

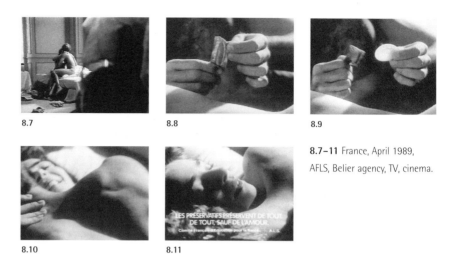

8.7   8.8   8.9

8.10   8.11

8.7–11 France, April 1989, AFLS, Belier agency, TV, cinema.

explain why in high prevalence countries such as France, it has been possible to mount more forthright campaigns (**8.7–11**). The difficulty of handling sensitive health educational material in relation to sexual health in general, and AIDS/HIV in particular, is heightened in countries in which the prevalence of HIV is relatively low. Support for more controversial measures may decline further as the threat of a large scale epidemic of AIDS/HIV in the general population recedes in many European countries. A careful appraisal of tactics which have successfully been used to deflect opposition will be needed.

Progress made

Despite the difficulties, a good deal of progress has been made in a short time. Traditional barriers have been rapidly eroded. The softening of attitudes is also reflected in the tone of advertisements, which have become more light-hearted. What emerges most strikingly from a review of the campaigns is the rapidity with which traditional barriers have been eroded. The example of the 1988–89 UK Health Education Authority press campaign (**8.5, 6**) demonstrates the different standards of acceptability of less than a decade ago. Compare also **Plates 13** and **14** with **15**. This has taken place alongside a general relaxation in standards of what is permissible.

A further example of such progress can be made by contrasting the UK Health Education Authority's 1988 TV spots (which were suggestive rather than informative) (**8.12–15**) with their pragmatic and direct 1993 magazine ad, the text of which asks the reader, 'How far will you go before you mention condoms?... How about when you're still wearing your knickers?' (**8.16**).

Major progress has been made by social marketing in creating a more accepting climate in which condoms can be discussed. Advertising of condoms and advice on how to use them have proved particularly problematic in AIDS public education, with constant claims from the moral lobby that their promotion undermined moral values. In the pre-AIDS period, attitudes towards condom

8.12–15 UK, 1988, HEA, TBWA agency, TV.

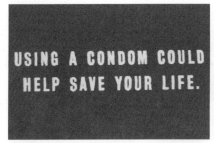

8.12

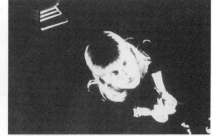

8.13

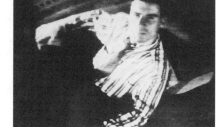

8.14

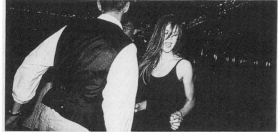

8.16 UK, 1993, HEA, BMP DDB Needham agency, women's magazines.

Things have moved a long way, as demonstrated in a comparison between these two UK advertisements.

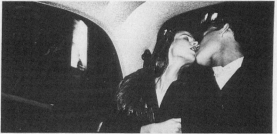

8.15

HOW FAR WILL YOU GO BEFORE YOU MENTION CONDOMS?

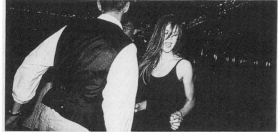

THIS FAR?

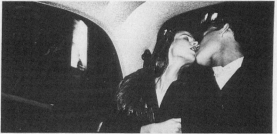

THIS FAR?

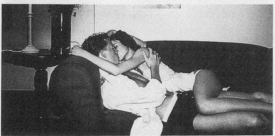

THIS FAR?

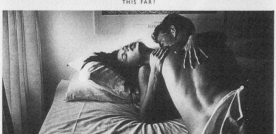

THIS FAR?

Today, no one can ignore the need to mention condoms. Have sex with someone without using one and not only could you risk an unwanted pregnancy, but you also risk contracting one of the many sexually transmitted diseases.

Like Herpes, Chlamydia, Gonorrhoea, and of course HIV, the virus which leads to AIDS.

So the question isn't if, but when you mention condoms. You could mention them at any moment leading up to sexual intercourse. In reality, it's not quite so easy.

Mention them too early and you might feel you look pushy or available. Leave it too late and you risk getting so carried away you might not mention them at all.

When is the easiest moment to say you want to use one? How about while you're still wearing your knickers? In this instance it would be picture three.

By now you've gone far enough to make it obvious that you both want to have sex. But not so far that you're in danger of getting emotionally and sexually carried away.

It's a perfect opportunity. So take it. Say you want to use a condom.

Say he hasn't got one? Well have one of your own at the ready just in case. It really doesn't matter whose you use.

And then you can go just as far as you like.

FOR MORE INFORMATION OR ADVICE ABOUT AIDS OR HIV PHONE THE FREE NATIONAL AIDS HELPLINE ON 0800 567 123. IT'S OPEN 24 HOURS A DAY AND IS COMPLETELY CONFIDENTIAL.

8.16

promotion were considerably more censorious. The AIDS/HIV epidemic has opened doors which no one thought possible. Because mass media work aims to help change the social environment, the measurement of such outcomes is a legitimate part of evaluation. This social advocacy function is important. In the long term, changing the wider social environment, as opposed to changing individual behaviour, may turn out to be the principal contribution social marketing can make in AIDS public education (Wellings 1992).

In the UK for example, the British Broadcasting Corporation refused to screen a 1985 Grand Prix because Durex sponsored one car, and TV advertising condoms was forbidden. Yet only two years later, in July 1987, this ban was lifted and the first TV condom commercial was screened. The ban on TV condom advertising was also lifted in Belgium in 1987; in Ireland, legislation restricting the sale of condoms was amended in 1992 and 1993. In 1993 the Irish Health Promotion Unit launched its first condom promotion campaign, in which personalities talked openly to the audience about condoms and safer sex. Although there has been some criticism of this campaign for not warning people of the dangers of sex, the pressure for moral messages has eased considerably.

Campaign strategies

The use of humour

Major progress has been made in deflecting opposition through the use of humour. Research shows that explicit imagery does not necessarily increase recall (Alexander and Judd 1978). The skilful use of jokes, puns and cartoons has bypassed possible criticism that campaign components are too frank, allowing the use of material which might otherwise have brought the charge of overexplicitness.

While virtually no European country has escaped some political difficulty in transmitting the condom message, varying degrees of success have been achieved in circumventing the sources of opposition. Some countries have done unexpectedly well in this respect. As mentioned above, in Spain for example, the use of cartoon characters depicting safe and unsafe sex helped deflect possible opposition (8.17) (see Chapter 2, '*SiDa NoDa*' campaign). In Germany and Norway too, the use of humour has helped ease the passage of some of the more explicit campaign components (8.18–21 and 8.22–5).

8.17 Spain, 1987–90, Ministry of Health, TV.
A whole series of actions depicted by round cartoon figures are presented with a play on words, with '*SiDa*' representing both AIDS and having the meaning 'can give', along with the antithesis '*NoDa*' – 'can't give'. Both the poster and the TV spot have the endline 'Don't change your life because of AIDS!'

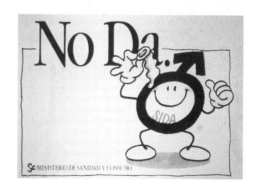

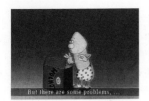

8.18

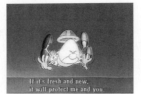

8.19

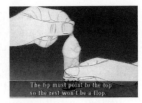

8.20

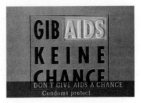

8.21

8.18–21 Germany, 1989–94, BZgA, TV, cinema.

Little Rolf

I'm so wild, I break everybody's heart

I'm full of passions, that's why they love me.

Little Rolf really likes to boast a little.

But there are some problems...

...one can't deny it would be a big lie.

If you don't care it's a frown...

...you put it on upside down.

If it's fresh and new it will protect me and you.

Little Rolf, don't be a fool. Let's start again, keep cool.

This one's new, it's our luck so we're not stuck.

The tip must point to the top so the rest won't be a flop.

Now little Rolf knows how easy it goes and how well it shows.

The moral is: we like each other so we don't mind using them

O, little Rolf.

Don't give AIDS a chance

Condoms protect

In this example from the German campaigns, the popular cartoon character Rolf is used to demonstrate the correct use of the condom.

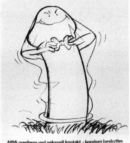

8.22

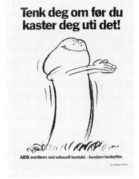

8.23

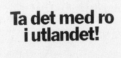

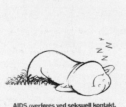

8.24

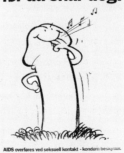

8.25

Norway, 1986, Directorate of Health, all media.

8.22 *Are you properly dressed for the occasion?*

8.23 *Think before you take the plunge!*

8.24 *When you're abroad – take it easy!*

8.25 *Think before you act!*

Technical approaches

Presentational strategies

Much possible criticism may be deflected by the tasteful presentation of more explicit scenes. In France in 1989, one of the first tasks for the newly created Agence Française de Lutte Contre le SIDA (AFLS) was to develop a public education intervention with the aim of normalizing condom use to make the condom everyday, commonplace, ordinary (*'banaliser'*) using a direct and explicit style of communication.

A new TV spot (April 1989) was developed by the Belier agency showing a couple making love (**8.7–11**). The tone conveyed is natural, and one of tenderness, harmony and desire, avoiding any suggestion of vulgarity. The feeling is one of satisfying lovemaking without impairing love and pleasure. Just before actual intercourse takes place, the man opens the condom, the bodies touch, and the action is harmoniously completed. The film seeks to be explicit rather than hiding things, allowing the public to feel involved and to identify themselves in the situation.

The candour of the film was conveyed partly by means of an absence of sophisticated artifice and an emphasis on naturalism. This was achieved by the choice of sober black and white, the use of a hand-held camera and by the selection of actors looking like ordinary people. All this was stated explicitly by the advertising agency in their treatment. The artful use of metaphor as advertising device was deliberately avoided for the explicitly stated reason that this could confuse the issue and distort the image of condoms and therefore hide the message. The photos for the press campaign were created in the same spirit. An earlier version of this film used the sounds of lovemaking as the background to the action and these were replaced by classical music in the final version.

Distancing devices

The aim of the Swedish state AIDS Delegation's 1989 campaign (**8.26–9**) was to be sex positive but mindful of sensitivities this might arouse. A strategy was devised which would minimize offence. A positive campaign was created, with images of life and lust dominating the posters – love scenes from a Japanese painting, a picture from Seriestarlet 1989 (a romantic comic book with illustrations redolent of the 1950s), a drawing after Matisse and an etching from 1792 depicting Casanova. The use of illustrations in both colour and black and white from another time (the eighteenth century) and another culture (Japan) provides distance and helps to desensitize the audience. The old-style italics font used for the headlines does the same. These distancing devices enabled the advertisements to be more sex positive than might have been possible using contemporary imagery. The campaign encourages love, lust and the use of condoms, and depends less on information, containing only the advice to make love sensibly.

Two semantic points need to be raised in the context of these advertisements. First, the Swedish word for love incorporates the words 'love' and 'game').

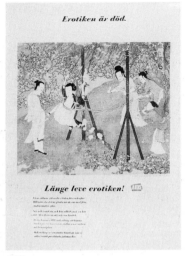

8.26

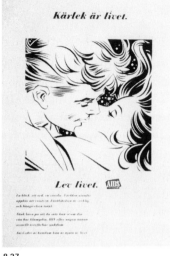

8.27

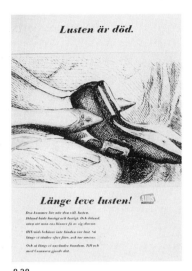

8.28

Sweden, spring 1989, State AIDS
Delegation, Ted Bates agency, posters.
8.26 *Erotica is dead. Long live erotica*
8.27 *Love is life. Live life*
8.28 *Lust is dead. Long live lust*
8.29 *Love is life. Live life*

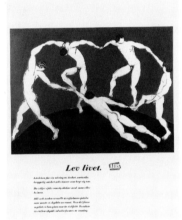

8.29

Second, the word 'lust' in Swedish has less negative connotations than in English; it is more connected with 'appetite', though with some sexual overtones.

This campaign also featured a cartoon on TV and cinema (May 1989). Two pairs of intertwined shoes are seen, one belonging to a man, the other to a woman. Background sounds of lovemaking are heard, squeaks, kisses and 'kiss kiss', 'hug hug'. Then the woman's voice says 'Wait, wait a little…there is something…', the male voice replies 'I know, I know.' Next a pause, and the woman's voice is heard saying 'You're not just handsome, you've got something in your head.' The endline is: 'Call for the AIDS hotline number and get information. You can be anonymous. Long live lust.'

Exchanging perspectives

Countries can clearly learn from one another but must always be aware of the cultural, social and political constraints in each. Local campaigns may avoid causing offence where similar ones at central level would run into difficulties. Health educators in western Europe often forget that in the West progess in changing public attitudes has been gradual and incremental rather than radical and revolutionary, and it may be necessary for countries in eastern and central Europe to follow this process.

Experience in this respect cautions against transferring materials developed in the West automatically to the East. For example, orthodox Catholics oppose most of the AIDS education interventions in Poland and it is impossible to use the mass media in relation to condom messages. A gay leaflet for gay men on safer sex translated from the French original was seen as dangerous and as encouraging homosexuality. Problems are also encountered in relation to the use of methadone in Poland, where it is seen as unethical to exchange one drug for another. In Romania a visitor from the Netherlands brought a text on the use of condoms to be used with factory workers, but the translator refused to translate the most explicit sections (Curtis 1992).

In western European countries, the assumption is often made that more sensitive work can be handled by NGOs, so as to relieve the government of embarrassment and harmful controversy. But it should not be taken for granted that all countries are well provided with such an infrastructure. The Czech Republic, for example, is lacking in this respect and institutions are highly medicalized. Alternatively, there may be an established framework of NGOs, but the problem lies in how to utilize it (Curtis 1992).

Nevertheless, experiences of coping with unfavourable conditions in one country may be extremely valuable to another. Certainly health educators in different European countries can learn from one another, and should do so increasingly if possibly diminishing resources are to be best used. Every effort should be made to exchange information about successes and failures. Some of the mistakes made in earlier campaigns in the West are in danger of being repeated. For example, in the Czech Republic, campaigners are reportedly using high levels of fear and there is little or no promotion of sexual enjoyment.

SUSTAINING PUBLIC AWARENESS – 'AIDS IS STILL WITH US'

A major challenge in AIDS public education has been that of maintaining levels of public awareness, interest and concern (Töppich and Christiansen 1993). The problem of keeping AIDS/HIV on the public agenda, while ensuring a level of activity which is manageable in terms of resource allocation, faces every European country but, paradoxically, most particularly those in which preventive efforts may have been most successful in averting greater disaster.

Delays in setting up preventive initiatives created problems, but expediting campaigns on the basis of the most pessimistic contemporary predictions at the outset has also produced problems in maintaining subsequent levels of public concern. One identifiable difficulty is that the goal of sustainability is often in opposition to establishing authenticity. Exaggerating the level of risk will destroy credibility, while honestly stating it may not be sufficient to motivate people. The challenge for many countries has been how to maintain a constant presence for AIDS/HIV in public education campaigns, at the same time as attempting to 'normalize' the disease, moving away from a concept of acute crisis to one of chronic public health problem.

The problem is compounded by the threat of shrinking resources. Relatively generous budgets continue to be dedicated to AIDS/HIV preventive activities. Strong government approval for preventive work exists, but there is no guarantee that this situation will continue, and indeed there are already signs of diminishing and declining interest at some levels. There is therefore a need to have structures in place now which will maintain a constant presence for AIDS, in anticipation of and preparation for possible cutbacks later.

In such circumstances the need to avoid *ad hoc*, uncoordinated interventions lacking in continuity, and instead to implement sustainable approaches is paramount. A major problem of AIDS/HIV public education in some countries has been its disjointed and uneven pace. Interventions need to be paced to avoid short, intermittent and apparently unconnected bursts of publicity. A further difficulty in this respect derives from the media used (Wellings and McVey 1990). Difficulties of sustaining public awareness have been exacerbated in those countries in which there was heavy reliance on television at the start of the campaigns, a medium which has helped to create peaks and troughs despite its initial effectiveness in achieving high impact. Television campaigns are expensive and take some time to develop, creating delays and gaps in public information. The problem has also been heightened in countries in which high impact, fear-inducing messages have been used; it has proved difficult to maintain concern at initial levels (for further discussion of this, see Chapter 6).

Possible approaches aimed at achieving sustainability

Public education campaigns in some countries have achieved considerable success in keeping AIDS/HIV on the public agenda and have helped guard against the 'here-today-gone-tomorrow' spirit which seems to be generated by high profile hyperactivity followed by periods of relative inactivity.

Creating continuity

One means by which continuity has been achieved has been by incorporating what has been termed a synergistic element into the campaign format, by employing a continuing theme, logo, leitmotif or slogan which unites and links campaign components. This serves simply to remind people of the ongoing threat of AIDS/HIV. A notable example of the synergistic approach is to be found in the advertisements of the Swiss 'Stop AIDS' campaigns, in which the ubiquitous condom image has appeared in a number of guises: as the O in 'Stop AIDS', in 'OK', in 'Tonight', as the moon above Geneva, Zurich, Berne or Montreux, and so on **(Plates 21–7)**.

An ingenious method of evaluating this aspect of the campaign was devised. Travellers through various airports in Switzerland were asked to say what they perceived the condom to be, in selected examples of the advertisements they were shown. Generally, and in most cases, the Swiss native travellers replied that the objects they saw were condoms, while the non-Swiss travellers in the airports identified them as the moon over Geneva, the sun in the sky, the letter O and so on, demonstrating effectively how successful the Swiss campaign had been in familiarizing the public with the condom (F Dubois-Arber, personal communication 1990).

In Germany, the slogan 'Don't give AIDS a chance' **(8.33–44)** has continued throughout the campaign. In Denmark, a two-tone whistle in the 1988–89 'Think twice' campaign served to unite campaign components. In Italy, too, although each campaign has addressed different themes, certain techniques have been used to achieve continuity: the endline 'If you know about it you can avoid it. If you know about it, it won't kill you' was used throughout four national campaigns run between 1988 and 1993; all the Italian AIDS campaign materials bear the logo of the National Commission – a thistle in a square in an octagon – over the words National Commission for the Fight Against Aids, Ministry of Health, using the same typography and the use of a yellow and blue colour scheme helped to introduce a coherence into the separate campaign components.

Condensing messages

After continued exposure to advertisements, a high level of public absorption of information can be assumed, and the problem is then rather one of providing reminders that AIDS remains a threat. Shortened, condensed messages which presuppose a familiarity with previous campaign components can be effective, serving simply to remind people of the presence of AIDS/HIV. Such techniques accommodate decreasing budgets better, since the development of each new wave of the campaign is more a continuation than a fresh beginning.

The strategy has also been put to good effect, although in a more limited way, in the minimalist Swedish advertisement using the Swedish Black Jack condom itself as the building block for a number of images signifying risk **(Plates 28–39)**.

The AIDS 'red ribbon' is a further example of such an approach and has been used on a crossnational scale **(8.30–2)**.

Pooling campaign components

In Germany, campaign components have been 'pooled', and a selection made from a central and accumulating store of executions mixed and matched differently for different audiences and at different times **(8.33–44)**. The repeat use of campaign components which have worked well presents a cost-effective solution to the twin problems of 'burn out' and funding difficulties, and will appeal to fresh audiences

8.30 Spain, 1993, Federación Anti-SIDA España posters.
8.31 UK, 1993, World AIDS Day Steering Group, leaflets.
8.32 Ireland, 1993, Dublin AIDS Alliance, brochure.

These examples from Spain, UK and Ireland illustrate how the red ribbon has been adapted and used as a way of 'condensing' the AIDS prevention message.

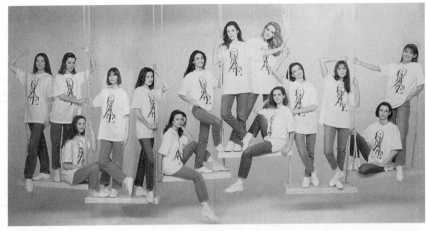

8.30

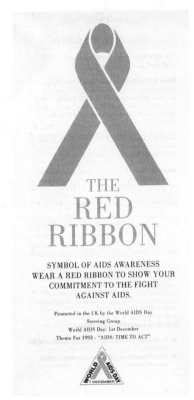

THE
RED
RIBBON

SYMBOL OF AIDS AWARENESS
WEAR A RED RIBBON TO SHOW YOUR
COMMITMENT TO THE FIGHT
AGAINST AIDS.

Promoted in the UK by the World AIDS Day
Steering Group
World AIDS Day: 1st December
Theme For 1993 - "AIDS: TIME TO ACT"

8.31

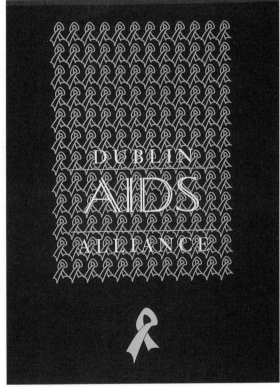

8.32

as new populations enter the pool of people at risk. This allows agencies to select successful strands of campaigns to be extended and expanded, and for agencies to capitalize on the advertisements which have worked best.

From their inception, the various interventions incorporating different messages have been combined and interchanged to appear repeatedly at regular intervals. This strategy obviated the need to develop novel approaches at each new

Germany, 1990–92, BZgA, TV, posters.

8.33 *Being faithful protects both of us*

8.34 *I think responsibility is necessary*

8.35 *Protecting ourselves is not old hat*

8.36 *On holiday did you think of everything?*

8.37 *Sick people belong to us*

8.38 *Man to man*

8.39 *Whether Jack or a Queen, safety is rule number one*

8.40 *Customer, only with...*

8.41 *Wanderlust has too high a price*

8.42 *Not every relationship is a stable one*

8.43 *Fixing? I'm not stupid*

8.44 *You don't share hot needles*

'Gib AIDS keine Chance', 'Don't give AIDS a chance', appears in every component. It unites and links campaign components designed for different audience groups.

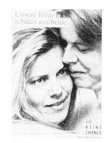
8.33

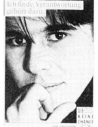
8.34

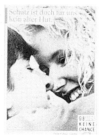
8.35

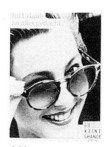
8.36

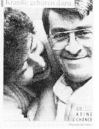
8.37

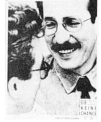
8.38

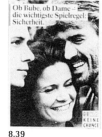
8.39

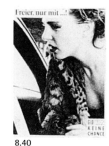
8.40

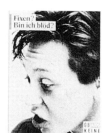
8.41

8.42

8.43

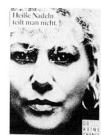
8.44

wave of public education, at the same time repeatedly serving to remind people of messages and to provide information to new audiences hearing it for the first time.

Exploiting seasonality

Summer vacations

Holiday campaigns have been used in most countries, and campaigns aimed at travellers have been a consistent annual feature of AIDS public education work in many countries. They have managed to escape controversy and are a good example of the use of seasonality to maintain continuity. The crossnational Europe against AIDS summer campaign is a good example of this (for further discussion of this campaign, see the final part of this chapter).

Other, perhaps less obvious, opportunities for exploiting seasonality include:

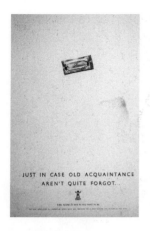

JUST IN CASE OLD ACQUAINTANCE
AREN'T QUITE FORGOT...

8.45 UK, 1989/90 New Year's
Eve, HEA, BMP DDB Needham
agency, press.

Christmas period

Since alcohol is implicated in unsafe sex, the link with Christmas festivities is an obvious one to exploit in AIDS public education. Abortion rates have been shown to increase each spring, and this has been linked with this phenomenon. The obvious parallel here is with drink-driving campaigns which similarly appear seasonally, and though a killjoy no-sex/no-alcohol message from the health educational agencies is clearly to be avoided, the New Year advertisement from the UK HEA illustrates how this link with condom use might lightly be achieved **(8.45)**. Figure 8.1 suggests that the Christmas period may offer opportunities for exploiting seasonality, since alcohol is implicated in unsafe sex and Christmas parties present opportunities for sexual liaisons. In spite of the evidence, no campaign has yet suggested the condom as a Christmas stocking-filler.

Figure 8.1 Practice of condom use in the UK: indexed condom sales April 1989–June 1990

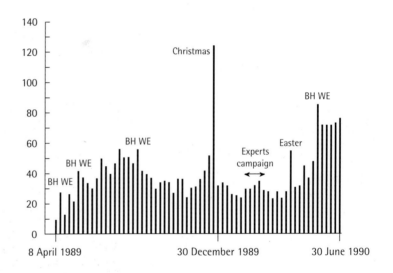

(Source: HEA) BH WE = Bank holiday weekend

Start of academic term

A high proportion of young people in Europe go on to higher education and the start of the academic year in autumn is a further example of an opportunity to introduce AIDS-related sexual health messages. This is the time when young people are leaving home for the first time and experiencing greater sexual freedom. Many universities and colleges around Europe have introduced condoms into 'fresher packs' aimed at students starting their courses **(8.46, 47)**.

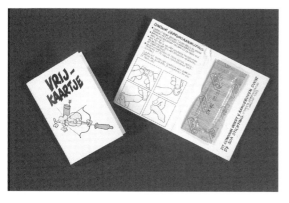

8.46 The Netherlands, 1992, STD Foundation, packs.

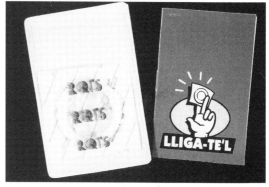

8.47 Spain, 1993, Department of Health and Social Security (Catalonia), packs. *'Lliga-te'l'* is a play on words either meaning 'get yourself one' or 'keep it with you' (referring to the condom); the verb *lligar* can also mean 'to chat up'.

World AIDS Day

An opportunity has been created in World AIDS Day to use calendar events to keep AIDS on the agenda. Illustrated examples are provided here from Greece (8.48–52).

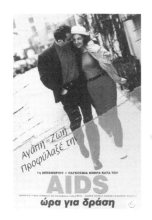

8.48 Greece, 1993, Hellenic Centre for the Control of AIDS and STDs, posters.
Love = life, look after it

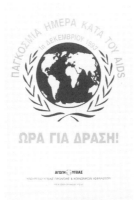

8.49 Greece, 1993, Ministry Of Health, posters.
Time for action

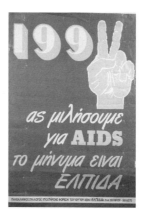

8.50 Greece, 1992, ELPIDA (NGO), posters.
Let's talk about AIDS. The message is hope

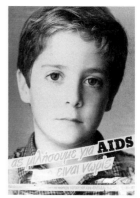

8.51 Greece, 1993, ELPIDA (NGO), posters.
Let's talk about AIDS. It's time

8.52 Greece, 1993, Hellenic Centre for the Control of AIDS and STDs, posters.

If you love you do not forget

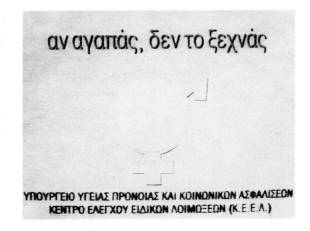

Learning from others

Such techniques have enabled countries to cope more easily with decreasing budgets and the consequence of decreasing scale of activity. This is potentially most effective as a strategy for those countries in which AIDS public education work is at an early stage of development. For those European countries which have now accumulated a long tradition of AIDS public education it is clearly too late to introduce suddenly an element of synergy in the form of a common logo into the campaign where none has previously existed.

Nevertheless, even in countries in which campaigns are well established, there exist opportunities for echoing particular features of earlier campaigns. In the Netherlands, for example, the phrase 'AIDS and understanding make a great team' used in the 1994 solidarity campaign recalled and reinforced the earlier message 'A little bit of understanding (never gave anyone AIDS)' from the solidarity campaign of 1990–92.

Because of continued uncertainty in predicting the future course of the AIDS epidemic, there will remain a need for the public to be kept reminded of the need for protection. Even in countries in which a unifying approach has not been used, opportunities for coping with budgetary constraints have been exploited.

Eastern and central Europe

The problem of sustainability is not, of course, applicable as yet to eastern Europe, where AIDS public education is just beginning. Not only is the duration of the AIDS epidemic shorter in these countries, but the lack of established health promotion structures has delayed response to it in terms of public education. Given the unstable economic and political situation, and the lack of networks to use for the purpose, it is not surprising that AIDS-prevention activities have been slow to get off the ground.

Recent experience in these countries cautions against the instant transfer of tried and tested strategies from the West, and calls for a respect for cultural, political and economic national constraints. Campaigns are necessarily culturally specific to some extent, so that what works in one country or with one group may not in another. In many eastern European countries a biomedical approach to public health is dominant; screening and testing have been seen as more appropriate interventions than information, education and communication. The National AIDS Federations in Hungary, Bulgaria and Russia, for example, have invested major efforts in mandatory screening with special emphasis on groups such as travellers, prostitutes, etc.

The move in these countries from biomedical approaches to prevention towards a greater reliance on health promotion has been slow so far. Medicalization of health issues is likely to put the perceived responsibility for health and illness in the hands of physicians rather than those of the public. An established dependence on medical approaches to stop the spread of disease is, as a consequence, problematic for AIDS prevention, where medical approaches have only limited use.

INTEGRATION INTO SEXUAL HEALTH

Increasingly, the future of AIDS prevention is seen by many as belonging to the domain of sexual health as a whole. The move both nationally and internationally (in organizations such as the World Health Organization and the International Planned Parenthood Federation), is towards the integration of AIDS/HIV with other sexual health programmes. The focus is broadening from work based solely on AIDS/HIV to encompass sexual health more generally, incorporating contraception, STD control, abortion, cervical cancer, etc.

The trend to integration is driven by:

- shrinking budgets
- the recognition that worst fears with regard to AIDS are unlikely to be realized in many countries
- the recognition of the need for positive approaches to sexual health
- the need to place AIDS/HIV on the agenda of a broader range of agencies.

Motives for integration

One reason for this shift has been economic. The plan to stop treating AIDS as a special case is the result of the possible phasing out of dedicated AIDS funding. The integration of AIDS into other areas of health promotion is now generally accepted as essential in view of the more equitable distribution of resources. To date a number of features have justified making AIDS a special case in terms of resourcing. The disease is fatal, transmittable, has the potential to escalate, is concentrated in the young population and is characterized by a skewed geographical distribution. These unique features justified generous and dedicated funding for preventive activities.

Yet the worst scenario predicted for many European countries has not been realized. The prevalence of AIDS/HIV in most of Europe is not only lower than in other parts of the world, but also lower than originally feared. To what extent this is attributable to preventive action is not clear, but it is possible that features of policy and practice in Europe have helped avert the scale of the epidemic as experienced elsewhere.

In some countries in Europe the prevalence of AIDS is high enough to warrant further dedicated funding and AIDS-specific campaigns for the foreseeable future. In others, the threat of AIDS itself has receded, and the time may have come for a reconsideration of the separatist strategy. The move towards an integrated focus is more likely to be a feature of campaigns in countries in which the low prevalence of HIV makes it difficult to justify continuing funding expensive mass media campaigns.

A strong case can also be made for integration in terms of achieving a positive climate around sexuality generally. Issues around healthy sexuality are not simply to do with the avoidance of disease but the maintenance of health (Mahler 1981). A consequence of the domination of the sexual health agenda by HIV is a tendency to link sexual activity with morbidity and to see it as life threatening rather than life enhancing. Sexually transmitted diseases remain embarrassing to many people, having connotations of sexual promiscuity and unfaithfulness. In this context, the pathological aspects of sexuality should not be dealt with to the exclusion of pleasure. Reluctance to integrate STD and AIDS prevention into

Sweden, 1993, RFSU, posters.
8.53 *Factor six/sex!* [same word in Swedish] *Love with condoms!*
8.54 *For even safer sex!*

Broadening the discussion to other sexual health issues makes it easier to place AIDS/HIV education on the agenda of a range of different groups in society with long experience in safer-sex education, in this case the RFSU.

The emphasis in advertisement **8.53** is on risk-reduction behaviour – hence the analogy with suntan cream and the focus on the protective factor.

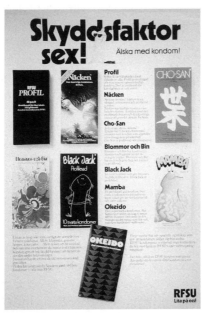

8.53

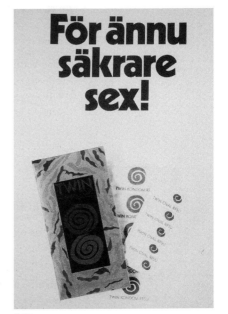

8.54

family planning programmes on the grounds that stigmatization might negatively affect use of contraception, has been shown to be unfounded (Elias 1994). It seems more likely that continuing to treat AIDS as a special area might lead to the stigmatization of affected individuals.

Widening the discussion to other sexual health issues also makes it easier to reach different groups in society (Bottomley 1993). Agencies concerned with the prevention of STDs and unplanned pregnancy have long experience in safer-sex education, and an integrated approach allows them to be brought in from the periphery. STD clinics and family planning clinics are useful settings for disseminating messages about sexual health. People attend such services voluntarily, present with a sexually related concern and therefore expect relevant advice. It then becomes a relatively easy task to broaden that advice to other aspects of sexual health **(8.53, 54)**.

The benefits of including AIDS/HIV education within sexual health should be reciprocal. AIDS/HIV has hastened progress in many countries in terms of sexual health education, and it would be a mistake not to take advantage of this development. In the past, opportunities to get across messages about sexual health have been missed because sex education has been neglected. AIDS/HIV offers a good chance to remedy this in the wider context of sexually transmitted diseases, psychosexual issues, and control of fertility and infertility.

Practical aspects of integration

The simplest way of effecting the transition to sexual health generally is to extend a strategic direction which has already begun. As communication strategies have developed, there has been a decreasing emphasis on the disease category, and an increasing emphasis on the underlying health-related behaviour. The risk of HIV infection is now largely recognized, and efforts can be directed towards promoting methods of protection from infection. The focus now is on condoms rather than AIDS; away from the disease towards the preventive action, i.e. from *health outcome* to the *preventive behaviour* or *risk-reduction strategy* itself, e.g. condom use, adoption of safer sex, reduction in numbers of partners, HIV testing, STD clinic attendance, etc.

This approach finds parallels in other areas of health promotion: cancer or coronary heart disease is not always mentioned specifically in support of recommendations to stop smoking, cut down drinking or eat sensibly; the benefit of staying healthy is promoted. This approach stresses not the avoidance of illness but the maintenance of good health, and has still more rational appeal in the context of increasing evidence that people exhibit a consistent risk profile across different behaviours. People who have higher numbers of sexual partners are also more likely to smoke and to drink more (Wadsworth and Johnson 1994).

Broadening the scope of interventions also has the potential to help solve problems relating to perception of risk. Although STDs may not be publicly perceived as being as serious as AIDS, larger numbers of people are affected even if the outcome is less grave. While HIV infection can be devastating, the actual probability of infection is so low that it is difficult to persuade people to change their behaviour due to the long odds of being affected (Fineberg 1988; Job 1988).

Disadvantages of integration

Caution needs to be exercised when assuming transfer of messages from disease prevention and protection from pregnancy. In terms of behaviour there is clearly a link between HIV, other STDs and sexual health. That condom use protects against other STDs is well known (Judson *et al.* 1989). Yet condoms may be less effective in protecting against pregnancy than other methods of contraception, so that advice to use them as protection from disease could potentially have an adverse effect on unplanned pregnancies (Bromham and Cartmill 1993a,b; Taylor 1993).

A further possible disadvantage of the generic approach is that, without the association of AIDS, the impact of advice on risk-reduction strategies related to sexual health may be diminished. STDs, pregnancy, infertility, etc. may be generally regarded as minor issues compared with the perceived magnitude and severity of the threat of AIDS. STDs and HIV are perceived very differently, and it may be difficult to develop a credible and relevant message which embraces the risk of both.

Broadening AIDS/HIV programmes to incorporate not just other STDs, but also issues relating to fertility has therefore advantages and disadvantages. As interest in AIDS/HIV wanes, however, it clearly makes sense to widen the health issue. On the other hand, in so doing we must guard against the risk of mixing messages and confusing the public.

The campaigns

Some European countries have been able to make the transition to a general sexual health programme more easily than others. In France the emphasis of condom advertisements has, from the beginning, been on the behaviour and not the disease. The endline of the 1990–91 French condom campaign, 'Condoms protect against everything, everything except love', encapsulates the move away from AIDS and towards a broader concept of sexual health, and also a positive attitude towards sexuality. Other countries, such as Switzerland, in which the condom has been an integral part of AIDS campaigns specifically, have greater difficulties in this respect. But in both these countries the prevalence of AIDS is high enough to warrant further specific AIDS prevention campaigns for the foreseeable future.

As part of the Spanish '*Póntelo, pónselo*' campaign, a poster was produced featuring a yellow condom over which was written the words: 'unwanted pregnancies, gonorrhoea, AIDS, fungal infection, hepatitis B, vaginitis, trichomoniasis, genital herpes, syphilis, candida', and other STDs lightly scratched out (8.55).

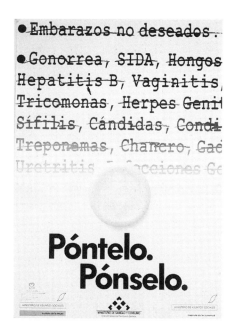

● Embarazos no deseados .

● Gonorrea, SIDA, Hongos
Hepatitis B, Vaginitis,
Tricomonas, Herpes Genit
Sífilis, Cándidas, Condi
Treponemas, Chancro, Gac
Uretritis ~ ~ccciones Ge

Póntelo.
Pónselo.

8.55 Spain, Ministry of Health
and Consumer Affairs, Ministry
of Social Affairs, Institute for
Women, Institute for Young
People, 1990–91, posters, TV,
radio.
This Spanish poster, part of the
'Póntelo, pónselo' ('Put it on,
put it on him') campaign,
appeared in the subway and
on street hoardings. It
associates the use of a
condom with prevention of
other STDs and pregnancy.

*The Netherlands 'Three steps to heaven' campaign 1993: a case study in the integration of
AIDS/HIV into sexual health*

In the Netherlands, the planned integration of AIDS into other sexual health issues is seen as a way in which the normalization of AIDS as an issue will occur. The AIDS public education campaign strategy between 1987–91 used the mass media for two separate campaigns: the Safe Sex Campaign for young people was run by the STD Foundation, thereby relieving the government-linked National Committee on AIDS Control of the need to be associated with more controversial national advertising; the National Information Campaign (knowledge of HIV and solidarity) was run by the National Committee on AIDS Control Sub-committee for HIV Prevention, in close collaboration with the Ministry of Health, Welfare and Culture. The Dutch STD Foundation had always been in favour of broadening the focus of campaigns to sexual health, principally because of a belief that the safer-sex message is fairly unpalatable, and that people therefore need to be given a range of reasons for practising risk reduction. The STD Foundation uses the expression 'Double Dutch' to describe the use of both condom and oral contraception, an approach now also being promoted by the commercial sector in other countries also **(8.56)**.

In 1991 the dual campaign strategy was combined into one working group responsible for safer sex, solidarity and general information campaigns, for reasons of economy and efficiency. This working group was responsible for the 1993 safer-sex campaign, 'Three steps to heaven', the aim of which was to empower young people to make choices relating to sexual health, to practise safer sex, use condoms and provide safer-sex advice relevant to each option. The campaign involved TV and cinema spots, set to the music and lyrics of the popular song 'Three steps to

8.56 UK, Schering Health Care Ltd, 1993, family planning clinics, GP surgeries.
An example from the commercial sector: Schering Health Care Ltd have produced a discreet black suedette pouch with space for both condom and oral contraceptive pills, to fit into a handbag. The pack was given out with prescriptions of Femodene.

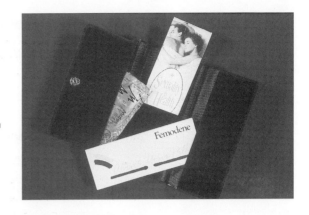

8.57–62 The Netherlands, February–June 1993, Ministry of Health, Welfare and Culture Working Group, TV, cinema. 'The three steps to heaven' safe-sex campaign.

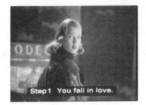

8.57

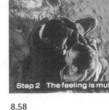

8.58

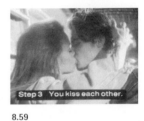

8.59

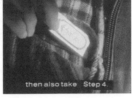

8.60

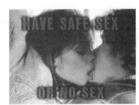

8.61

8.62

8.63 The Netherlands, 1993, Ministry of Health, Welfare and Culture Working Group, posters, booklet, TV.
The booklet accompanying the campaign describes HIV and some of the more common STDs, provides advice on safer sex, discusses issues concerning communication, and explains how to buy and use both male and female condoms.

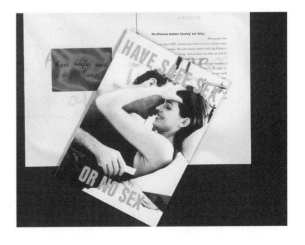

heaven' (**8.57–62**), the 'fourth step' being to use a condom. Posters, press advertisements and billboards were also used, featuring both heterosexuals and gay men (**Plates 40–2**). The campaign pleased the churches and appeased more conservative groups since the message 'Have safe sex or no sex' gave people the chance to say 'no' as well as giving 'tips' for safe sex (**8.63**).

Evaluation of the Netherlands safe-sex campaign, 'Three steps to heaven'

In September 1993 the effects of this campaign were assessed by means of research conducted routinely to prepare, adjust and evaluate campaigns, which has been a part of the AIDS programme in the Netherlands since 1987. 805 respondents were interviewed, using a face-to-face questionnaire (NSS/Marktonderzoek BV 1993).

Selected results

The campaign achieved high awareness: 60 per cent spontaneously recalled the television adverts and the same proportion, 60 per cent, did so when prompted. Those aged 18–24 were more likely spontaneously to recall the TV advertisements (77 per cent). Respondents were asked to complete the slogan 'I practise safe sex or…?' 62 per cent were able to do so in a way which reflected the aims of the campaign, 11 per cent gave incorrect answers and 27 per cent were unable to finish the sentence. 75 per cent found the slogan appropriate, 9 per cent had difficulty with it and 15 per cent failed to answer or were disinclined to do so. One of the posters shows a heterosexual couple making love, the man with a condom packet in his hand (**8.63**). Of those who were familiar with the campaign, 33 per cent were able to remember that one poster features a condom in a packet; 23 per cent were not; 43 per cent were unable to provide an answer to this question.

Asked to whom they thought the campaign was targeted, 50 per cent replied everyone, 48 per cent young people, 17 per cent people with multiple partners, 15 per cent homosexuals, 6 per cent heterosexuals, 8 per cent others, 3 per cent did not know. Half the respondents who recalled the campaign felt it was not targeted at them but at others, 45 per cent thought that this campaign was also aimed at themselves, 5 per cent gave no answer. Sub-group analysis showed that 18- to 24-year-olds and the highly educated shared the opinion that the campaign was targeted at themselves.

Respondents were asked whether or not they sympathized with homosexuals, and more specifically whether they thought it was good or bad if in a general sex campaign two homosexual men were portrayed. 47 per cent were in favour of portraying homosexual men, 24 per cent thought it neither bad nor good, 21 per cent were not in favour.

CONDOM NORMALIZATION

As AIDS has moved from acute crisis to chronic public health problem, the challenge facing health education has been one of establishing risk-reduction practices

Condom normalization campaigns have been driven by:

- a recognition that changing group norms is essential to changing individual behaviour
- the need for sustainable images
- a shift in emphasis from disease category to health behaviour
- the need to avoid particular target groups.

8.64, 65 Germany, 1993–95, BZgA, TV

Relationship

'Write to me?'

'Yes'

'Every day'

'I'm missing you already!'

'I love you'

'See you in two weeks'

'I love you'

'Sorry'

'Doesn't matter. It's okay'

'Sonja? It's been ages!'

'Alexander!'

'What are you doing here?'

'I'm jostling pretty girls'

'What's that?'

'What does it look like?'

'Give it to me!'

'You use condoms?'

'So what!'

'Aren't you going steady?'

'Nosy like a reporter!'

'The pill doesn't agree with me and Dirk's away on business so often'

'What's that to you?'

'Condoms protect and prevent!'

'Yes'

'Uli and I have both agreed'

'Uli he or she? Tell me!'

If you have any questions about AIDS, please call us. The

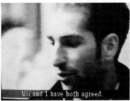

8.64

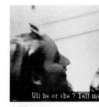

8.65

personal telephone conversation will name advisory centres in your area. Don't give AIDS a chance

In this advertisement from the German public education campaigns, the focus is primarily on the condom and not on the target group – which remains deliberately ambiguous, as in 'Uli he or she? Tell me!'

as a routine part of everyday life rather than as an emergency measure. One expression of this has been in the setting up of campaigns to normalize condom use and encourage its adoption as an everyday occurrence rather than as a practice specifically intended to meet an acute problem.

The move towards condom normalization is the clearest manifestation of trends described in previous chapters. The development of such campaigns has been motivated by increasing recognition of the importance of modifying the social context in which condom use occurs, and of establishing social norms determining individual behaviour. There is no obvious hint in many of the AIDS campaigns currently running throughout Europe of a link with AIDS. They make exclusive reference to neither disease category nor risk group, allowing integration of AIDS into sexual health, and including specific target groups as part of the general population **(8.64, 65)**. Such campaigns, in anticipating AIDS/HIV becoming part of a general programme of sexual health education on STDs, have considerable potential for sustaining awareness and concern. Because the message depends on image rather than text, they have the additional advantage of being able to transcend linguistic boundaries.

The new breed of condom advertisements which have become a feature of several European countries – light-hearted, minimalist – simply remind the public of the need for routine preventive action. They are more likely than were campaign components at the start of the AIDS epidemic to utilize humour than fear; the evidence is not that they will be less effective as a result (Dubé *et al.* 1993a,b).

Social context

The development of condom normalization campaigns reflects the success of efforts to change the social context in which AIDS public education has been carried out.

Considerable progress has also been made in reducing resistance to public discussion of condoms. In many countries this has, ironically, often partly resulted from the controversy created by the condom campaigns themselves. The airing of conflicting views over condom promotion has had the same effect in breaking down resistance to the open discussion of condoms as might more harmonious accounts. Examples are to be found in relation to the Spanish '*Póntelo, pónselo*' (Chapter 6) campaign and the French condom campaigns (Chapter 4), and Italy's controversy over *Lupo Alberto* (this chapter).

It is now possible, in many countries, to feature condoms openly on television and cinema screens where once advertising was banned, and they are increasingly to be seen outside their packets (**Plates 43–6**). The earlier discussion of **8.12–16** shows how much progress has been made.

Sweden

The Swedish AIDS public education campaigns featured what was to become the archetypal minimalist condom campaign in 1990. In that year, the BRO agency's first round of condom advertisements was launched, commissioned by the AIDS Delegation, consisting of a set of twelve different variants (see **Plates 28–39**). By spring 1992, four such sets had been produced. The advertisements show simple pictures built up from the brightly coloured condom packets of the Black Jack brand, which is so well known in Sweden that it is almost synonymous with the term 'condom'.

The condoms are arranged to compose simple pictures symbolizing events, situations, experiences and points in time in a humorous and playful way. Sometimes they have a double meaning; sometimes they function as ideogrammatic puzzles, riddles or puns, inviting the audience to decipher their meaning: the World soccer championships in Italy, for example, the unification of Germany ('when two become one'), or an electric guitar for music and celebrations. Allusion is made to specific situations and encounters which could involve risk rather than risk groups. Because of the absence of any dependancy on verbal text, the message can reach people of other nationalities than Swedes. Both the texts and the illustrations are highly condensed and the images suggestive rather than descriptive.

The campaign was not specifically targeted at any group, so the advertisements have broad appeal. Campaign components have been adapted to the different media in which they were presented. Some of the advertisements were better suited to magazines intended for female readers, others for magazines predominantly read by men, such as business or motor magazines, or soft-porn magazines. The open-air campaigns contained constant reference to holiday situations and targeted tourists – 2 million Swedes visit southern Europe on holiday

Figure 8.2 Condom sales figures (millions)

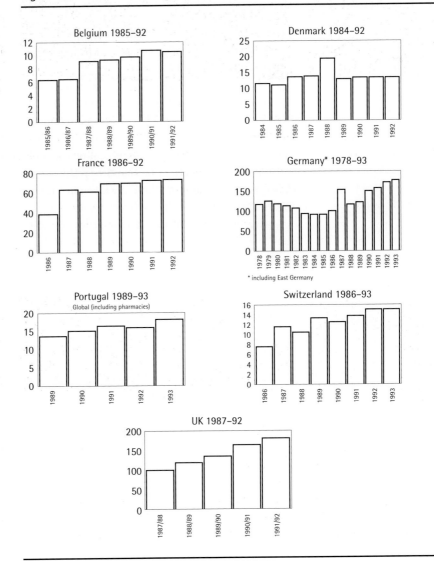

(Source: Goodrich *et al*. 1995)

each year. The 'Eiffel Tower' advertisement, for example, appeared in the holiday and tourist season. This drew complaints from the French ambassador for suggesting that French people presented increased risk.

This flexible approach provides opportunities for adding new messages incrementally as the need arises, thus furthering the goal of sustainability.

Research evidence

The effectiveness of the condom message has no doubt played a major role in helping to counter earlier resistance. Condom use, as represented by both survey

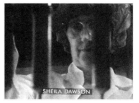

8.66

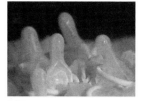

8.67

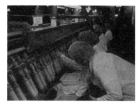

8.68

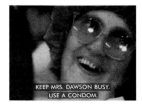

8.69

8.66–73 UK, July
1991–September 1992, HEA,
BMP agency, TV, cinema.
These were two popular
components from the UK
condom normalization
campaign, empowering young
people to use condoms.

8.66–9
Mrs Dawson: *Of course,
working here we're the first to
notice the change in people's
behaviour. We're making more
of these things than ever
before. Obviously it's down to
AIDS and HIV. Young people*

*can't afford to take chances
these days. Seems they've got
their heads screwed on though.
I've never been so busy.*

On a black background, the
caption reads 'A condom can
help protect against HIV and

other sexually transmitted
diseases'. The final shot shows
the Health Education Authority
logo.

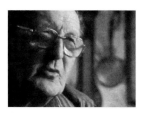

8.70

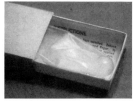

8.71

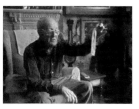

8.72

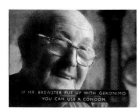

8.73

8.70–3
Voice-over: *Fred Brewster, 81*
Mr Brewster: *I just don't know
why young people complain
about having to wear condoms
against the HIV virus and AIDS,
look what we had to wear...I*

*called it Geronimo, my friend.
Compared with the condoms of
today, it was like wearing the
inner tube of a bicycle. It
wasn't like the modern
condoms, it was designed to be
used again and again. It was*

*like having a bath with your
socks on! But it never stopped
me, no way.*

The screen shows the words: 'If
Mr Brewster can put up with
Geronimo you can use a

condom'. On a black
background, the caption reads
'A condom can help protect
against HIV and other sexually
transmitted diseases'; final shot
of HEA logo.

results and commercial sales figures, shows upward trends in most countries for which data are available (Figure 8.2), while data relating to other changes in behaviour, e.g. numbers of partners, are sparse or inconclusive. This progress has been harnessed to campaigns attempting to encourage people to build on what has already been achieved.

This is illustrated in the UK by the condom factory advertisement which came to be known as 'Mrs Dawson' after the worker who commends young people for 'keeping her busy' (**8.66–9**). The advertisement again focuses on the risk-reduction strategy to be adopted, not disease to be avoided. In another an old man, Mr Brewster, talks cheerfully about the condoms he used to use (**8.70–3**). These UK condom normalization advertisements point on the one hand to the increased general responsibility of the young, with an up-beat motivational message (Mrs Dawson), and on the other to the revival of a tried and tested traditional prophylactic, helping to erode the barrier of loss of sensation (Mr Brewster). The juxtaposition of these two advertisements with those using personal testimonies of people who are HIV positive (UK, HEA, 1991–92), in which the emphasis is more on AIDS and how it can affect anyone, mirrors closely the French campaign, in which this formula has been used to good effect.

The Swiss campaign also uses the achievements made to date to motivate people to continue the good work. In this example the research data have been used to demonstrate progress, using condoms to illustrate graphically the rising trend (**Plate 47**).

Europe against AIDS summer campaign 1994–95: a case study in crossnational campaigns

The Europe against AIDS summer campaign (**8.74**) was an example of the move towards condom normalization advertisements in Europe. Originally a summer campaign of the Agence Prévention SIDA and INFORSIDA in Belgium, after 1994 it was financed by the European Commission and was the first *international* mass media AIDS prevention campaign. Run primarily as a seasonal campaign across Europe, its aim was to act as a reminder to young travellers in Europe of the importance of AIDS prevention during summertime, by the use of a visual code, the flying condom. It was used either as a supplement to national campaigns – an additional reminder to practise safe sex in the summer – or as a focus for national campaigns in some eastern European countries. This campaign encouraged a sustainable campaign, acting as a building block on which each country could build, and allowed adaptation of materials to the national context.

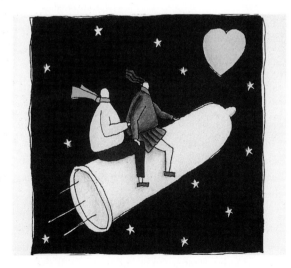

8.74 Europe-wide, 1994–95, INFORSIDA/EC, all media. The minimalist images used in the summer 'Flying condom' campaign allowed the advertisement to be used in all countries without problems of language barriers.

Description of the campaign

The launch of the different national campaigns in summer 1994 intended to show young people that the use of the condom is no longer taboo. The national launch events featured famous people, the message being 'Do as the stars do: use a condom.'

Communication tools produced by INFORSIDA were intended for free adaptation by each country: a standard press information file included a slide of the flying condom graphic for press/TV reproduction, and a TV/cinema spot which was a mix of images and languages set to modern music. It provided blank space to incorporate the 'national signature'. Elton John recorded two video messages intended to be shown at the national campaign launches. A particular feature of the campaign was the sixteen-page 'Passport against AIDS' which featured nine cartoons in the language of each EU country (with captions in English) and included information on condom accessibility in EU countries (where to buy, the cost, the word for condom in each language); the idea was that a young person outside their native country would be able to pick up the passport and be able to understand the preventive message. A mailing to 1,200 NGOs and to the 626 members of the European Parliament also took place to coincide with the launch of the campaign.

AIDS organizations in 25 European countries participated in the 'Flying condom' campaign in summer 1995 – EU: Austria, Belgium, Denmark, Germany, Spain, Finland, France, Greece, Ireland, Italy, Luxembourg, Portugal, Sweden, UK. Non-EU: Switzerland, Tunisia, Malta. Eastern Europe: Bulgaria, Estonia, Latvia, Lithuania, Croatia, Czech Republic, Macedonia, Slovenia. The Youth Hostel Federations participated in 21 countries, the Youth Card Associations participated in 18 countries and Interrail participated in 11 countries.

At the crossnational level INFORSIDA attempted to ensure the consistency of the campaign and the exchange of information between partners. The national AIDS body (either the Ministry of Health or an NGO) attempted to ensure optimal appropriation of the message and adaptation according to cultural sensitivities. The crossnational coordination involved liaison with Interrail, the International Youth Hostels Association and the International Youth Card Association. The national coordinators tried to get sponsorship for the campaign on a national level and establish partnerships with AIDS/health/youth/travel/leisure organizations.

Evaluation of the summer 1995 crossnational 'Flying condom' campaign

Questionnaires evaluating the passport were distributed to the international youth networks (youth hostels, Youth Card, Interrail); the international TV stations were sent questionnaires evaluating the TV spot.

The use of the Youth Card network to distribute questionnaires achieved a 95 per cent response rate. 70 per cent of young people were very interested in the passport, and 72 per cent had discussed it. More than three-quarters felt the information presented to have been useful. A high proportion of participating outlets expressed a desire to participate again the following year. Responses were similarly favourable for the youth hostel network (66 per cent) and Interrail (55 per cent).

The Europe against AIDS summer campaign, because of its international nature, effectively complemented national prevention activities; young travellers were exposed to the flying condom image in 25 countries. Some countries – for example France, Belgium and Luxembourg – developed the European campaign to help their national action. There was overwhelming enthusiasm for the passport; the flying condom visual was generally appreciated, but especially so in southern and eastern Europe and in Finland. The campaign caused some controversy in Malta and Tunisia, where the promotion of condoms is still taboo.

References

Alexander, M W and B Judd Jr 1978 Do nudes in ads enhance brand recall? *Journal of Advertising Research* **18**; 47–50

Bottomley, V 1993 *Address by Rt. Hon. Virginia Bottomley, Secretary of State for Health, UK Department of Health* report of the 1993 Conference of European Community Parliamentarians on HIV/AIDS, April 1993, British All-Party Parliamentary Group on AIDS, London

Bromham, D R and R S V Cartmill 1993a Knowledge and use of secondary contraception among patients requesting termination of pregnancy, *British Medical Journal* **306**; 556–7

Bromham, D R and R S V Cartmill 1993b Are current sources of contraceptive advice adequate to meet changes in contraceptive practice? A study of patients requesting termination of pregnancy, *British Journal of Family Planning* **19**; 179–83

Curtis, H (ed.) 1992 *Promoting sexual health, proceedings of the second international workshop on prevention of HIV and other sexually transmitted diseases*, Cambridge, 24–27 March 1991, British Medical Foundation for AIDS, London

Dubé, L, G B Reaidi and C Descombes 1993a *Comparing affective and cognitive responses to informational vs emotional messages on AIDS prevention: a field study among Canadian young adults*, PO-C22-3160 IXth International Conference on AIDS, IVth STD World Congress, Berlin 1993

Dubé, L, G B Reaidi and C Descombes 1993b *A field study on communication effectiveness in promoting condom use for AIDS prevention: fear may not be a good approach*, PO-C22-3161 IXth International Conference on AIDS, IVth STD World Congress, Berlin 1993

Elias, C J 1994 Family planning and AIDS prevention can be combined, *British Medical Journal* **308**; 790

Fineberg, H V 1988 Education to prevent AIDS: prospects and obstacles, *Science* **239**; 592–6

Goodrich, J, K Wellings and D McVey 1995 The use of condom sales data in assessing the impact of HIV/AIDS prevention measures, report for Health Education Authority, London (unpublished)

Hiv-Aktuellt 1993 Love power fick tre ägg, *Hiv-Aktuellt* 5; 8

Huybrechts, A 1995 *Europe against AIDS – summer campaign*, presentation at Joint Europe against AIDS Seminar, AIDS Public Education Information Exchange and Europe against AIDS Summer Campaign, Egham, England, 2–4 November 1995 (unpublished)

Job, R F Soames 1988 Effective and ineffective use of fear in health promotion campaigns, *American Journal of Public Health* 78 (2); 163–7

Judson, F N, J M Ehret, G F Bodin, M J Levin and C A M Reitmeijer 1989 In vitro evaluations of condoms with and without nonoxynol 9 as physical and chemical barriers against chlamydia trachomatis, herpes simplex virus type 2 and Human Immunodeficiency Virus, *Sexually Transmitted Diseases* 16 (March); 51–6

Levy, S and L Posner-Körösi 1993 *Resultat från en kvalitativ undersökning avseende attityder till den pågående Love Power kampanjen*, Stockholm: Folkhälsoinsitutet-Garbergs

Mahler, H 1981 The meaning of world health for all by the year 2000, *World Health Forum* 1 (1); 5–33

NSS/Marktonderzoek BV 1993 *Evaluatie Aidscampagne1993*, Gravenhage: NSS/Marktonderzoek

Rubery, E 1993 *UK prevention policy*, Medical Research Council AIDS Programme Workshop, 12–15 September 1993

Taylor, C 1993 Increasing patients' knowledge of secondary contraception, *British Medical Journal* 306; 931

Toppich, J and G Christiansen 1993 *Is the AIDS education campaign wearing out?* PO-C22-3141 IXth International Conference on AIDS, IVth STD World Congress, Berlin, 1993

Wadsworth, J and A M Johnson 1994 Physical health and sexual behaviour. In K Wellings, J Field, A M Johnson and J Wadsworth (eds) *Sexual behaviour in Britain*, London: Penguin, pp. 275–324

Wellings, K 1992 Selling AIDS prevention, *Critical Public Health* 3 (1); 4–13

Wellings, K and D McVey 1990 Evaluation of the HEA AIDS press campaign: December 1988–March 1989, *Health Education Journal* 49 (3); 108–16

9 Evaluating AIDS public education campaigns

Attempts to assess the effectiveness of AIDS public education are beset by a number of difficulties. Not least of these is the scarcity of data with which to gauge public response. Because of the precipitate nature of the epidemic and the shortage of time in which to react, early AIDS public education campaigns were often steered more by art than science, and their success was determined more by luck than judgement. The speed with which preventive measures had to be implemented left little time to set in place the necessary evaluative procedures. The cautionary note of Fishbein and Middlestadt (1989), that 'the AIDS epidemic is much too serious to allow interventions to be based on some communicator's untested and all too often incorrect intuitions about the factors that will influence the performance or non-performance in a given population', went largely unheeded at the start of the epidemic.

The WHO defines evaluation (in a public health education context) as 'the determination of the effectiveness, efficiency and acceptability of a planned intervention in achieving stated objectives'. The term 'acceptability' refers to the public perception of a campaign; mention has been made to this throughout the descriptions in the previous chapters. Evaluation of the effectiveness and efficiency of campaigns also requires the use of indicators by which the outcomes of interventions and programmes can be assessed. The selection of these reflect campaign objectives, and since the ultimate aim of AIDS preventive interventions has been to prevent further spread of the Human Immuno-deficiency Virus (HIV), the primary outcome to be measured, ideally, is the incidence of new HIV infection. Outcome measures related to morbidity and mortality have not been appropriate to evaluation of the AIDS epidemic partly because of the nature of the virus – in particular the long time lag between infection and the appearance of symptoms of HIV-related illness – and partly because of deficiencies and inconsistencies in the surveillance data. Attention has instead turned to the outcomes most relevant to reducing HIV transmission: the adoption and maintenance of behaviours which protect uninfected individuals against infection with HIV, and which protect those already infected against discrimination and isolation.

Knowledge, attitude and behaviour surveys

These behavioural indicators have been chiefly measured by means of survey investigation. The stock-in-trade of evaluation of public education in relation to the general population, particularly interventions using the mass media, is the knowledge, attitude and behaviour (KAB) survey. Typically, KAB surveys investigate exposure to, recall and comprehension of campaign messages, and self-reported behaviour change. KAB surveys have limitations in the extent to which they can monitor changes brought about in the social context since their focus is on the individual. They also present problems of validity and reliability.

Most surveys use quota samples which, like all surveys using this selection method, are potentially unreliable, since those most likely to be willing to disclose details of their personal opinions and behaviour cannot be taken to be representative of the population as a whole. Reliance on retrospective accounts of behaviour and attitudes also suffers from the biases introduced by the desirability response (a tendency to report what is considered socially acceptable), by recall difficulties and by a lack of specificity in terms of meaning. Pre- and post-test surveys and tracking surveys (involving repeating the same set of questions at intervals of similarly selected samples) offer some improvement but provide no assurance that what is being measured is the effect of a particular intervention and not a generalized response to the AIDS epidemic. Again, these difficulties were exacerbated in relation to the assessment of AIDS/HIV preventive strategies, because of the sensitive nature of behaviour under investigation.

Nevertheless, these investigative tools are the mainstay of evaluation procedures in AIDS public education and have been used to measure knowledge of routes of transmission, risk-reduction strategies and behaviour change. As a check on self-reported data, more objective measures, for example proxy indicators of safer sex in the form of condom sales data, have also been used to monitor response to the AIDS epidemic.

Attributing outcome to intervention

A major challenge relating to assessing the efficacy (whether one type of intervention works better than another in achieving desired ends) of mass media approaches to AIDS/HIV prevention is that of attributing outcome to intervention (that is, ensuring that the apparent observed effects are truly the outcome of public education campaigns and not the result of heightened awareness of the issues through some other source, such as the mass media generally or local preventive interventions). The necessity for this is widely held to be essential to the evaluation of public health interventions (Heyman and Biritwum 1990).

Attributing an outcome to a specific intervention is difficult where mass communicational techniques are used to reach the general population. An effective campaign will have an effect far beyond its original remit, creating media discussion, providing the impetus for local efforts, and so on, so that the effects of the original campaign may not easily be distinguished from subsequent events triggered by it. This is particularly relevant in the case of AIDS, where an explicit objective of many campaigns was to help create a social climate in which interventions could be favourably received.

The most reliable method of ensuring that a particular outcome is the unique consequence of a particular campaign is to use an experimental design, comparing one group who have been exposed to the intervention with a control group who have not. Such designs are difficult to apply to mass media campaigns because ideally, and by definition, virtually everyone is exposed to them. Experimental methods of assessing mass media campaigns which have been applied in other areas of health promotion – the use of phased implementation, randomized field experiments, the application of media weight bias, or simple random assignment of individuals to one group or another – have not been feasible in the case of AIDS preventive strategies. There were practical, ethical and, in some cases, economic obstacles to the implementation of these strategies. The urgent need for information made it indefensible to deny people (in the interests of scientific accuracy) interventions which could benefit them by offering protection against a deadly virus.

The success of the experimental approach depends on being able to ensure that observed differences in outcomes between treatment and control group do not arise from any other factors than the intervention under investigation. In the case of the AIDS epidemic, however, the usual problem of interference or 'background noise' was heightened. Public knowledge was accumulating, through media coverage, commercial advertising, etc., at such a pace that even a short time lag could result in a change in attitudes or behaviour with or without intervention. Not only has it been difficult to separate out the effects of national campaigns from the effects of national news coverage, but overspill between countries has made it difficult to separate out the effects of one national campaign from another. In Ireland, for example, 75 per cent of households receive British TV and so had been heavily exposed to British campaigns before the start of their own in 1987 (Harkin and Hurley 1988).

Crossnational comparisons

Crossnational comparisons present potentially ideal opportunities in terms of comparing different approaches to AIDS public education among the general population, across different timescales and different geographical and epidemiological contexts. Europe might, at first sight, seem to provide an ideal experimental setting for the purposes of assessing AIDS prevention strategies. An investigation of public response to the AIDS epidemic as reflected in surveys of attitudes, knowledge and behaviour has the potential to provide insights into the differential effects of social contexts, public health strategies and approaches used in AIDS public education.

Yet in practice the potential for this is limited. Direct crossnational comparisons of the effectiveness of interventions are difficult because of methodological differences between surveys conducted in different countries – in particular, wording – and because fieldwork is carried out at different times. They are also limited in many cases by the absence of data. There have been budgetary constraints on the capacity to conduct evaluative research. Mass media campaigns are expensive, and extensive evaluation was seen by some as an unnecessary luxury, or as an opportunity for cost-cutting. Not surprisingly, those countries in which lavish resources have been allocated to interventions will also be those in which adequate resources have been made available for monitoring and evaluation studies. Such countries may be more affluent, perhaps they may have a higher prevalence of HIV, or they may have a stronger tradition of evaluative empirical work. Whatever the reason, it follows that selection for evaluation on the basis of accessibility and availability cannot be relied upon to be free from bias.

As a result, extreme care needs to be exercised in making comparisons between countries on the basis of existing data. International comparative research has a powerful tendency to produce some kind of rank ordering which may be complimentary for some countries and less so for others. For this reason, extreme care must be taken to ensure that the results obtained are a function of factors relating directly to interventions and their outcomes, and not a result of the methodology or timing of the studies used to evaluate them. Even when there is a common research protocol and a shared language, when one has good access to the data available, and when one has a good overall knowledge of the national cultures, the problems of comparison are seemingly formidable. The difficulties of examining differences between countries and the impossibility of holding constant all other variables save the intervention itself are obvious. The multiplicity of different social, political and health factors operating in different countries rules out any kind of controlled analysis.

Although the common aim of European KAB surveys was to monitor public response to the AIDS epidemic, in some countries they were set up to evaluate the preventive programme as a whole in that country, while in others their aim was specifically to monitor response to public education campaigns, particularly those using the mass media. The aim of the Swiss evaluation programme, for example, is to assess the overall AIDS prevention strategy in Switzerland. The aim of the Irish survey, on the other hand, was to assess knowledge and attitudes towards AIDS as a direct consequence of public education campaigns and hardly features behavioural outcomes at all.

Throughout the preceding chapters results of campaign-specific evaluations have been included where campaigns have been used as case studies; these analyses are more properly defined as attempts to monitor campaigns rather than evaluate them, i.e. to look at their general effects rather than at whether they achieved intended goals. This chapter attempts to provide a broader overview of public response to the AIDS epidemic than is possible by reference to the pre- and post-tests provided by evaluations of individual campaigns. The focus is, as far as possible, on the public response to the AIDS epidemic across Europe as a whole.

Risk perception

Perceived seriousness of the disease

In order to gauge how serious a problem AIDS was considered to be by the public, evaluation surveys most commonly listed AIDS alongside other major health problems warranting concern and compared the results. Concern for the AIDS problem was clearly high in those countries for which there are relevant data (Figure 9.1), ranking alongside such major causes of mortality as cancer and cardiovascular disease. This high level of public concern is perhaps as much a consequence of prior sensitization to the issue than the interventions themselves.

Figure 9.1 Perceived seriousness of AIDS compared with other diseases

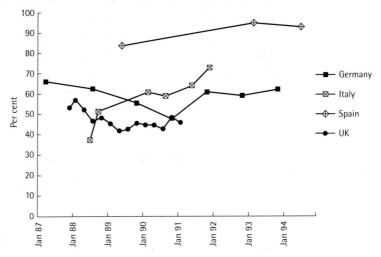

Germany *In your opinion, which are the most dangerous diseases at the moment in Germany?*
per cent mentioning 'AIDS' among most dangerous diseases, spontaneous answers
n = 2,295 (16–65 years) (BZgA 1993)

Italy *In your opinion, which are the most health-threatening diseases today?*
per cent answering 'AIDS', spontaneous answers
n = 1,011 (15–64 years) (Telecontatto 1990, 1992)

Spain *I'm going to read out a series of health problems that exist today. In your opinion, which do you consider to be very serious, serious, or not very serious?*
per cent answering 'AIDS, very serious'
n = 1,555 (15–60 years) (Ministerio de Sanidad 1993, 1994)

UK *Thinking just of diseases or infections that people can get, which ones might seriously affect the health of people in the UK?*
per cent answering 'AIDS', spontaneous and probed
n = 2,073 (13 years and over) (HEA/BMRB 1989, 1992a)

In most countries, the advent of the AIDS epidemic in the early 1980s was accompanied by a great deal of publicity, media coverage and public alarm; public perceptions of seriousness seemed to peak in early 1987, irrespective of the nature of campaigns.

The seriousness with which AIDS is perceived seems to be related more to the scale of the epidemic than to the intensity of national campaigning efforts. Perceived seriousness continues to rise in those countries in which the incidence of AIDS is increasing most rapidly. The proportion of French people who believed a large number of people in France were dying from AIDS increased from 69.5 per cent to 77.9 per cent between 1990 and 1992. In Italy, the proportion of respondents perceiving AIDS to be currently one of the most health-threatening diseases rose from a third in 1988 to more than two-thirds in 1992. In Spain, the proportion believing AIDS to be a very serious disease has been continuously high, yet rose still further, from 80 per cent to 90 per cent in the five years between 1989 and 1994. Figure 9.2 illustrates the actual incidence of AIDS in European countries. The apparently high proportion of the German public seeing AIDS as a serious threat reflects the wording of the question, which asked respondents to list all the major health problems facing the country instead of singling out the most serious.

Figure 9.2 AIDS incidence rates per million population by year of diagnosis, for selected European countries, 31 March 1995

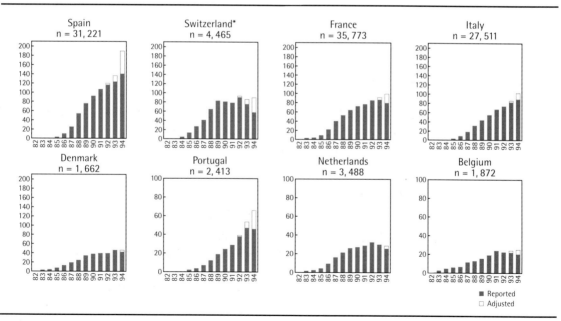

*Since around 20 per cent of all AIDS cases are reported through a parallel surveillance system based on death certificates (with longer delays between diagnosis and report), adjusted numbers are probably too low.

(Source: European Collaborating Centre)

Survey data show considerable variation between countries in the extent to which members of the public consider themselves to be at personal risk (Figure 9.3). To some extent the degree of personal concern might be expected to reflect the actual numbers affected in each country. To some extent, too, it is a function of question wording. Clearly though, there have been very real differences in the extent to which the public in different countries have been able to engage personally in a perception of risk.

Sources of AIDS information

The most important source of AIDS information in all countries is television, followed by newspapers; between half and two-thirds of people across Europe report having obtained their information from this source (Matthews *et al.* 1995). Surveys showed that people considered themselves to have been adequately informed in all those countries represented. This testifies to a high degree of success in providing adequate levels of information. It is not possible to infer to what extent differences between countries are real or a result of the methodology or question wording; such differences are anyway not substantial, and all the graphs show a stable or slightly upward trend over time. Personal adequacy of AIDS information is an important yardstick with which to assess the need for continuation of public education, though on its own, it gives no indication of whether people are accurately informed.

Knowledge of routes of transmission of HIV

Despite the recognition that knowledge alone will not lead to behaviour change, there is general agreement that it is a necessary precondition to action. Evaluation surveys in most countries contained questions probing knowledge of ways in which the virus was most commonly transmitted as well as the extent of misinformation, including fears relating to casual contact.

Surveys revealed a high level of knowledge, across most countries, of the major transmission routes. Indeed knowledge of transmission routes of HIV may well be higher than for almost any other disease. It is doubtful whether, if asked, most people would know whether viruses causing common infectious diseases like pertussis, rubella or even influenza are airborne, waterborne or passed on through exchange of bodily fluids. Clearly, knowledge is more important in the case of AIDS/HIV because of the behavioural implications.

The vast majority, nine out of ten respondents in most countries for which data are available, were aware that HIV could be transmitted via blood contact, unprotected sexual intercourse and exchange of contaminated needles (Matthews *et al.* 1995). Such a high degree of awareness, however, generally predated the start of official general population public education campaigns in many countries. The public had gained much of their information from other sources,

Figure 9.3 Personal susceptibility to AIDS

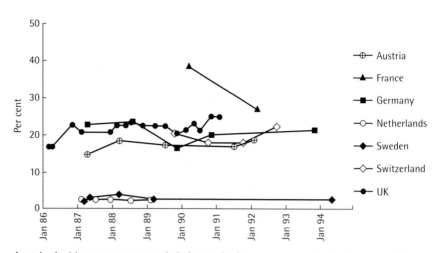

Austria *And have you ever worried about whether you yourself could become infected with AIDS?*
per cent answering 'yes'
n = approx. 1,400 (14 years and over) (IFES 1992)

France *Do you think that: (circle one answer only)*
You are more at risk of contracting the AIDS virus than the average person
You have the same risk of contracting the AIDS virus as the average person
You have less risk of contracting the AIDS virus than the average person
You have absolutely no risk of contracting the AIDS virus
per cent answering 'more at risk' or 'same risk of contracting AIDS than the average person'
n = 916 (1990), n = 1,927 (1992) (18–69 years) (Moatti *et al*.1992)

Germany *Have you ever worried that you yourself might get AIDS?*
per cent answering 'yes'
n = 2,295 (16–65 years) (BZgA 1991, 1994)

The Netherlands *And how about you? How threatening do you find AIDS for yourself?*
per cent answering 9 or 10 on a 10-point scale
n = approx. 1,000 (15–65 years) (Intomart July 1987a, b, 1988, 1989)

Sweden *How big do you suppose the risk is for you to become infected?* [with HIV]
per cent answering 'very big' or 'quite big'
n = 2,369 (16–44 years) (Brorsson 1989, 1994)

Switzerland *Do you sometimes worry about contracting AIDS?*
per cent answering 'yes' or 'on the whole yes'
n = 2,602 (17–45 years) (Dubois-Arber 1993)

UK *I don't think I'll ever get the AIDS virus*
per cent answering 'tend to disagree' or 'disagree strongly'
n = 2,073 per quarter (13 years and over) (HEA/BMRB 1987, 1990, 1992a)

particularly press and television reports. By the time public knowledge was assessed, the main transmission routes were familiar to more than three-quarters of respondents in most countries. The high level of knowledge limited the further improvements which could be achieved by means of mass media campaigns and also – more negatively – limited the extent to which entrenched myths relating to transmission could be dislodged. Nevertheless, official campaigns may well have fulfilled a valuable function in authoritatively confirming knowledge of the modes of transmission.

There has been considerable confusion in most European countries over whether HIV can be transmitted via casual social contact, and also over the distinction between contagion and infection. A sizeable proportion of people in all countries for which there are data believed that the virus can be passed on through kissing, shaking hands, using public swimming pools, and – more seriously, in terms of the social and public health consequences – the donation and receipt of blood (Matthews *et al.* 1995).

Data from tracking surveys show how persistent these myths have been, albeit in a minority of the population. A belief in casual transmission has been eroded to some extent, most significantly in the period of intensive public education between 1986 and 1987, when many countries mounted campaigns specifically addressing this issue, (the '*SiDa NoDa*', campaign in Spain, for example, and the 'No catch' campaigns in Britain and in Switzerland). Nevertheless, among a minority, mistaken beliefs about ways in which HIV can be passed on remain entrenched.

The persistence of beliefs relating to risk associated with blood transfusion is possibly the most striking example of misinformation. Confusion over receiving blood has persisted in the face of constant campaigns aimed at eliminating this false belief. In Germany and France the high figures are more understandable, perhaps, because of the well-publicized controversy over blood supplies (Crawshaw 1993; Dorozynski 1995). Yet the proportion of Irish respondents who believed blood transfusions presented a risk of transmission has also remained high. Only one in twenty believed the statement 'the HIV/AIDS virus can be passed on by receiving a blood transfusion' to be false despite the fact that almost two-thirds of respondents knew that steps had been taken in Ireland to make blood transfusions safe from infection (Irish Health Promotion Unit 1994).

Knowledge of risk-reduction strategies

What is the influence of official messages on familiarity with risk-reduction strategies? Knowledge of the protective effects of condoms seems to have been extremely high. In the UK, 95 per cent were aware that using a condom reduces the risk of HIV transmission (DHSS and Welsh Office 1987); in the Swiss survey it was 90 per cent (Dubois-Arber 1993) and in the survey used in the Netherlands it was 97 per cent (Dinglestad *et al.* 1992). It may be that the controversy generated in certain countries by the message to use condoms brought them to public attention as effectively as did deliberate attempts to promote them. Over the period of the most intensive campaigning efforts in Ireland, perhaps the European country most influenced by the Catholic church, the number of people spontaneously mentioning condom use as an effective preventive measure increased from less than a half to more than two-thirds, while the proportions mentioning monogamy and avoidance of casual sex decreased slightly.

Table 9.1 compares data from surveys in three countries conducted at roughly the same point in time. The selective emphases on different messages in different countries are to some extent reflected in (spontaneous) responses for each country. In all three countries, using a condom is the risk-reduction strategy which was most commonly seen as constituting 'safer sex', but the proportion of respondents mentioning it is highest in Switzerland, where the condom message was dominant; slightly lower in the Netherlands, where a more diversified message was broadcast; and lowest in the UK, where more ambivalence attended the condom message. Nevertheless, nearly half the Swiss respondents and a third of Dutch respondents also mentioned restricting the numbers of partners, and a quarter mentioned choosing a partner more carefully.

Table 9.1. Definitions of safer sex (per cent)

	Netherlands	Switzerland	UK
	October1988[1] What does the term 'safer sex' mean to you?	October1988[2] Methods of preventing AIDS infection	July/October1988[3] What does the term 'safer sex' mean to you?
Reducing number of partners	33	48	61
Using condoms	82	92	75
Careful choice of partner	n.m.[4]	25	31

[1]de Vroome *et al.* 1990 [2]Wellings 1992 [3]Dubois-Arber *et al.* 1991 [4]not mentioned

Reducing numbers of partners, avoiding casual sex and being faithful have also been promoted as risk-reduction strategies in some countries, though these seem not to have had the impact of the condom messages (Table 9.2).

Table 9.2 Familiarity with risk-reduction strategies (per cent)

Condoms

	1987	1988	1989	1990	1991	1992	1993	1994
Austria (with casual partners)	54	69	68		75	79		
Ireland	48[1]		66					
Italy		34[2]		42[2]	46[2]			
The Netherlands[3]		43	63	71	73	96	97	
Spain		89	87					89
Switzerland	62[4]	92	90	88	90	91		
UK	93	94	93	93				

[1]Pre- and post-surveys in February and September 1987 [2]Pre- and post-surveys July and October 1988, March and September 1990 and June and December 1991 [3]Two measurements taken every year (May and October) [4]Two measurements taken in first year of survey (January and October 1987)

Reduce number of sexual partners

	1987	1988	1989	1990	1991	1992	1993	1994
Austria		59	54		60	68		
France				68.9		60.1		
Ireland	12[1]		10					
The Netherlands[2]	14	40	39	25	8	7		
Spain		73					67	61
Switzerland					6.5	6.5		
UK	76	74	74	75				

[1]Pre- and post-surveys in February and September 1987 [2]Two measurements taken every year (May and October)

No casual sex

	1987	1988	1989	1990	1991	1992	1993	1994
Austria	67	73	69		67	75		
Ireland	20[1]	16						
Italy					32[2]	32[2]		
Spain			87	85				82

[1]Pre- and post-surveys in February and September 1987 [2]Pre- and post-surveys March and September 1990 and June and December 1991

Careful choice of partner

	1987	1988	1989	1990	1991	1992	1993	1994
France				76.1		65.6		
Switzerland	42[1]	25	15.5	15	12.5	9		
UK	83	80	80	80				

[1]Two measurements taken in first year of survey (January and October 1987)

Monogamy

	1987	1988	1989	1990	1991	1992
Austria	62	67	64		66	69
Ireland	54[1]		50			
Switzerland	18[2]	48	53.9	40.4	39	32.5

[1]Pre- and post-surveys in February and September 1987 [2]Two measurements taken in first year of survey (January and October 1987)

Sterilizing/using disposable needles

	1987	1988	1989	1990	1991	1992	1993	1994
Italy (use disposable syringes)				11[1] 18	18[1] 20			
Spain (sterilize non-disposable syringes)		88					77	73
Switzerland (clean syringes)	18[2]	25	11.1	12.6	13.6	11.6		
UK (clean/sterilized needles)	76	76						

[1]March and September 1990 and June and December 1991 [2]Two measurements taken in first year of survey (January and October 1987)

Sources of surveys and question wording

Austria *With the exception of drug use, today AIDS is transmitted primarily through sexual intercourse. Which of the following preventive measures against AIDS infection do you think are effective [read out, circle if yes]?* (IFES 1992)

France *I will read out some possible ways of protecting oneself against AIDS. For each one can you tell me whether it is an effective means of protection against AIDS?* (ANRS/AFLS 1992)

Ireland *Given that sexual intercourse is a common method of spreading HIV/AIDS, what do you think are the most effective things sexually active people can do to reduce their risk?* [spontaneous answers] (Harkin 1989)

Italy *In your opinion, what are the precautions that should be taken to avoid contracting AIDS?* [spontaneous answers] (Telecontatto 1990, 1992)

The Netherlands *Which types of safe sex do you know?* [spontaneous answers] (Dingelstad *et al.* 1992)

Spain *Of the following precautions to avoid the contraction of AIDS, could you tell me which you believe to be effective, not very effective or not at all effective...* (Ministerio de Sanidad 1993)

Switzerland *Can you tell me some ways to protect oneself from AIDS?* [spontaneous answers] (Dubois-Arber *et al.* 1993)

UK *Next I'd like you to look at a number of things people have said about AIDS, and tell me how much you agree or disagree with each one. People are having fewer sexual partners these days because of AIDS...People are more careful about who they sleep with now, because of AIDS...Using a condom reduces the risk of getting the AIDS virus...If [drug users] are not going to give up taking drugs, what is the most important thing they could do to avoid AIDS?* (HEA/BMRB 1991a)

Barriers to action

Surveys included questions on the perceived barriers which might militate against the implementation of safer-sex strategies. Of interest were the responses in countries in which campaigns had deliberately addressed the barriers to the adoption of risk-reduction strategies, the 'condom excuses' campaigns in the Netherlands, France and Britain, for example. The evidence is that there was a slight shift in public opinion in favour of condom use over the period of these campaigns.

In France, where a major goal was the erosion of negative beliefs about condoms, attitudes proved largely favourable, though the cost, the fact that they are not natural and the diminishment of sexual pleasure were mentioned as disadvantages by a sizeable section of the sample (Moatti *et al.* 1990). In addition, a large proportion of the French believed condoms not to be completely effective in preventing AIDS, higher than in the Netherlands and in the UK. Nevertheless, achievements in France, where vigorous condom campaigns were mounted, were considerable.

The trend in all countries has been towards decreasing proportions of people seeing embarrassment as a problem associated with condom use, suggesting that progress has been made in shifting opinion on this issue. In France, for example, the proportion agreeing that they would be ashamed to buy a condom was halved over the two-year period from 1990 to 1992 (ANRS/AFLS 1992).

Behaviour change

As noted in Chapter 4, the data relating to numbers of partners – whether expressed in terms of multiple partners, casual partners or exclusivity – fluctuate within fairly narrow bands. It would seem that few changes in terms of numbers of sexual partners have occurred as a result of the AIDS epidemic. The proportions of people reporting more than one partner in the last year has remained remarkably static, more or less irrespective of country.

By contrast, figures for condom use show some remarkable achievements over the period of the most intensive campaigning, namely 1986–89. At the aggregate level, the proportion of the population who claim to have used condoms in the recent past is small; between a quarter and a third of people across Europe claim to have used a condom in the recent past. Interpretation of such results has led in some cases to a criticism of campaigns for not having achieved their objectives. Yet, as has been pointed out elsewhere (Wellings 1988), although large scale changes in behaviour are often assumed to be necessary, the actual numbers of people who needed to make changes in their behaviour in order to reduce the risk of HIV transmission is still relatively small. The proportion of people who report having had more than one partner in the past year in the UK, for example, is around 10 per cent. If the 4 to 6 per cent reporting homosexual relations and the 1 per cent who inject drugs are added, the proportion at risk is relatively small (HEA/BMRB 1992a).

The data on condom use at the general population level are shown in Chapter 4. What is most striking about these data is that, despite differences in question wording relating to different time periods, frequencies, etc. – and despite all the variations in methods of data collection, sample selection, etc. – results are remarkably consistent across Europe. Indeed in many cases the differences between countries are difficult to discern since the lines representing trends are so close as to be, in some cases, virtually superimposed on one another. Those reporting condom use will include those for whom the condom has been the mainstay of their contraceptive practice as well as the smaller proportion who have more recently adopted condom use as a way of preventing infection.

It is at the level of subgroup activity that achievements really become apparent. Figure 9.4 shows a marked upward trend in the proportion of respondents with casual partners who reported condom use for most countries, but especially for Germany and Switzerland. The increase in reported condom use by young people and those with multiple partners is equally noticeable (Figures 9.5 and 9.6). (The marked increase in the UK data between 1990 and 1992 may in part be attributable to a change in the survey methodology.) When the data for young people were further disaggregated into consistent and occasional users, the results are even more impressive (Matthews *et al.* 1995), given that an important aim of AIDS public education is to maintain as well as initiate protective behaviours.

Cross-validation of survey data with more objective measures of behavioural change, such as condom sales data (as noted above, Chapter 4), has broadly confirmed these results. Changing prevalence of sexually transmitted infection in many European countries also suggests an impact of increased condom use (Renton and Whitaker 1992), though no claims may be made that this is a direct consequence of AIDS public education.

Figure 9.4 Condom use for respondents reporting casual partners

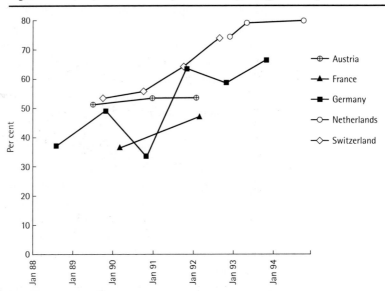

Austria *If you had casual sex in the last twelve months, did you use a condom on that occasion?*
per cent answering 'yes'
n = n.a. (14 years and over and had casual sex in last twelve months) (IFES 1992)

France *In the last twelve months have you used condoms with a casual partner?*
per cent answering 'systematically' or 'once in a while'
n = 105 (1990), n = 279 (1992) (18–69 years with more than one sexual partner in last twelve months) (ANRS/AFLS 1992; J P Moatti, personal communication 1995)

Germany *Did you use a condom in those situations* [one-night stand]?
per cent answering 'always' or 'sometimes'
n = approx. 93 (16–65 years and had casual sex in last year) (BZgA 1994)

The Netherlands *How often have you used condoms in the last six months with casual partners?*
per cent answering 'always', 'almost always', 'sometimes' or 'rarely'
n = 88 (1992), n = 61 (1993), n = 73 (1994) (15–45 years and had casual sex in last six months) (E M M de Vroome, personal communication 1995)

Switzerland *Did you use a condom with this partner?* [last casual partner]
per cent answering 'always' or 'sometimes'
n = approx. 305 (17–45 years and had casual sex in last six months) (Dubois-Arber *et al.* 1993)

Figure 9.5 Condom use by young people – occasional use

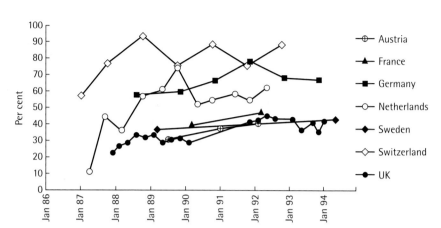

Austria *During sexual encounters do you use condoms always, most of the time, or now and then?*
per cent of young people answering 'always', 'most of the time' or 'now and then'
n = n.a. (14–19 years) (IFES 1992)

France *In the last twelve months have you used condoms?*
per cent of young people answering 'yes'
n = 121 (1990), n = 193 (1992) (18–24 years and sexually active in last twelve months) (Moatti *et al.* 1992; J P Moatti, personal communication 1995)

Germany *In the recent past, how often have you used a condom when having sexual intercourse?*
per cent of young people answering 'always', 'often' or 'occasionally'
n = 205 (16–20 years) (BZgA 1994)

The Netherlands *How often have you used condoms in the last six months?*
per cent of young people answering 'always', 'almost always' or 'rarely'
n = 93 (15–20 years) (Dingelstad *et al.* 1992)

Sweden *Have you or your partner ever used a condom during the last month?*
per cent of young people answering 'yes'
n = 230 (1989), n = 200 (1994) (16–17 years) (Brorsson 1994)

Switzerland *Did you use a condom with this partner?* [last casual partner]
per cent of young people answering 'always' or 'sometimes'
n = approx. 60 (17–20 years and had casual sex in last six months) (Dubois-Arber *et al.* 1993)

UK *Was a condom used at all?* [last sexual experience]
per cent of young people answering 'yes'
n = 344 per quarter (18–24 years and sexually active) (HEA/BMRB 1990, 1991a, b, 1994)

Figure 9.6 Condom use by young people – consistent use

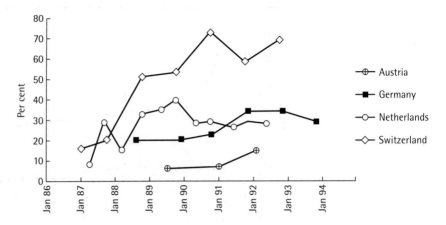

Austria *During sexual encounters do you use condoms always, most of the time, or now and then?*
per cent of young people answering 'always'
n = n.a. (14–19 years) (IFES 1992)

Germany *In the recent past, how often have you used a condom when having sexual intercourse?*
per cent of young people answering 'always'
n = n.a. (16–20 years) (BZgA 1994)

The Netherlands *How often have you used condoms in last six months?*
per cent of young people answering 'always'
n = 93 (15–20 years) (Dingelstad *et al.* 1992)

Switzerland *Did you use a condom with this partner?* [last casual partner]
per cent of young people answering 'always'
n = approx. 60 (17–20 years and had casual sex in last six months) (Dubois-Arber *et al.* 1993)

Other measures of control

Since the creation of a social context which would facilitate the prevention and treatment of HIV infection was an explicit objective of AIDS public education, measures of tolerance were also important indicators of campaign achievement. Survey results suggest that the majority of people in most European countries prefer to control AIDS through voluntary measures relying on individual responsibility rather than more coercive measures. Only a minority in different countries favour isolationist strategies (Figures 9.7 and 9.8). What is interesting is the size of the minority in favour of more repressive methods, how it has

Figure 9.7 Views on treatment of people with AIDS – those advocating avoidance of contact

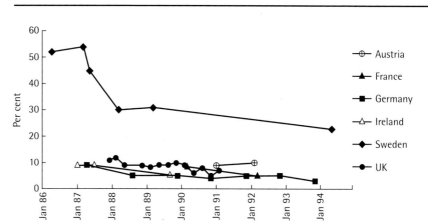

Austria *Assuming that one of your colleagues at work is infected with AIDS, what would you do?*
per cent answering 'would try to stay away from him/her'
n = approx. 1,400 (14 years and over) (IFES 1992)

France *If you knew that someone was HIV positive would you agree to continue seeing them?*
per cent answering 'no'
n = 916 (1990), n = 1,927 (1992) (18–69 years) (ANRS/AFLS 1992)

Germany *What advice would you give to someone whose boyfriend or girlfriend was infected with AIDS, should they withdraw from that person, should they carry on as usual, or should they look after him or her more?*
per cent answering 'withdraw'
n = 2,295 (16–65 years) (BZgA 1994)

Ireland *Which if any, of the following do you think would be your reaction if you met someone with HIV/AIDS? Please read out the appropriate letter. You can choose as many or as few as you wish.*

a) Surprise   b) Sympathy   c) Disgust and physical revulsion
d) Fear   e) Uneasy/uncomfortable f) Would react just as I would with anyone
g) None of these h) Don't know

per cent answering 'disgust and physical revulsion'
n = 973 (18 years and over) (Irish Health Promotion Unit 1994; Harkin 1989)

Sweden *How would you react if you were told that for example one of your colleagues or school friends was HIV infected?*
Avoid close contact...
per cent agreeing
n = 2,369 (16–44 years) (Brorsson 1989, 1994)

UK *And now I'd like to get some idea of how you personally would feel if a close rela-*
tive, like a brother or sister, developed the disease AIDS.
I'd think I might stop seeing them...
per cent agreeing
n = 2,073 (13 years and over) (HEA/BMRB 1990, 1992a)

**Figure 9.8 Views on treatment of people with AIDS – agreement with
isolation from community**

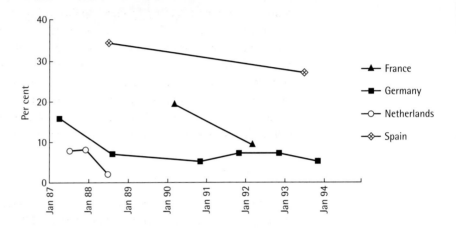

France *One should isolate AIDS patients from the rest of the population*
per cent agreeing
n = 916 (1990), n = 1,927 (1992) (18–69 years) (ANRS/AFLS 1992; J P Moatti,
personal communication 1995)

Germany *Do you think it is right or not right to prevent AIDS patients from coming
into contact with anyone other than medical staff and relatives?*
per cent answering 'right'
n = approx. 2,295 (16–65 years) (BZgA 1994)

The Netherlands *AIDS patients should be banned from public places, such as schools,
canteens and the like. Do you think that would be excellent, good, reasonable, poor or
bad?*
per cent agreeing 'excellent', 'good'
n = 1,000 (15–65 years) (Intomart 1987a, b, 1988)

Spain *AIDS sufferers should be isolated from everyone else to prevent others contracting the disease*
per cent answering 'agree'
n = approx. 1,555 (15–60 years) (Ministerio de Sanidad 1993)

changed over time, and in relation to which factors. It is difficult to determine to what extent expressed beliefs are unique to each country, but as Figures 9.7 and 9.8 suggest, major gains in terms of the liberalization of attitudes have been achieved.

This may have been the result of the partial removal of some of the irrational fears about transmission caused by misinformation about the virus, or it may be attributable to increased information from a variety of sources. Improvements occurred to a greater or lesser degree in all countries, irrespective of whether it was an explicit intention of the campaign to improve the social climate in which interventions took place. However, in some countries in which persistent and sustained efforts were made to achieve solidarity in the population, continued improvements can be seen in public attitudes towards people with HIV and AIDS. In Germany, for example, more than a third of respondents favoured isolation of people with AIDS in 1985, a proportion which had fallen to 6 per cent by 1989 (Matthews *et al.* 1995). Energetic efforts invested in the long-running 'testimonial' campaign in France may also have contributed to the downward trend in the numbers endorsing isolationist measures for people affected. In the Netherlands, the minority of people in favour of coercive methods was reduced still further during the period of the campaigns.

Conclusion

Crossnational comparisons seem to offer valuable opportunities for the assessment of different intervention strategies. Theoretically, if all other factors could be held constant except the intervention itself, a comparison of effects in different European countries would yield valuable information on efficacy. In practice, Europe is not like a laboratory. Attempts to achieve comparability in terms of evaluation meet a variety of problems. For the reasons detailed above, it has not been possible to carry out a systematic controlled investigation of the factors which collectively determine the relative success or failure of public education initiatives. There are too many variables – the social and political context in which campaigns are conducted, the scale of the epidemic, the nature of the agencies involved, and so on – and there are no two European countries in which the social, political and economic context (not to mention the shape of the epidemic itself) are so exactly similar as to warrant attributing differences in effect to differences in AIDS public education.

Nevertheless some generalizations can be made in relation to the interventions, albeit at the level of untested and, for the reasons mentioned above, possibly untestable observation. Some of these seem merely to confirm, in the context of AIDS prevention, existing health educational tenets. Despite the fragility of the data and the frustrations of dealing with data resulting from differently designed and conducted surveys, it is difficult to avoid the conclusion that the campaigns which set out singlemindedly to educate the public about safer sex (particularly condom use) and in which those responsible for public education were most resolute in countering resistance, seem to have made greater progress in achieving their goals than the campaigns in which there was a greater degree of hesitancy over the condom message. The apparently greater compliance with the condom message compared with advice to restrict numbers of partners tends to reinforce the view that the most striking examples of response to information are in areas in which alternative choices are available so that changes in behaviour require no significant change in lifestyle.

In broader terms, there seem to have been advantages for AIDS public education in those countries in which external influences – the media, the activities of different interest groups – have confirmed rather than contradicted official messages; in which there has been consensus rather than conflict at the level of operational interaction; in which responsibility has been vested in fewer hands, thus avoiding competing claims on the content; in which the design and execution of campaigns was chiefly delegated to professional groups with expertise and experience in health promotion, who were able to operate at some distance from government; and in which efforts have been made to maintain and sustain an even pace and profile for AIDS and HIV public education, avoiding peaks and troughs of activity.

References

ANRS/AFLS 1992 *Evaluer la prévention du sida en France*, Paris and Vanves, France

Brorsson, B 1989 *Allmänheten och HIV/AIDS: kunskaper, attiyder och beteende 1986–1989*, Uppsala Universitet, Sweden

Brorsson, B 1994 *Allmänheten och HIV/AIDS: kunskaper, attiyder och beteende 1986–1994*, Uppsala Universitet, Sweden

BZgA 1991 *AIDS in öffentlichen Bewußtsein der Bundesrepublik: Wiederholungsbefragung 1990*, Cologne: BZgA

BZgA 1993 *AIDS in öffentlichen Bewußtsein der Bundesrepublik: Wiederholungsbefragung 1992*, Cologne: BZgA

BZgA 1994 *AIDS in öffentlichen Bewußtsein der Bundesrepublik: Wiederholungsbefragung 1993*, Cologne: BZgA

Crawshaw, S 1993 When fear flows like blood, *Independent* 18 November

DHSS and Welsh Office 1987 *AIDS: monitoring response to the public education campaign February 1986–February 1987*, London: HMSO

de Vroome, E M M, M E M Paalman, T G M Sandfort *et al.* 1990 AIDS in the Netherlands: the effects of several years of campaigning, *International Journal of STDs and AIDS* 1; 268–75

de Vroome, E M M and T G M Sandfort 1994 Increase in safe sex among the young and non-monogamous: knowledge, attitudes and behaviour regarding safe sex and condom use in the Netherlands from 1987 to 1993, *Patient Education and Counselling* **24**; 279–88

Dingelstad, A A M, E M M de Vroome and T G M Sandfort 1992 *Safe sex and condom use in the general Dutch population*, Gay and Lesbian Department, University of Utrecht

Dorozynski, A 1995 Report of French 'blood scandal' is leaked to press, *British Medical Journal* **310**; 959

Dubois-Arber, F, A Jeannin, G Meystre-Augustoni, F Guet and F Paccaud 1991 *Evaluation of the AIDS prevention strategy in Switzerland, third assessment report 1989–1990*, Lausanne: IUMSP

Dubois-Arber, F, A Jeannin, G Meystre-Augustoni, F Guet and F Paccaud 1993 *Evaluation of the AIDS prevention strategy in Switzerland, fourth assessment report 1991–1992*, Lausanne: IUMSP

Fishbein, M and S E Middlestadt 1989 Using the theory of reasoned action as a framework for understanding and changing AIDS-related behaviours. In V M Mays, G W Albee and S F Schneider (eds) *Primary prevention of AIDS*, Newbury Park, CA: Sage

Harkin, A M 1989 *National survey of public knowledge of, and attitudes to AIDS*, Dublin: Health Promotion Unit and Irish Marketing Surveys

Harkin, A M and M Hurley 1988 National survey on public knowledge of AIDS in Ireland, *Health Education Research* **3** (1); 25–9

HEA/BMRB 1987 *AIDS advertising campaign: report on four surveys during the first year of advertising 1986–1987*, London: BMRB

HEA/BMRB 1989 *AIDS strategic monitor: report on the survey period November 1987–December 1988*, London: BMRB

HEA/BMRB 1990 *AIDS strategic monitor: trends to January/February 1990*, London: BMRB

HEA/BMRB 1991a *AIDS strategic monitor: report on the survey period November 1987–December 1988*, London: HEA

HEA/BMRB 1991b *AIDS strategic monitor: report on the survey period January–December 1989*, London: HEA

HEA/BMRB 1992a *AIDS strategic monitor: report on the survey period January 1990–February 1991*, London: BMRB

HEA/BMRB 1994 *Communications monitor: AIDS update*, presented to HEA, unpublished

Heyman, D L and R Biritwum 1990 *Evaluation of the effectiveness of national AIDS programmes*, Geneva: GPA WHO

IFES 1992 *Verhalten und Wissensstand der Bevölkerung nach der Aufklärungskampagne*, Vienna: IFES

Intomart 1987a *AIDS onderzoek 1 – meting*, Amsterdam: Intomart and NAC

Intomart 1987b *AIDS onderzoek 2 – meting*, Amsterdam: Intomart and NAC

Intomart 1988 *AIDS meting 3 – voorlichting AIDS*, Amsterdam: Intomart and NAC

Intomart 1989 *AIDS meting 4 – voorlichting AIDS*, Amsterdam: Intomart and NAC

Irish Health Promotion Unit 1994 *AIDS awareness survey July 1994*, Dublin: Health Promotion Unit

Matthews M, K Wellings and E Kupek 1995 *AIDS/HIV KAB surveys in the European Community (general population)*, London: LSHTM

Ministerio de Sanidad 1993 *Actitudes sociales ante el SIDA, informe de resultados población general*, Madrid

Ministerio de Sanidad 1994 *Actitudes sociales ante el SIDA, informe de resultados población general*, Madrid

Moatti, J P, 1992 Impact on the general public of media campaigns against AIDS: a French evaluation *Health Policy* **21**; 233–47

Moatti, J P, W Dab, M Pollak, P Quesnel, A Anes, N Beltzer, C Ménard and C Serrand 1990 Les attitudes et comportements des Français face au SIDA, *La Recherche* **223**; 888–95

Renton, A and L Whitaker 1992 *Using STD occurrence to monitor AIDS prevention. Report for the EC.* London: Academic Department of Public Health, St Mary's Hospital Medical School

Telecontatto 1990 *Advertising test AIDS pre-campagna*, Milan: Telecontatto

Telecontatto 1992 *Indagine AIDS pre-post campagna 1991*, Milan: Telecontatto

Wellings, K 1988 Do we need to change sexual behaviour, should we and can we? *Health Education Journal* **46**; 57–60

Wellings, K, J Wadsworth, A M Johnson, J Field and R Anderson 1990 Sexual lifestyles under scrutiny, *Nature* **348**; 276–8

Wellings, K 1992 *Assessing AIDS prevention in the general population, report for the EC concerted action 'Assessment of AIDS/HIV preventive strategies'*, Lausanne: IUMSP

Country reports

To ensure that they all refer to a similar timespan, the following country reports describe general population AIDS education from its inception in the early mid-1980s until the end of 1993.

For all country reports, surveillance data for each transmission group may not sum exactly to the totals stated because of missing data.

These reports do not necessarily reflect the views of the organizations or individuals consulted.

AUSTRIA

Context

Epidemiology

According to the European Centre for the Epidemiological Monitoring of AIDS, by 31 December 1994, the cumulative total of AIDS cases was 1,293, with an incidence rate (per million population) of 16.8 (n = 133). The cumulative total of AIDS cases by transmission group (percentages in parentheses) was as follows: homo/bisexual male 518 (40.9); injecting drug user (IDU) 353 (27.9); homo/bisexual IDU 6 (0.5); haemophiliac/coagula-

tion disorder 60 (4.7); transfusion recipient 27 (2.1); heterosexual contact 155 (12.2); other/undetermined 148 (11.7).

The first AIDS case was recorded in 1983. The total number of HIV-infected people in Austria is estimated to be between 10,000 and 15,000.

Social and political background

Austria is a federal country with nine Länder. The Catholic church is a significant influence in political and social affairs.

Issue	Legislation	Date of legislation	Services provided
Homosexuality	Age of consent 14 (same as for lesbians and heterosexuals). In some cases homosexual sex with an <18-year-old can be liable to prosecution	1989	
Abortion	After consultation with doctor, available on request ≤15 weeks, ≤6 months on grounds of risk to woman's life, physical/mental health, risk to foetal health/handicap. <14s need parental consent	1975	Yes, but not covered by normal health insurance
Drug use (non-medicinal)			
Prostitution	Illegal for <18s. Selectively forbidden, legal in private flats/ brothels. Male prostitution legal. Obligatory registration with police, fines if law not observed	1991	Yes
Contraception	Except oral contraceptives, sale of contraceptives not legally regulated. No free state provision		
Contraception for those under age of sexual consent	Conditional		

Health education

In the past ten years there has been public education about heart disease, contraception, pregnancy, dental health, smoking, abortion, road accidents, STDs (other than AIDS/HIV) and infant health.

Sex education

For the previous ten years sex education has been included in the school curriculum for 14-year-olds, as an interdisciplinary subject. However, in practice it is neglected and provision depends on individual teachers and schools; in most schools, no sex education is provided. This is thought to be mainly because no person or body actually bears responsibility for its implementation and the lack of training for teachers. Where it is taught, it is often covered as a part of biology lessons.

AIDS/HIV education is generally covered in natural science subjects and occurs as transmission of facts; little attention is paid to the personal and emotional aspects of disease and prevention.

Recently some innovative projects have begun such as a peer education project in public schools in Vienna, organized by the Red Cross. The Österreichische AIDS-Hilfe (ÖAH) 'AIDS kit' available from the Ministry of Health, Sport and Consumer Protection (hereafter referred to as the Ministry of Health or MoH) has been widely used in many schools.

AIDS/HIV public education

Aims and objectives

- To reduce the future spread of HIV infection;
- to inform the public about how HIV is and is not transmitted and about protection from HIV (through condom use);
- to ensure the non-discriminatory treatment of people with AIDS/HIV and increase solidarity with them.

Structure and organization

The AIDS Bill (1986, renewed 1993) states that the federal Ministry of Health is responsible for national information campaigns, epidemiological research, and AIDS policy coordination and implementation. A permanent AIDS Commission (comprising mainly epidemiologists and virologists) at the MoH was established in 1986 and acts as a primarily advisory body to the MoH on all topics relating to AIDS/HIV. No national institution is specifically concerned with AIDS; this is paralleled in the Länder.

The federal Ministry of Justice is responsible for AIDS prevention in prisons. The federal Ministry of Education and Art is responsible for the provision of information and materials in sexual education, AIDS/HIV drug-related prevention and the education of 'multiplicators' – teachers and approximately 3,000 school nurses/doctors.

In 1992 the ÖAH established the AIDS Information Centre to offer information and educational services, a documentation centre, psychosocial counselling, social support services (employment, housing, finance) and anonymous HIV tests.

Several other private organizations have emerged since 1990: the Austrian AIDS Committee is run by doctors, to educate doctors on the characteristics of HIV. The Austrian AIDS Society aims to stimulate AIDS research through scientific conferences, seminars and cooperation programmes. Live Positively and the Buddy Society provide psychosocial support for people with AIDS/HIV. Apart from these organizations and the various regional branches of ÖAH, no other structures for AIDS prevention exist.

Criticisms of AIDS prevention in Austria are that communication between the various agencies involved is poor and that the federal ministries with responsibilities for AIDS prevention work independently of others, with little communication between them.

Development of campaigns

Österreichische AIDS-Hilfe was founded in 1985, originating in the homosexual community; it was also partly managed by Health Ministry officials. The first ÖAH office was established in Vienna in 1985 and regional offices soon followed. The ÖAH, as an independent non-profit organization –

although exclusively financed by the state – developed new initiatives which were not always approved by the MoH. The ÖAH was closed down in 1990 and totally restructured. Since 1991, seven regional Austrian AIDS-Hilfen, each independent organizations, have been operating in seven of the nine provinces, mainly with MoH funding.

Campaign chronology

Date and agency	Campaign theme/title	Aims	Media	Main message/endline	Target groups	Tone and style
February 1987 MoH		Give basic and general information about AIDS, modes of transmission and methods of prevention	TV, brochures, press ads, seminars	AIDS concerns everybody	General public, young people, ethnic minorities, health professionals, civil servants	Informative
1987 ÖAH			Cinema	Prevention is better than fear	General public	Humorous
December 1987– January 1988 MoH		Continue to provide information and maintain knowledge of AIDS to increase personal awareness and so yield behavioural changes	TV, cinema, press ads	Non-transmission of AIDS through social contact, solidarity, condom use, danger of HIV infection at first use of drugs	General public, young people, parents. IDUs, prostitutes, travellers	Personal
September 1988 MoH		Provide information in schools	Brochure	AIDS also concerns you	Young people (7th and 8th grade)	Factual
July 1989 MoH		Improve information about routes of infection and prevention measures, decrease irrational fears and thus discrimination	Brochures, posters	AIDS doesn't know the difference; AIDS needs help; AIDS can have repercussions; AIDS from man to man; AIDS: drug use is at the top	General public, travellers, IDUs, gay men	
1991 MoH		Raise public awareness and concern to change public opinion	Press ads, radio, cinema, billboards	Protect yourself against AIDS	General public	Death imagery
1992 MoH		Change behaviour relating to discrimination and condom use	Radio, cinema, (1991 repeats), TV, brochure	Protect yourself against AIDS	General public	Personal (TV)
Summer November–December 1993 MoH		Promote anti-discrimination and condom use	Cinema, brochure	AIDS concerns us all, the condom protects against AIDS; Have a good trip: tips for travellers	General public, travellers	

The events of 1990–91 led to the virtual disappearance of what could be called the 'national AIDS community'. Whereas this community was politically active and visible between 1985–90, since then AIDS/HIV organizations appear to be struggling along more individual paths without raising much public awareness.

Tone and style

Generally, Austrian advertisements have been open and candid in tone, although posters prepared by ÖAH which portrayed two gay men were forbidden by the authorities. German and Swiss campaigns are seen by many of the Austrian population.

Messages

Government campaign messages have covered information about transmission routes and condom use; solidarity and non-discrimination towards people with AIDS/HIV have also been promoted. Messages have generally not been moralistic; abstinence and exclusive partnerships have not featured as messages, rather the message has been that with various partners, the risk increases. In terms of drug use, messages have not been to avoid drugs completely, but if you do use drugs, don't share needles.

The ÖAH has tried not to use frightening messages. Instead, messages have generally aimed to encourage the use of services provided, to make clear that informative material is available, to advertise the helpline, counselling services, and the availability of free and anonymous testing.

Target groups

In addition to the general population, AIDS information campaigns have been directed towards gay men and covert homosexuals, IDUs, sex workers (particularly from former Eastern bloc countries) and their clients, sex tourists and travellers, truck drivers, and workers.

Other measures of prevention and control

HIV testing and surveillance

Since March 1983 it has been obligatory to notify the federal Ministry of Health of all AIDS cases. Safeguards for confidentiality exist. There is no notification of HIV positive persons.

Anonymous testing has been available in Austria since 1985.

All registered prostitutes have been tested for HIV since June 1985 and are obliged to visit the Health Office every week where they are tested for HIV every four weeks. It is estimated that 30 per cent of prostitutes are registered. The licence of an HIV positive prostitute is not renewed. This policy has been controversial in Austria.

Needle exchange schemes

There are approximately twenty needle exchange programmes in Austria. The first needle exchange programme was opened in 1985 by ÖAH in Vienna. The sale of needles and syringes has always been unrestricted in pharmacies. Although methadone treatment has been available since 1986 on prescription, it is not universally available throughout Austria.

In some prisons – depending on the director and the prison's doctor – needles can be sterilized and condoms are made available. There has been political debate about this issue.

Condoms

The availability of condoms has never been restricted and they are available from vending machines and pharmacies.

Evaluation

Although no systematic evaluation has taken place, the 1993 AIDS Informations und Präventionskonzept report assessed the Ministry of Health's AIDS education strategies.

Country visit: Detlef Liche 1993

Report preparation: Becky Field

Individuals and organizations contacted:

Dr Helga Halbich-Zankl
National AIDS Coordinator, Federal Ministry of Health, Vienna

Dr Judith Hutterer
Österreichisches AIDS-Komitee, Vienna

Dr Patrick Kenis, Dr Christiana Nöstlinger
European Centre for Social Welfare Policy and Research, Vienna

Dr Wolfgang Svoboda
AIDS Informationzentrale, Vienna

Bibliography

AIDS Informations und Präventionskonzept March 1993, Dr Halbich, Dr Klein and M Podorgski, Bundesministerium für Geshundheit Sport und Konsumentenschutz Sktion Geshundheitwesen Abteilung II/A/2

AIDS surveillance in Europe, quarterly report no. 40 31 December 1993, European Centre for the Epidemiological Monitoring of AIDS

Context of sexual behaviour in Europe, selected indices relating to social, cultural and demographic variables May 1993, Becky Field and Kaye Wellings, EC Concerted Action 'Sexual behaviour and the risk of HIV infection'

Managing HIV/AIDS. Organizational responses to HIV/AIDS in Austria. In P Kenis and B Marin (eds) *Managing HIV/AIDS. Organizational Responses in Six European Countries*. Aldershot: Avebury

Translation of documents: Richard Reithinger

BELGIUM

Context

Epidemiology

According to the European Centre for the Epidemiological Monitoring of AIDS, by 31 December 1994, the cumulative total of AIDS cases was 1,792, with an incidence rate (per million population) of 17.7 (n = 178). The cumulative total of AIDS cases by transmission group (percentages in parentheses) was as follows: homo/bisexual male 716 (42.2); injecting drug user (IDU) 113 (6.7); homo/bisexual IDU 16 (0.9); haemophiliac/coagulation disorder 5 (0.3); transfusion recipient 88 (5.2); heterosexual contact 738 (43.5); other/undetermined 21 (1.2). Most people with HIV live in Brussels.

The first AIDS cases were registered in Belgium in 1983. More than half of those with AIDS/HIV whose place of residence is known live in the Brussels area; the others mainly come from the big urban areas such as Antwerp, Ghent and Liège. The estimated figure of HIV positive people in Belgium is approximately 15,000.

Social and political background

A marked feature of Belgium, politically and socially, is the division of the country into three linguistic blocs. Revisions of the Belgian constitution during the 1970s replaced a unitary system of government with a federal system of communities and regions: the communities were established according to the three predominant cultures and languages, Flemish, French and German; the regions established were Flanders (Flemish-speaking), Walloon (French-speaking) and Brussels. The country is further divided into ten provinces and 589 local communities. The reforms have meant that

Issue	Legislation	Date of legislation	Services provided
Homosexuality	Legal. Age of consent 16 (same as for heterosexuals)	1985[1]	Yes
Abortion	Legal <12 weeks on grounds of 'distress/emergency'. No time limit if grounds are risk to women's/foetal health. Obligatory counselling. <18s need parental consent	1990	
Drug use (non-medicinal)	Illegal		Yes
Prostitution	Prostitution legal but third-party involvement, use of accommodation and soliciting illegal. Illegal for client		Yes
Contraception	Legal, GP charges reimbursed through national health insurance		Yes
Contraception for those under age of sexual consent	Permitted		Yes

[1]Prior to this the age of consent for homosexuals was 18.

government is shared between the various government bodies at different levels, each of which have equal legal status.

Another important division exists between Catholics and non-Catholics. The influence of the Catholic church on the moral climate is significant.

Abortion is a major political issue. It was legalized in 1990, after a twenty-year debate, but significant anti-abortion activity continues. Homosexuality is still far from accepted in Belgium. There have been several instances of discriminatory practices in relation to the treatment of those with AIDS/HIV, particularly in the workplace.

Nine per cent of the total population are non-Belgian, the majority of whom live in Brussels and the Walloon region; they are from other European and North African countries.

Little reliable data exist on the number of injecting drug users (or other drug users) in Belgium, though police estimates range from 10,000 to 20,000 illegal drug users. Needle exchange and harm-reduction programmes are being promoted, although generally harm-reduction prevention measures meet with some opposition.

Health care services are funded by a system in which contributions are made directly by workers as a proportion of earnings, by employers, and by national government. At time of use patients pay 20 per cent and the government 80 per cent.

Belgium Flemish (Flanders) community

Health education

Public health education campaigns have mainly been the result of NGO efforts – the Red Cross, for example, and other voluntary organizations – acting as and when a health problem has arisen.

In 1991, largely as the result of criticisms that health education in Flanders was unplanned, the Flemish Health Promotion Institution (VIG), based in Brussels, was established as a collaboration centre between several officially recognized preventive health organizations. AIDS has been a catalyst for action in this area.

The Flemish Minister of Education is responsible for health education in schools.

Sex education

In the Flemish-speaking community, health and sex education in schools are not obligatory; sex education in schools is a sensitive issue and provision is piecemeal. Attempts have been made to provide guidelines for teachers in the state schools since the 1950s but lack of political continuity, with successive replacements of Ministers of Education, has militated against coherent policy measures. The Catholic school administration has pursued guidelines with some vigour but all resulting curricula conform essentially to the teachings of the church, particularly with respect to contraceptives. This was reflected in the reaction of the director general of the National Secretariat for Catholic Education to the 1987 information campaign on AIDS; a letter circulated to all school governors and head teachers labelled the campaign as too permissive.

The Flemish Ministry of Education commissioned the development of a strategy on sex education in schools, but has no power to enforce a sex education curriculum in all schools.

AIDS/HIV public education (Flemish-speaking community)

Aims and objectives

AIDS prevention policy in Flanders has been somewhat fragmented. Until 1993, IPAC (Flemish AIDS Coordinating Centre) had no AIDS strategy with clear objectives. In 1993–94 policy documents were published with the aim of establishing a comprehensive strategy. These documents reflect the wish to implement an effective interdisciplinary and intersectoral policy based on the work already started by professional and numerous semi-governmental organizations.

Structure and organization

At federal level the Ministry of Public Health and Environment is responsible for policy on blood screening, HIV testing, pharmaceutical regulations and condoms. The state-funded Institute of Hygiene and Epidemiology is responsible for disease surveillance and epidemiological studies. The Ministry of Social Affairs is responsible for the organization of health care provision. The body responsible for implementing public health finances is INAMI/RIZIV (the National Health Insurance Institute), which also directly finances the nine national HIV reference laboratories. Research is a matter for both federal and community Ministries. Important national AIDS/HIV policy issues can be raised at the interministerial committee on public health.

At the regional level, regional health ministries are principally responsible for local applications of federal laws, especially local health care provision and staff e.g. family planning and health promotion centres. The running of harm-reduction interventions such as methadone programmes is also part of their responsibilities, the costs of the relevant medicines being met through the health insurance system.

Most AIDS/HIV activities are coordinated at community level, and each community has developed an AIDS/HIV preventive strategy. Thus there are Flemish and French community authorities and organizations involved in AIDS/HIV prevention and care at federal, community and regional level. The major NGOs are structured along similar lines. There is no comprehensive AIDS/HIV public education mass media strategy at federal level, but the Flemish- and French-speaking communities have developed their own separate campaigns.

The absence of a tradition of health education meant there was little expertise or experience on which to draw when AIDS emerged, nor any agency which could immediately take on the task.

At community level, between 1986 and 1992 the Minister of Public Health was responsible for preventive health policy. Since 1992 the Minister for Employment and Social Affairs has been responsible for preventive health policy in general and AIDS/HIV programmes in particular. The Flemish AIDS Coordinating Centre (IPAC), a private institution designated by the Minister to coordinate AIDS-related activities, facilitates the work of NGOs by assisting in planning coordination and policy development. It has developed a large public information, documentation and resource centre.

In Flanders more than 40 organizations are

involved in AIDS/HIV-related activities, for the general population and specific groups. The NGO StAG (AIDS and Health Care Foundation) was established in 1985; it runs the AIDS hotline for the general public and conducts information campaigns for the general population. In addition, the health education departments of the Belgian Red Cross, family planning centres, the Federation of Centres for Birth Control and Sexual Education, and the Federation of Centres for Family and Life Problems also make significant contributions to general population AIDS education.

In 1987 IPAC established an informal AIDS advisory body (AIDS Overleg) in which approximately 30 relevant research and implementation organizations are represented. It acts as an information exchange platform for fieldworkers and scientific researchers.

Development of campaigns

In 1985, the AIDS campaign in Flanders was set up from the Ministry of Employment and Social Welfare.

The original impetus to preventive efforts in relation to AIDS in Flanders came from the Institute for Tropical Medicine in Antwerp. At a fairly early stage Africans – from the Belgian Congo, etc. – were visibly affected by the disease and this prompted action. The Institute for Tropical Medicine also started initiatives among prostitutes. Homosexuals organized themselves around the AIDS Team and began preventive activities.

The first government initiative, in September 1987 was a national leaflet drop, designed by a commercial agency. The government gave 1 million Belgian francs to a publicity company to mount a campaign between October and December 1989. In

Campaign chronology

Date and agency	Campaign theme/title	Aims	Media	Main message/endline	Target groups	Tone and style
September 1987 FMESW	National leaflet drop	Inform public about AIDS/HIV	Leaflet to all households	Nature of disease, routes of transmission, etc.	General public	Informative, slightly frightening
1988 AIDS Team	AIDS bus	Inform public about AIDS/HIV	Bus tours in Flanders		General public	Informative
1989 StAG			TV, posters	AIDS. Talk about it beforehand. AIDS Telefon number	General public, young people	Informative
1990 StAG	AIDS Telefon campaign	Advertise AIDS Telefon	TV, posters	AIDS. Talk about it beforehand	General public	Plasticine figures
September 1992 FMESW	National leaflet drop	Correct misconceptions about transmission, give prevention advice, warn against risky behaviour	*TV, †leaflet to all households, posters	*Inform public leaflet is coming	General public, young people	†Grave
February 1993 StAG/ FMESW	Condom campaign	Promote condom use and advertise new AIDS Telefon phone number	TV, radio	Put it on. AIDS Telefon number	General public	Humorous

1989 AIDS Telefon translated clips from other countries' campaigns and obtained free space from the media to show them. In 1993 the Flanders Ministry of Employment and Social Welfare (FMESW) set in place plans for media campaigns over several years. In 1993 a condom campaign began, in cooperation with AIDS Telefon, and was backed up with regional/local actions by the various AIDS organizations.

Tone and style

Despite expert advice which cautioned against the use of scare tactics, fear was used as a motivator in the 1987 leaflet drop. Subsequent more subtle attempts have been made to motivate young people and these have been lighter and more stylish. There was some opposition to the 1993 condom promotion TV spot – a man free-falls from an aeroplane, erotic noises accompanying him, his parachute goes up at the last moment, and the words 'Put it on' come on to the screen. Some parents complained it was inappropriate for it to be shown at a time when children could see it.

Messages

The principal messages of AIDS public education have been: 'Stay with one partner' (1987) and 'Use a condom' (1993). The Catholic constituency has favoured the first of these as the single dominant message; some parliamentarians, especially those from the Catholic party, reacted against the 1993 condom campaign, on the ground that the campaign incited young people to have sex. The Minister publicly defended the campaign several times on TV.

Target groups

In addition to the general population, AIDS information campaigns have been directed towards men who have sex with men, and sex workers in Flanders.

Belgian French-speaking community

Health education

A network of local and community coordinators for health education covers the French-speaking community and is responsible for programmes promoting healthy lifestyles, nutrition, prevention of drug abuse, domestic accidents, smoking and alcohol abuse, as well as AIDS prevention.

In 1989 the budget for health education was 80 million Belgian francs, including AIDS prevention. In 1990 the allocation for activities (excluding AIDS) was 84 million Belgian francs, and for 1991, 120 million.

Sex education

Provision of sex education in the French-speaking community varies according to individual teachers and schools. More than 50 per cent of pupils attend Catholic schools. At the end of primary school or at the beginning of secondary school, the psycho-medical centres usually organize a visit to a family planning centre and/or organize special talks. These interventions mostly take place in the context of biology, ethics or religious studies classes.

A coordinated policy on the promotion of sexual health within formal education curricula is being addressed. Negotiations are taking place between the Agence Prévention SIDA, CEDIF (the NGO responsible for education and training) and the French community's Ministries of Health and Education. However, effective implementation of the training programme depends on the practical support of the relevant authorities. For example, the cooperation of the community Ministry of Education is vital for ensuring that time off is granted to teachers wishing to take part in CEDIF's training, but it is unclear whether this is the case.

The role of the media

Generally the French community press has been responsible in its reporting of AIDS, although there have been some instances of sensationalism. The French-speaking community is also influenced by the French press.

AIDS/HIV public education (French-speaking community)

Aims and objectives

The main aim of primary prevention is to avoid the infection of healthy people. In terms of secondary prevention, the French-speaking community Ministry of Health and Social Affairs state that finding out who is most at risk of infecting others (i.e. to avoid them infecting others) is important. In terms of tertiary prevention the Ministry aims to lessen the psychological, social and physical effects of the disease.

Another objective is to integrate AIDS into health education more fully, and in areas where health education structures exist, to include AIDS in their programmes.

Structure and organization

At community level, the Ministry of Health and Social Affairs is responsible for prevention and health promotion, care and other public health issues which do not have implications for the social security insurance system. The Ministry of Education is responsible for health education and health promotion in the formal education sector. However, coordination between different government administrations tends to be informal.

In 1991 the French-speaking community Minister of Health and Social Affairs created the Agence Prévention SIDA (APS) to plan, coordinate and manage a decentralized AIDS-prevention strategy for the French-speaking community. APS is responsible for implementing prevention campaigns, administering budgets for various AIDS organizations within the community, coordinating prevention and research in private and public organizations and evaluating these actions, and for trying to obtain financial support from the private sector. The

Scientific and Ethical Council was also established in April 1991, to advise the Council of the French community about prevention priorities, ethical and legal matters. The APS subcontracts INFORSIDA to run information campaigns (mass media, the production and distribution of educational materials) for the general population. INFORSIDA is an NGO which quickly became the official body in charge of prevention for the general population.

The APS is also potentially a central reference point for the exchange of information on epidemiological trends and evaluation and research findings (e.g. via the Institute of Hygiene and Epidemiology as well as via NGO and local organizer activity feedback).

Regional health authorities are principally responsible for local applications of federal laws, especially local provisions, structures and staff, e.g. family planning and health promotion centres and social assistance. Local AIDS prevention coordinators operate in Liège, Libramont, Brabant Wallon, Charleroi and Namur.

Development of campaigns

The French community Ministry of Health and Social Affairs commissioned a commercial advertising company (TBWA) to design the first TV spots, aired in 1988. Once established in 1991, the Agence Prévention SIDA took over responsibility for general population AIDS public education and commissioned and coproduced the spots with various commercial agencies. More recently the pattern has been for a general population campaign to take place in the summer, and a solidarity campaign to take place in the run-up to World AIDS Day in December.

Tone and style

Over time, the tone and style of campaigns has changed. The first TV spot in 1988 was slightly imposing and asked the viewer to read the leaflet, without actually stating where it was available. In contrast, the 1991 spot featured a young couple,

Campaign chronology

Date and agency	Campaign theme/title	Aims	Media	Main message/endline	Target groups	Tone and style
1988 FMHSA/ TBWA	'Open your eyes if you don't want AIDS to close them'	Raise awareness, inform public about AIDS	TV, leaflet	Read this leaflet, talk to your friends about it; AIDS/HIV can affect anyone	General public	Serious, sombre
December 1989–January 1990 FMHSA INFORSIDA/ Télé Bruxelles	'To fight AIDS you must talk about it'	Raise awareness, encourage solidarity	TV	Be honest with your partner; talk about AIDS	General public	Personalities, b/w, serious
June 1991 APS/INFORSIDA To Do Today/ Lowe Troost	'There are some words of love you must dare to say'	Promote condom use	TV, posters, cinema, press	'We are stronger to protect ourselves against AIDS when we are two'	General public, young people	Romantic, sex positive
December 1992 APS/MdeWP/ Forum	'AIDS, I act'	Encourage solidarity, promote condom use	TV, brochure (in libraries)		General public	Documentary style, emotive, pragmatic
March 1993 APS/MdeWP/ Forum	'AIDS and testing'	Promote testing for those at risk	TV	'AIDS. Feel free to talk to your doctor'	General public	Documentary style

[1]Michel de Wourters Production

smiling, flirting and laughing, with no dialogue, just music. The 1992 spots were launched to coincide with World AIDS Day. Some were pragmatic in tone, for example, a manager is 'interviewed' about how he feels about employing an HIV positive person; in another a shopkeeper talks openly and enthusiastically about stocking and selling condoms, saying that 'saving one life' makes it 'worthwhile'. In another our sympathy is invoked as a parent talks about having an HIV positive child, emphasizing the importance of the child's quality of life.

Messages

The Agence Prévention SIDA (APS) has promoted three messages:

• solidarity – with the aim of reducing the social impact of AIDS;
• prevention of sexual transmission – with the intention of improving the acceptability of condoms through 'normalization';

• testing – campaigns aim to train doctors on when to do tests and how to use the opportunity for prevention.

Target groups

In addition to the general population, AIDS information campaigns have been directed towards sex workers, men who have sex with men, IDUs, teachers and youth workers, health care professionals and immigrants.

Other measures of prevention and control in both Flanders and the French-speaking community

HIV testing and surveillance

In Belgium as a whole the system in operation is based on voluntary testing. National insurance refunds the total cost of an HIV test. For those without national insurance, there are centres that will perform the test free of charge and anonymously. No money has been made available for seropositivity testing, on the basis that with such low prevalence it would not be cost-effective.

In 1990 the Ministry for Public Health estimated that more than 500,000 HIV tests had been carried out by general practitioners, specialists and hospitals (excluding blood transfusions). It was estimated that one-third of these were carried out without the informed consent of the person tested. Almost all antenatal women are tested on their first visit. In hospitals a large proportion of tests are also carried out without consent. Guidelines from professional medical associations are ambiguous: for example the National Council of Medical Practitioners Association advises informed consent as 'advisable' but in the case of no consent, the practitioner is 'free to refuse further consultation except in emergencies'. Reports suggest that testing is still mandatory for entry applications for short- to long-term stays by students from endemic countries; medical checks of asylum seekers prior to residence in a few cities; and medical check-ups of Belgian UN soldiers returning from missions.

HIV screening for blood transfusions is well organized and effective. Belgium has the lowest HIV prevalence among blood donations in Europe.

In the French-speaking community any doctor can carry out an HIV test, and tests are also available at family planing centres and other specialist centres. Confidentiality is guaranteed.

Needle exchange schemes

In Flanders, at the time of writing, there were no formalized needle exchange programmes although a feasibility study showed promising results. There were plans to introduce a needle exchange scheme in 1995. In one study of IDUs in the Flemish-speaking community almost half said they used only disinfected needles. Local needle exchange schemes exist but only in limited numbers at the time of writing. In the French-speaking community needles and syringes can be bought from pharmacies.

Condoms

Until 1987, condoms were sold only on medical prescription at pharmacies, as contraceptive measures. Since the advent of AIDS, the situation has relaxed considerably and condoms are easily obtainable without medical prescription.

In Flanders condoms are sold in prisons but the lack of privacy hinders sales and work on promoting condom use. In the French-speaking community the Agence Prévention SIDA seeks to promote condom 'normalization', to present the condom as part of youth culture, and to increase availability. Condoms can be bought from sex shops, pharmacies, vending machines and supermarkets, tending to be cheapest in supermarkets.

Evaluation

At national level, by 1992 the Institute of Hygiene and Epidemiology had developed an initial set of prevention indicators: epidemiological indicators for STD and AIDS/HIV surveillance; and knowledge, attitude, behaviour and practice indicators for measuring the effectiveness of HIV prevention.

In Flanders, the first government campaign in September 1987 (a leaflet drop) was evaluated by a telephone survey conducted by Antwerp University three and six weeks after the leaflets were posted. Research also investigated the reactions of young people in order to investigate more effective ways of reaching them.

The 1993 condom (parachute) campaign was evaluated by a telephone survey.

In the French-speaking community, the Agence Prévention SIDA evaluates its campaigns.

Belgian German-speaking community

There are no official statistics for the German-speaking community owing to the lack of a specific reference centre. Nevertheless, according to informal statements from GPs and hospital doctors, the AIDS helpline in Aachen, Germany and from those in charge of the reference centre at the University of Liège, the number of HIV positive people in the community is estimated to be around ten.

The German-speaking community comprises 67,000 people, and is part rural, part urban; some parts are more affiliated to Holland, others to Germany and Luxembourg.

The church is not regarded as an obstacle to AIDS education in the German-speaking community. Indeed some young priests are supportive.

Sex education in schools is not mandatory.

The German-speaking Community Ministry for Family and Health (MFH) is responsible for AIDS public education campaigns.

The AIDS Commission is a working group, established by the MFH in 1987, with the purpose of preventing AIDS. It is in close and steady contact with the reference centre in Liège; the Agence Prévention SIDA in Brussels; and (in Germany) AIDS-Hilfe, the city and regional health authorities in Aachen and the Federal Centre for Health Education.

The main focus of the AIDS Commission's work is AIDS prevention and sexuality education. Issues about sexuality, including AIDS, are taboo in the German-speaking community, which is generally conservative.

In summer 1993 the AIDS Commission re-ran AIDS radio spots from previous years. Discos and cafes were provided with posters, informative material, stickers, postcards and flyers advertising the helpline number. In autumn 1992 proprietors were sent letters from the AIDS Commission urging them to install condom vending machines in their establishments. At least five followed this up and asked for further informative materials. An article entitled 'AIDS - advice for travellers' was published in the local press. Condoms and informative materials were distributed at concerts and festivals.

One of the activities in which the MFH has been instrumental was the setting up of a team to go into schools and talk to 15-year-olds. In December 1993 the AIDS Commission agency and the Agence Prévention SIDA brought together teachers and headteachers at a symposium to discuss teaching

about AIDS in schools. The AIDS Commission has run 'action days' for older pupils in secondary schools when there is a general lecture given, then boys and girls are separated into two groups for questions and answers. There is no obligation for schools to run these action days. There was some parental protest about them, which received media coverage. A lack of willingness on the part of teachers to participate in AIDS and sex education is reported.

The AIDS Commission also offers advice and help to affected people.

There is an AIDS helpline operating in the German-speaking community on Mondays 7 p.m. to 9 p.m. and Thursdays 10 a.m. to 12 noon, as well as the Centre for Help on AIDS (reference centre of the University of Liège) open Monday to Friday 8 a.m. to 5 p.m. In 1992 31 calls were registered, and sixteen personal consultations resulted from this.

The AIDS Commission plans to continue providing public education and information in order to change attitudes and behaviours, through for example, radio spots, initiatives to install condom vending machines in discos and cafes, etc. The AIDS Commission has planned a street work programme involving HIV positive persons as a contact person. They will also circulate the comic JOE (produced by the Federal Centre for Health Education in Germany) to schools and youth clubs. The comic covers AIDS, drugs, sexuality and intergenerational conflicts.

A small budget means it is not possible for the German-speaking community to produce specifically tailored materials. Materials from the Agence Prévention SIDA, Deutsche AIDS-Hilfe and Bundezentrale für gesundheitliche Aufklärung (the Federal Centre for Health Education) in Germany are used. There has been little contact with the Flemish campaign.

This report was compiled from field visits completed in 1990 and 1993 and from the 'Review of the Belgian AIDS Programme 2–10 November 1994' by M Laubli Loud, E van Praag, F Varet and K de Vries of the WHO Regional Office for Europe,

Global Programme on AIDS, Copenhagen, Denmark.

Country visit: Kaye Wellings 1990; Claire Gibbons 1993

Report preparation: Becky Field and Kaye Wellings

Individuals and organizations contacted:

Flanders (Flemish-speaking community)
Dominique Caplin
IPAC, Antwerp

Dr Freddy Deven
Population and Family Studies Centre, Brussels

Rita de Mey
Independent consultant, Brussels

Marc van Daele
AIDS Telefon, Antwerp

Professor Eric van Hove
Institute of Hygiene and Epidemiology,
Department BSW VIA, Antwerp

French-speaking community
Michel Hubert, Luc van Campenhoudt
Centre d'Etudes Sociologiques
Facultés Universitaires Saint-Louis, Brussels

Pierre Moureaux, documentaliste
Patrick Petitjean, Directeur
Marianne Prevost
INFORSIDA, Agence Prévention SIDA, Brussels

Gris von der Auera
Ministry for Health and Welfare, Brussels

German-speaking community
Pascal Sarlette
Ministerium der Deutschsprachigen Gemeinschaft,
Familie, Gesundheit und Soziales, Eupen

Bibliography

AIDS in Flanders policy note 1993 (adapted February 1993 version), Minister of the Government of Flanders for Employment and Social Affairs, Leona Detiege
AIDS – Prävention immer noch notwendig?
AIDS surveillance in Europe, quarterly report no. 44 31 December 1994, European Centre for the Epidemiological Monitoring of AIDS
Die AIDS-Kommission in der DG oder Über die Schwierigkeiten, die Scheuklappenmentalität in Ostbelgien zu überwinden
La Lutte Contre le SIDA en Communauté Française de Belgique December 1991, Communauté Française

Translation of documents: Greet Peersman, Lola Martinez and Isabella Aboderin

---

DENMARK

Context

Epidemiology

According to the European Centre for the Epidemiological Monitoring of AIDS, by 31 December 1994, the cumulative total of AIDS cases was 1,604, with an incidence rate (per million population) of 40.6 (n = 210). The cumulative total of AIDS cases by transmission group (percentages in parentheses) was as follows: homo/bisexual male 1,146 (71.9); injecting drug user (IDU) 111 (7.0); homo/bisexual IDU 14 (0.9); haemophiliac/coagulation disorder 33 (2.1); transfusion recipient 25 (1.6); heterosexual contact 221 (13.9); other/undetermined 43 (2.7). Approximately half of female heterosexually transmitted AIDS cases are African

Issue	Legislation	Date of legislation	Services provided
Homosexuality	Legal[1] Age of consent: 15[2] (same as for heterosexuals) Discrimination on grounds of sexuality legally outlawed Civil partnerships	1933[1] 1976[2] 1987 1989	Yes
Abortion	Legal on request ≤12 weeks; >12 weeks legal on social, socio-medical or socio-economic grounds; as result of sex crime/incest; or on foetal grounds. >12 weeks conditions have to be verified by authorized committee. Parental consent needed for 15–18s	1973	Yes
Drug use (non-medicinal)	Illegal. Possession of cannabis for personal use unlikely to be prosecuted		Yes
Prostitution	Legal but if sole occupation prosecution under penal law possible	1930	Yes
Contraception	Public Hygiene Act integrates family planning into National Health Service. Consumers pay for all the contraceptives. Oral and postcoital contraception on prescription	1966	Yes
Contraception for those under age of sexual consent	Legal. Confidentiality guaranteed by law. Youth clinics in each county	1970	Yes

[1]On legalization in 1933, the age of consent was 18. [2]Law revised by private members Bill.

women, and approximately a third of male AIDS cases are African men.

The first AIDS case in Denmark was diagnosed in 1980, and reported in 1983 when AIDS became a mandatory notifiable disease, as with other communicable diseases. A female surgeon, who had worked in Africa and died in 1979, was in retrospect considered the first Danish AIDS case.

It is estimated that there are between 3,500 and 4,000 HIV positive men who have sex with men and 700 to 1,000 who have been infected with HIV heterosexually. It is estimated that fewer than one person per 1,000 is HIV positive in the Danish population.

Social and political background

Danish society is marked by a high level of social and political consensus. In contrast to Sweden, with its highly centralized social welfare administration, Denmark is extensively decentralized; domestic decision making takes place at the community level.

Denmark shares with other Scandinavian countries a relatively relaxed attitude towards sexuality, and is known for its liberal tradition. A mark of this was the provision made to permit registration of homosexual partnerships (both men and women) in a civil marriage.

Tradition in relation to contraception is similarly liberal. Denmark was the first country to legalize contraception for those under the age of sexual consent and guarantee confidentiality. In 1993 the Christian People's Party successfully opposed a Bill that would have ended the need for parental consent to abortion for women aged between 15 and 17, although this issue has been brought before Parliament again.

Prostitution is legal in itself, but is criminalized where it is the sole occupation. As a result it can be difficult to reach prostitutes with services.

There have been isolated instances of discrimination against those with AIDS/HIV, as in one controversial and highly publicized case of a cook with HIV who was sacked from his job after cutting his hand at work. Otherwise, the medical profession are extremely anxious to avoid discrimination.

Sex education

Denmark has a long tradition of sex education, which began with some schools teaching hygiene after the turn of the century. In the 1950s publications of the Swedish National Commission on Sex Education, and increasing public concern about numbers of unwanted pregnancies, particularly among adolescents, spurred the Danish government to appoint a similar commission. Irrespective of these events, sex education is believed to have become widespread by the 1950s due to the initiative taken by school teachers themselves.

The role of the media

There has been some sensationalization of sex in the Danish press, in *Ekstra Bladet*, for example, the biggest-circulation newspaper in the country. The more serious newspapers are more responsible in approach, and treat sexual issues positively.

AIDS/HIV public education

Aims and objectives

The two main goals of the Danish HIV public education campaign have been to show how AIDS is and is not transmitted, and how to protect against infection; and, secondly, to eradicate discrimination against those with HIV and AIDS.

Guidelines on how AIDS prevention campaigns should be conducted were agreed during a preliminary debate in Parliament on 31 March 1987. Discussion from the beginning clarified that the objective of mass media work should be to raise awareness and not to change behaviour. The belief was that requisite changes in attitudes and behaviour were better achieved through face-to-face and small group work at community level.

Structure and organization

In 1986 the Ministry of Health established a National AIDS Committee with overall responsibility for formulating general policy and implementation of measures to reduce AIDS prevalence. On 1 November 1986, the AIDS Secretariat (AS) was established within the National Board of Health – the advisory board to the Ministry – to initiate and coordinate measures to combat AIDS.

A nationwide AIDS hotline, responsible to the National Board of Health, was opened in 1986 and receives about 15,000 calls each year. In addition, two local AIDS hotlines operate.

Local AIDS committees exist to coordinate and initiate activities within the communities. The 'Cenloc' system was instituted to ensure that regional organizations were better coordinated, whereby the AS takes the initiative for mass media work, coordinates the campaigns from the centre and centrally produces and distributes all materials but does not dictate local activities.

Among the many voluntary groups involved in AIDS public eduction, the National Organization of Gays and Lesbians has been the most important.

Development of campaigns

An early problem in Denmark, in common with some other countries, was that there existed no pre-existing structure in which AIDS/HIV preventive activities could obviously be located. The National Board of Health was officially responsible for health promotion, but its closeness to the government was considered problematic for the development of an effective campaign. As a result, early efforts were set up haphazardly, with the most effective initiatives being taken by the gay organizations whose constituents were most affected.

In 1983 the first booklet was distributed to the gay community and the National Board of Health sent out guidelines concerning AIDS to health care personnel. A film for health care personnel caring for

HIV positive patients was produced, together with other films for use in the educational system. In 1985 the national campaign began at community level, with a leaflet drop late that year to all households.

As in other countries, key personnel emerged in Denmark with a crucial influence on the shape and spirit of public education efforts. They were few in number and included heads of department in an AIDS hospital and in the Department of Epidemiology in the State Serum Institute. The National Board of Health formed an advisory group, with gay representation and epidemiologists from the State Serum Institute, to advise them on initiatives. The first national campaign was

created in close collaboration with a professional advertising agency – Jersild, which was renowned for its success in the area of attitude formation – and with the National Organization of Gays and Lesbians.

In August 1986 the government decided to allocate special funds for AIDS information. By November the AIDS Secretariat had been established to execute, initiate and coordinate campaigns with money from the Ministry of Health.

In 1990 the 'Cenloc' system of collaboration with county AIDS coordinators began, and campaigns have followed this format since.

Every year new materials are produced for

Campaign chronology

Date and agency	Campaign theme/title	Aims	Media	Main message/endline	Target groups	Tone and style
1985 NBH[1]	National leaflet drop	Raise public awareness	Leaflet		General public	
1987 NBH/ JS[2]/SIS[3]	*'Only you' (cinema) †'AIDS letters' (TV) 'Supermarket' (TV)	Encourage condom use and provide accurate information about transmission	5m posters on buses, cinema, TV, posters	*Sex is beautiful †A condom protects both of you also against AIDS/ Don't exaggerate	General public	Sex positive, life orientated †humorous *romantic/ erotic
1988 NBH/ DR-TV	'Think twice'	Encourage condom use and provide accurate information about transmission	TV, radio, press, posters, leaflets, videos	Ways in which HIV is and is not transmitted; Use a condom	General public, young people (15-25s)	Sex positive, humorous, life orientated
1989 NBH/NFC[4]	Cinema campaign – 'Petrol station' (2) and 'Ugh'	Encourage condom use	Cinema, posters		General public	Humorous
1989 NBH/DR-TV/ TV-Cruppen	1988 TV campaign repeat	As 1988	As 1988	As 1988 Remember the condom when the going gets hard on	General public, gay men	Sex positive, humorous, life orientated
1990 Cenloc NBH	Solidarity campaign	Counter discrimination	Press and magazine campaign, central and local	'You shouldn't think, you should know'; Ways in which HIV is and is not transmitted; HIV concerns us all	General public	Empathetic, authoritative, serious
1990 Cenloc NBH/SIS	Interrail campaign	Encourage condom use	TV, press, magazines, money belt	Get a leaflet and two free condoms when you buy...Have a safe journey	Young people	Light-hearted, humorous

1991 Cenloc NBH	AIDS/HIV in the workplace	Encourage companies and others to introduce AIDS policy as part of general personnel policy to counter discrimination in the workplace	Newsletter, video ('Cenloc' system)	It is safe to work with HIV positive persons; AIDS/HIV should be treated as other life threatening diseases	Employers, employees	Informative, guidelines for policy
1992, 1993 NBH and DoT[5] Cenloc	Travellers' campaigns	Encourage condom use	Posters, magazines, youth, business and airline magazines, travel catalogues	Take no chances; Use a condom; AIDS knows no borders	Young people, travellers, gay/bisexuals, business people	Direct
1992 Cenloc NBH			Magazines, local and national press	Every day there's a new HIV infection; AIDS can't be cured, only avoided	General public, young people, gay/bisexuals	B/w photos
November/ December 1993 Cenloc NBH			Magazines	Show respect for AIDS; It's too late to think about it afterwards; There are some things which should be stopped in time	General public	Confrontational
1993–94 NBH	Sports campaign		Posters, T-shirts, leaflets	Sports give you life not HIV	Active sports people, trainers and leaders	Documentary

[1]National Board of Health [2]Jacob Stegelmann. This agency was responsible for the 'Only you' campaign. [3]State Information Service. The SIS worked on the 'Supermarket' campaign. [4]Nordisk Film Commission [5]Department of Travel

November/December, in the run-up to World AIDS Day.

Tone and style

The 1985 leaflet carried a front cover picture of an iceberg intending to convey the suggestion that the epidemic was scarcely visible currently but had great latent potential for harm. Subsequent interventions have been characterized by a lighter and more humorous approach. Attempts were made to give the spots a life enhancing rather than death orientated tone, to design materials deliberately as sex positive rather than anti-sex. In 1987 posters and a TV spot featured a series of full-body pictures of naked couples embracing, with the message 'Sex is beautiful!' Under the slogan, the text read: 'It should stay that way. When you know how AIDS is transmitted and is not transmitted, you can keep it that way. When you use a condom, you don't have to be afraid of AIDS. Protect yourself.' In 1988 a well-known Danish pop group sang an AIDS/HIV prevention message to the tune of a popular pop song. The accompanying video showed disco scenes intercut with film of young people having sex. The images are explicit and positive about sex.

Some attempt has been made in the Danish campaign to use synergistic techniques to provide continuity over time and across different campaigns. For example, a short whistle was associated with the early TV spots.

Messages

Campaigns have not featured advice to avoid sex or reduce numbers of partners; rather messages have been couched in terms of continuing to enjoy sex, but safely. The same approach has been used in relation to injecting drug use, the emphasis being on minimizing harm rather than eliminating the habit. In this sense the objectives of the Danish campaign have much in common with those of the Norwegian campaign, the focus is on promoting achievable messages.

Target groups

In addition to the general population, AIDS information campaigns have been directed towards gay men, sex workers, drug users, immigrants, young people in schools, health care professionals and GPs.

Other measures of prevention and control

HIV testing and surveillance

By government order, all doctors who diagnose an AIDS case are required to report this information to the State Serum Institute (SIS). People with high risk behaviour are asked not to donate blood, and from January 1986 all blood has been routinely screened for HIV. All blood and plasma products have to undergo inactivating steps during production, and imported products have to fulfil the same criteria as Danish products. No unlinked anonymous testing for surveillance purposes takes place.

Free and anonymous screening for HIV is readily obtainable from general practitioners, STD clinics, or special public screening clinics spread across the country. Guidance and counselling are provided primarily at public screening clinics, although two-thirds of tests are carried out by GPs.

From 1 August 1990, a national HIV reporting system was introduced obliging doctors to report HIV seropositives to the SIS, analysed by age, gender, risk group and geographical area. In addition, all laboratories are obliged to report on the total number of HIV tests and numbers of seropositive results. There is a nearly 100 per cent reporting of HIV tests. In 1990 100,000 tests were carried out, and in 1994 140,000, a high rate for a small (approximately 5.5 million) population.

The use of legislation in regard to testing is generally seen as unwise. The strategy of 'voluntary participation, anonymity, open direct and honest information' was confirmed by an almost unanimous vote in Parliament (177 out of 179 votes) in March 1987. As a result, information and education have been accorded highest priority. Discussions in Parliament led to the abolition of the 1973 Act concerning measures to prevent STDs and its replacement with guidelines for all STDs, including AIDS/HIV on 1 June 1988 (previously AIDS/HIV and other STDs had been regarded separately). These guidelines made contact tracing recommended rather than mandatory. Contact tracing is part of the national prevention strategy. The 1988 guidelines require the establishment of opportunities for the dissemination of both general and specific information to individuals about STDs and contraception, free examinations and treatment, and case tracing and treatment to break the cycle of infection.

Needle exchange schemes

The relatively high level of recreational drug use in Denmark necessitated reconsideration of existing drug treatment programmes in the light of AIDS. Easy access to hypodermic syringes and needles, increased information activities, and new and expanded treatment programmes using methadone as well as psychological and social support systems were recommended. The AIDS Secretariat established guidelines for IDU AIDS prevention and took responsibility for implementing services, ensuring availability of needles and syringes at community level.

Needle exchange schemes were first established in 1986-87 and now exist in every big city. No exchange, bleach or clean needle schemes exist in prisons. Discussions continue but the fear is that needles could be used as weapons, and that such initiatives could be seen as condoning drug use in prisons.

Condoms

Condoms have been the cornerstone of the Danish campaign, and are widely available from shops, supermarkets, chemists, tourist shops and bars. Attempts to promote usage have included enclosing free condoms with packs sent out to young people using youth hostels. In the Copenhagen gay community condoms and water-based lubricants are widely and freely available in bars and gay meeting places. Sales of condoms, at least as represented by the six main manufacturers, increased from 11 million in 1987 to between 14 and 15 million in 1988, but returned to the pre-campaign level in 1989 and 1990.

Evaluation

The 1988 'Think twice' campaign has been the only one to be subjected to systematic evaluation as part of a general evaluation of strategy. This involved a survey monitoring knowledge, attitudes and behaviour prior to the campaign, directly after it finished, and again one year later. Focus groups, personal in-depth interviews with representatives from key target groups, a retrospective mass media content analysis, and a review of public opinion data and other data on knowledge, attitudes and sexual behaviour were conducted.

Other campaigns have been evaluated, but in a more limited way; every year since 1986–87 the AIDS Secretariat (AS) has commissioned a market research agency to administer a survey of about ten questions, designed by the AS, covering attitudes and knowledge. If a campaign has taken place, recall questions are included. Otherwise the AS tends to carry out qualitative or focus groups research, which is intended as formative and process (rather than outcome) evaluation of campaign effectiveness.

The 'Stop AIDS' campaign began in 1984 and was evaluated for the first time in 1992–93.

Other tools of evaluation have been of a biomedical nature (i.e. STD rates as proxy measures of sexual behaviour).

Country visit: Kaye Wellings 1990, Becky Field 1995

Report preparation: Becky Field and Kaye Wellings

Individuals and organizations contacted:

Jakob Bjrner, Gerd Winther, Bo Mohl
Sexological Clinic, Rigshospitalet, Copenhagen

Anker Brink Lund
Department of Communication Studies, University of Roskilde

Bent Hansen
Gay and Lesbian Association, Stop AIDS Campaign and AIDS Line, Copenhagen

Bjørn Knudsen
AIDS Secretariat, National Board of Health, Copenhagen

Professor Mads Melbye
Danish Epidemiological Centre, Copenhagen

Nell Rasmussen, Andreas Christansen
Family Planning Association

Dr Else Smith, Henrik Zoffman
State Serum Institute, Copenhagen

Bibliography

AIDS surveillance in Europe, quarterly report no. 44
31 December 1994, European Centre for the Epidemiological Monitoring of AIDS
HIV and AIDS in Denmark epidemiology, the Danish national AIDS policies and health education programmes January 1995, National Board of Health
More emphasis on local prevention of AIDS through 'Cenloc' July 1992, National Board of Health
Indasatsen MOD AIDS i Danmark materialer 1983–1993 Sundhedsstyrelsen

Translation of documents: Natasha Hansjee and Robert Badura

FINLAND

Context

Epidemiology

According to the European Centre for the Epidemiological Monitoring of AIDS, by 31 December 1994 the cumulative total of AIDS cases was 196, with an incidence rate (per million population) of 9.2 (n = 47). The cumulative total of AIDS cases, by transmission group (percentages in parentheses) was as follows: homo/bisexual male 135 (69.2); injecting drug user (IDU) 8 (4.1); homo/bisexual IDU 0; haemophiliac/coagulation disorder 1 (0.5); transfusion recipient 7 (3.6); heterosexual contact 37 (19); other/undetermined 7 (3.6).

The first AIDS case was reported in Finland in 1982.

Social and political background

Finland is a fairly conservative country although it is becoming more liberal. The church has no real influence and adopts a fairly neutral stance on most issues.

The enactment of a clause in the law (Clause RL20) which prohibits the 'public encouragement of fornication between members of the same sex' has had a negative effect on homosexuals.

People with AIDS in Finland are well provided for in terms of care and support services and enjoy certain protective rights. It is possible, for example, to obtain a full pension from the start of symptomatic infection. At the same time there have been instances of illegal dismissals, prejudiced attitudes and reported cases of deportation of foreigners found to have HIV.

Health education

Finland is rightly renowned for some innovative health promotional interventions, notably in the area of cardiovascular disease.

Sex education

The National Board of Education makes general recommendations although the actual content of sex education is determined locally by school boards. The concentration to date has been on physiological

Issue	Legislation	Date of legislation	Services provided
Homosexuality	Age of consent for gay men 18 (14 for heterosexuals and lesbians)	1971	Yes[1]
Abortion	Legal ≤12 weeks if risk to woman's mental health; legal <20 weeks if risk to life/physical health of mother or child, result of sex crime, social/medical/economic circumstances. Recommendations of 2 physicians and State Medical Board needed	1970, 1978, 1985	Yes – free under national health insurance but daily hospital fee
Drug use (non-medicinal)	Illegal		
Prostitution	Prostitution legal, soliciting illegal		
Contraception	Legal	1972	First method free, free provision from municipal clinics
Contraception for those under age of sexual consent	Legal		Special services for young people

[1]Limited to SETA (Gay and Lesbian Organization) and AIDS centres.

and biological aspects of reproduction but there have been recent efforts to balance this with an increased focus on emotional aspects of relationships. During the last few years sex education teaching material has been prepared for teachers, and teachers are also offered in-service training for sex education.

The role of the media

After an early sensationalist phase the media now deal with AIDS/HIV in a more matter-of-fact way. Regular and precise information concerning the development of the epidemic is provided to the media by health authorities. This has helped reduce sensational reporting.

AIDS/HIV public education

Aims and objectives

The goals of the action to prevent AIDS are the prevention of new infections, and the provision of good care and humane treatment to those infected.

Structure and organization

According to the Communicable Diseases Act, the Ministry of Social Affairs and Health (MSAH) is responsible for planning and monitoring preventive action concerning communicable diseases, including AIDS. It is also the responsibility of the MSAH to ensure that the population has access to health education material on the prevention of communicable diseases.

The National Board of Health – an administrative office directly subordinated to the MSAH – is responsible for national AIDS information campaigns. In 1983 the National Board of Health set up an expert group on AIDS to study the spread of AIDS in Finland, which recommended measures to be taken to prevent its spread. In addition, the National Board of Health appointed an HIV monitoring group composed of policy makers, scientists, members of voluntary organizations, etc. and insti-

tuted a parliamentary AIDS group. The MSAH also established an expert group on HIV consisting of representatives from NGOs, research institutes and experts from the fields of medicine, psychology, sociology, social policy, pedagogics and legal science.

Local health authorities organize prevention campaigns with participation by community groups. The National Board of Health also cooperates with various NGOs (e.g. homosexual organizations) in planning AIDS public education campaigns. The MSAH also cooperates with voluntary organizations (e.g. the Finnish Red Cross, AIDS help centres, Folkhälsan (the organization for Finland's Swedish-speaking population)) in the prevention of AIDS. It finances research and health education programmes carried out by government bodies and NGOs.

Health care services are the responsibility of the public sector but private health care services are also available. Primary health care is the responsibility of the municipalities and federations of municipalities; a network of health centres covers the country. In addition, citizens' groups offer services, for example to those suspecting HIV infection.

Development of campaigns

The first medical AIDS committee was established in 1983, and a national AIDS committee was established in 1985. The earliest attempt at AIDS public education was made in 1985 by the National Board of Health, when a leaflet was delivered to every household.

In accordance with the recommendations of the National Board of Health expert group, specific health education programmes began in 1984 in collaboration with homosexual organizations. In 1985 educational material was sent to physicians and other health care staff. In 1986 general population AIDS campaigns, including outdoor advertising, advertising on radio, TV and in newspapers began. In 1987 all young people aged 16–21 were personally sent an information leaflet on AIDS and other STDs, with a condom enclosed. An expanded version of this leaflet has been sent every year to those attaining the age of 16.

Campaign chronology

Date and agency	Campaign theme/title	Aims	Media	Main message/endline	Target groups	Tone and style
1984	Information for homosexuals	Provide information about AIDS and methods of prevention	Brochure		Gay people	
1985		As above	Leaflet drop to all households		General public, physicians, health care staff	
1986	Helpline campaign	Provide information about helpline	TV, radio, videos, leaflets	Helpline number	General public, teachers, schoolworkers, pupils	
1986–87	AIDS today	As above	TV (once a week, 5 mins)	Helpline number	General public	
1986 onwards	As above	Continued awareness	Billboards		General public	
1987			Leaflet drop to 16–21s		Young people (16–21s)	

All campaigns have been produced by the National Board of Health.

Tone and style

It is characteristic of the Finnish AIDS campaigns that fear has been avoided and that humour often facilitates dealing with any difficult issue.

Messages

The advice to use a condom and reduce numbers of partners has featured among messages disseminated. Messages have generally been sex positive in tone, but have stated that unprotected sexual relations, in particular with unknown partners, increase the risk of getting AIDS or other STDs. The importance of condom use in such situations is stressed.

Target groups

In addition to the general population, AIDS information campaigns have been directed towards homosexual men, young people, travellers, health care professionals, teachers and social workers.

Other measures of prevention and control

HIV testing and surveillance

Since 1986, physicians have been required to report all AIDS cases and diagnosed HIV infection to the National Board of Health. In the case of symptomatic infection, identification is made additionally by name. A system of contact tracing is put into effect if the patient is willing to disclose how the infection might have been contracted and transmitted. No system of legal sanctions operates to force compliance. The law does not permit involuntary restraint or isolation of HIV-infected persons. HIV is dealt with under the Communicable Diseases Act which became effective in early 1987; notification of identified HIV cases to the health authorities is mandatory both for the laboratory and for the physician, together with an identification of the person by social security code in the case of symptom-free infection. Based on these reports, an anonymous HIV register is compiled by the National Public Health Institute and used for analysis of the epidemic.

Anonymous testing is carried out in the five largest towns. Cases detected via these tests are also reported to the National Board of Health, but those concerned are not identified.

The National Board of Health stresses that testing is on a voluntary basis. In practice, however, hospitals are free to perform tests considered necessary by the medical personnel; there are some indications that the nature and purpose of tests are not always fully explained by doctors to their patients. Some patients have been tested for HIV if they exhibit certain symptoms or if they fall into specific risk groups.

STD clinics, primary health care centres, AIDS support centres and private laboratories offer free anonymous HIV testing. Consented testing is encouraged and frequent among visitors for rehabilitation of drug misuse nationwide, for pregnant women in some municipalities (including Helsinki) and for STD clinic attenders. Since 1987, army recruits have been offered a test in Helsinki. Voluntary and consented contact tracing is endorsed in most STD clinics and other sites where HIV positive persons are counselled and treated.

National surveillance programmes, conducted by the National Public Health Institute, include unlinked anonymous testing of all pregnant women, which began in 1986 in Helsinki and 1987 elsewhere (blood is collected for other purposes), medico–legal autopsies and suspects of drunken driving.

In spite of strong public opposition, some employers in Finland have adopted a compulsory test as part of the selection process for employment.

Needle exchange schemes

The number of injecting drug users is relatively small in Finland. Methadone replacement therapy is limited. Needles can be bought in pharmacies.

Condoms

Several campaigns have had the aim of increasing condom use and in general they have been well accepted by the public. A newsletter on sexually transmitted diseases containing a condom was mailed to all 16- to 20-year-olds in Finland. Television advertising of condoms is permitted. Condoms have been widely distributed, e.g. in supermarkets and petrol stations, and their correct use has been taught, especially in the campaigns for young people.

Evaluation

The national AIDS programme has not been evaluated by independent experts but individual campaigns have been evaluated on several occasions.

No country visit was made to Finland.

Report preparation: Kaye Wellings and Becky Field

Individual and organizations contacted:

Olli Haikala
Medical practitioner, Helsinki

Olli Salstrom
Helsinki

Tarja Tamminen
Ministry of Social Affairs and Health, Helsinki

Timo Ylonen
Information Secretary, National AIDS Committee, Helsinki

Bibliography

AIDS Asiallisesti. AIDS Tukikeskus 1989, O Salstrom

AIDS and the media in Finland, 1987, H Palousa, paper presented at the Conference on Social Science and Medicine, Leuwenhourst, the Netherlands

AIDS surveillance in Europe, quarterly report no. 44 31 December 1994, European Centre for the Epidemiological Monitoring of AIDS

FRANCE

Context

Epidemiology

According to the European Centre for the Epidemiological Monitoring of AIDS, by 31 December 1994, the cumulative total of AIDS cases was 34,287, with an incidence rate (per million population) of 67.5 (n = 4,002). The cumulative total of AIDS cases by transmission group (percentages in parentheses) was as follows: homo/bisexual male 16,149 (47.9); injecting drug user (IDU) 8,048 (23.8); homo/bisexual IDU 484 (1.4); haemophiliac/coagulation disorder 425 (1.3); transfusion recipient 1,452 (4.3); heterosexual contact 5,307 (15.7); other/undetermined 1,881 (5.6).

The first AIDS case was registered in France in 1981.

In 1993 official estimates of the number of people infected with HIV were between 80,000 and 120,000.

Social and political background

Although France is a staunchly Catholic country and traditionally attitudes towards abortion and contraception in France have been hostile and restrictive, there have been few political problems over the representation of issues relating to sexuality or condoms. Contraception was legalized only in 1967.

Homosexuality is rarely discussed in the official arena and is tolerated rather than accepted.

Anonymity is guaranteed for those registered as having AIDS. Employers are not allowed to subject an applicant to an HIV antibody test, nor to ask about antibody status. Nevertheless, there has been unofficial discrimination against people with AIDS/HIV in the context of employment, and breaches of medical secrecy do occur.

Health education

Health education in France has been underfunded and ineffective in the past, a fact which may be partly

Issue	Legislation	Date of legislation	Services provided
Homosexuality	Legal. Age of consent 15 (same as for heterosexuals). Although not explicit in law, protection from discrimination as 'moeurs' interpreted to include homosexuality	1982	Yes
Abortion	<10 weeks available on request, <6 months if grounds are risk to woman's life/physical health/risk to foetal health/handicap. Certificate needed from 2 recognized doctors. <18s need parental consent	1975, 1979	Yes
Drug use (non-medicinal)	Illegal. Treatment for addiction can be imposed on convicted drug users. Penalties for trafficking: 2–10 years in prison and/or fines; penalties for users: 2 months to 1 year and/or fine	1970	Yes
Prostitution	Prostitution itself legal; soliciting, procuring and running as a business civil offences		Yes
Contraception	Those not covered by social insurance get 70 per cent of cost of some pills, IUD and diaphragm reimbursed	1967	
Contraception for those under age of sexual consent	<18s entitled to free contraception and anonymous treatment, no lower age limit.[1] Age of sexual consent 15 but sex not illegal before then	1990	Yes[2]

[1]Parental consent previously needed [2]Varies geographically

attributable to the strong national emphasis on the rights of the individual to freedom and autonomy. The Comité Français d'Education pour la Santé (CFES, French Committee for Health Education) is responsible for public health education campaigns and executed the first AIDS prevention campaigns in France (1987–89).

Sex education

A 1973 circular outlined recommendations for sex education in schools; anatomy and the physiology of human reproduction were included in the secondary school natural science syllabus. STDs and contraception are included in biology courses for 13- to 15-year-olds, and a compulsory chapter on contraception has been introduced into the set textbooks. In 1985 sex education was introduced into the primary syllabus, under the title 'life education'. All schools organize a talk about AIDS at least once a year for all pupils over 11.

The role of the media

Initially some media reports were unhelpfully sensationalist in tone, but coverage has been more balanced since. Generally the press has been supportive of official health educational efforts although there were criticisms about the long time taken in getting campaigns started. Even when a communication strategy was in place, the national press attacked the authorities for delays ('AIDS: ignored for too long by official institutions' Liberation 16 May 1989). The television channels give a 20 per cent reduction in cost for off-peak AIDS prevention spots but none for those shown at prime time.

AIDS/HIV public education

Aims and objectives

Since 1987, prevention policy in France has followed two objectives: to fight against the spread of the epidemic through information and condom use campaigns, and to prevent the social consequences of

HIV infection through solidarity campaigns with HIV positive people.

AIDS public education campaign objectives are to reduce the risks of infection by helping people to feel responsible about the real risks they are exposed to or that they can expose their partners to, and by reinforcing solidarity with HIV positive people.

Structure and organization

In 1986 the National AIDS Committee was established to advise the Minister of Health, assisted by 23 regional reference centres. Until early 1989, the CFES, under the control of the Minister of Social Affairs and Health, was responsible for AIDS public education.

In 1988 growing concern over the increasing number of AIDS cases coincided with a change of government and a reappraisal of health policies. Late in 1988 Claude Evin, the new Health Minister, commissioned Professor Got to examine AIDS prevention in France. The resulting document was critical of past efforts and recommended the replacement of existing mechanisms with a tripartite structure of organizations, to focus on the social, scientific and preventive aspects of the epidemic. In February 1989, the Health Minister, on this advice, created the Conseil National de SIDA (CNS, National AIDS Council), a body whose role was to concentrate on the social and ethical impact of the disease; the Agence Nationale de Recherches sur le SIDA (ANRS, National Agency on AIDS Research) was founded as a committee to oversee medical and social research; and the Agence Française de Lutte Contre le SIDA (AFLS, French Agency for the Fight Against AIDS) was to be in charge of prevention campaigns under the authority of the Ministry of Social Affairs and Health. The AFLS's role was to coordinate all public education efforts, a task which it shared with the CFES before assuming total responsibility in May 1989.

In 1993 the Minister of Health commissioned Dr Luc Montaigner to examine the management of AIDS in France. Largely as a result of his recommendations the AFLS was dissolved in February

1994, and its duties taken over by the AIDS Division, Direction Générale de la Santé, Ministry of Health. Responsibility for the design, implementation and evaluation of AIDS general population prevention campaigns has been returned to the CFES. The Comité Interministériel de Lutte Contre le SIDA has been created, whose president is the Prime Minister.

The NGO AIDES was established in 1984 with volunteers and 100 staff in 72 towns in France and the French territories. It established a 24-hour AIDS helpline, now run by the SIDA Info Service and paid for by the government. AIDES also carries out preventive work and a care service for people with AIDS.

Campaign chronology

Date and agency	Campaign theme/title	Aims	Media	Main message/endline	Target groups	Tone and style
April–May* July–Aug[†] October–November[‡] 1987 CFES	Information campaign	Raise awareness	*[†]TV, radio, *Minitel, *leaflets, [†]posters, [†]regional newspapers, [‡]cinema	'AIDS won't happen to me'	General public	Plain, informative
November–December 1988 CFES	Condom campaign	Remove barriers to condom use and encourage their everyday use	TV, cinema, brochures	'Condoms protect you from everything, even ridicule'	General public	Humorous, light
April–May, December 1989 January 1990 CFES/AFLS	Condom campaign	Remove barriers to condom use, encourage and eroticize their everyday use	TV, press	Condoms protect you from everything, everything except love'	General public	Erotic, life enhancing, sex positive
June, November 1989 AFLS	Solidarity campaign	Encourage solidarity and empathy with people affected by AIDS/HIV	TV, helpline, brochures	'Through the prevention of illness and the understanding of those who are ill, you can fight AIDS. AIDS. Every one of us can meet it'	General public	Testimonials, documentary style, serious, emotive
July–August 1989* July–August 1990[†] AFLS	Condom campaign	Raise awareness of need for condoms on holiday	*Cinema, *radio, [†]posters at airports and railway stations, [†]video on certain trains, [†]shopping malls, [†]TV	'Condoms wish you a happy holiday'	General public, travellers	Light, romantic
May 1990 AFLS	Condom campaign	Encourage condom use	TV, press	Condoms are easily available	General public, gay men	Light, sex positive, romantic
June 1990 AFLS	Solidarity campaign	Encourage solidarity and empathy with people affected by AIDS/HIV	TV, press	'Today there are thousands of people who are HIV positive or ill with AIDS. Today every one of us can help them to live'	General public	Testimonials, documentary style, serious, emotive

November–December 1990 May 1991–January 1992 AFLS	SIDA Info Service campaign	Inform about helpline and information service	TV, radio, national, gay and medical press		General public, gays, health professionals	Informative
Summer 1991 AIDES	Condom promotion	Increase acceptability of condoms	Posters	'The condom: for our protection against AIDS'	General public	Commercial, stylish
July–August 1991 AFLS	Solidarity campaign	Encourage solidarity with and empathy for people affected by AIDS/HIV	Posters, posters on buses	'Tell me yes'	General public	Positive, plain, direct
June 1991–January 1992 AFLS	Condom campaign	Encourage condom use	TV, posters	'Why wait any longer?'	General public, gay men	Sex positive, light, humorous
April 1992 AFLS	Testing campaign	Encourage those at risk to take a test	Posters, Paris region press	'What if I think I've taken a risk?' 'What if I want to get it off my chest?' 'What if I haven't always used condoms?' 'What if I've just begun a big love affair?'...Talk about it to your doctor, he'll give you advice about the test	Those at risk	Plain
July–August* October–November* September–December† 1992 July–October* 1993* AFLS	Condom campaign	Encourage condom use	*TV, *posters, †cinema	'The condom. Today everyone says yes'	General public, gay	Positive, light, humorous, stylish (b/w)
January 1993 onwards SIS	Helpline campaign	Increase awareness of the freephone service	Radio, press, posters		General public	
1993 AFLS	Solidarity campaign	Encourage solidarity and empathy for people affected by AIDS/HIV	Posters	'Why should someone who is HIV positive be any different from you?'	General public	Plain, direct

Development of campaigns

At the beginning of the AIDS epidemic there was no national body with the proven expertise, a sufficiently high public profile and the financial resources to undertake AIDS/HIV public education. The lack of government effort in relation to health education in general, and AIDS in particular, was heavily criticized.

In 1987 the CFES aimed to raise awareness of AIDS and fulfilled this with high public recall of the first campaign. The budget, however, was inadequate to the task of providing continuous high profile campaigns. There was no visible campaign activity from November 1987 to November 1988, when the then new Rocard government and the health authorities stepped up their AIDS action; a more generous budget was allocated, a system of free and anonymous testing was established, centres in the most affected areas were opened, there was a doubling of staff and the establishment of the above-mentioned agencies to coordinate action. A coherent communication strategy began when the AFLS took over responsibility in February 1989.

Specific problems addressed in the campaigns were twofold, namely, resistance to condom use and possible hostility to people with AIDS. A condom promotion campaign was launched in March 1989, by the CFES and the AFLS, which aimed to improve the image of the condom and normalize its usage. After two condom campaigns (December 1988 and May 1989), the AFLS turned to the issue of AIDS itself and in June 1989 began a solidarity campaign using a testimonial approach.

A distinctive feature of the French campaigns, and a departure from the strategy adopted in any other European country, is the disassociation of AIDS from the recommended action for risk reduction; the campaigns have been developed along two separate lines.

Tone and style

The French advertisements have been stylishly filmed and are positive in outlook and in tone towards sexuality. The advertisements are life, rather than death, orientated. Overt humour is not used but advertisements are light-hearted. They also tend to be impressionistic rather than informational, relying on images and associations rather than hard facts to get a message across. Likewise, the tone of the solidarity advertisements, showing people affected – either people with AIDS, seropositive people or those close to them – are positive and optimistic in tone, focusing on quality of life, support and communication.

Since the beginning the AFLS was of the view that use of fear and violent emotions could not usefully serve the cause of AIDS prevention, contending there is no certainty of the desired outcome.

Messages

The dominant messages have consistently been that condoms are to be used as part of everyday practice; and that we should show empathy with and understanding of those with AIDS/HIV.

The separation of AIDS information campaigns from those promoting condoms makes no negative associations with a fatal and sexually transmitted disease.

The condom message, although well received by the public, has not been without its critics, in particular in relation to the appropriateness of the social marketing approach to AIDS/HIV prevention.

Other messages of the French campaign relate to tolerance and caring for people with AIDS/HIV, and have relied heavily on the testimonial approach. There is no mention of how the virus was contracted, with the intention that viewers did not distance themselves.

Target groups

In addition to the general population, AIDS information campaigns have been directed towards gay men, IDUs, sex workers, young people, migrants, the African community, social workers, community leaders, tourists and travellers, workers, prisoners and health care professionals.

Other measures of prevention and control

HIV testing and surveillance

Systematic screening has been performed for blood, sperm and organ donors since 1985.

In 1988, the French government established free and anonymous HIV testing and counselling sites. Little counselling is given apart from at the specialist centres. Contact tracing is not carried out. The number of tested clients increased from 35,844 in 1988 to 58,914 in 1989, 59,948 in 1990, 75,595 in 1991, 125,169 in 1992 and to 139,520 in 1993. The percentage of seropositive clients has decreased over time: in 1988 it was about 4.7, in 1989 3.5, in 1990 3.0, in 1991 2.2, in 1992 1.6 and in 1993 1.0.

The blood contamination scandal, much covered by the press between late 1991 and July 1992, revealed that hundreds of people had received blood contaminated with HIV. When biological testing of donors became compulsory in August 1985 it established that the ratio of contaminated blood donations in France was about 30 times higher than in England. By March 1993 France accounted for over half (57.6 per cent) of the total number of cases of AIDS acquired by transfusion (over 2,000) for the twelve countries of the then European Community.

Obligatory prenatal, premarital and military service testing have been proposed at various times. In 1991, when a CNS report totally opposed any form of mandatory testing or screening, the debate was so heated that the president and vice-president of the CNS sought audience with the President to explain what they felt was at stake in terms of public health. In a parliamentary debate, few MPs voted in favour of mandatory testing or for changing the law in relation to confidentiality (protected by law in France). Thus all testing remains voluntary. A testing campaign organized by the AFLS was developed.

Notification of AIDS cases has been compulsory since June 1986. It is not mandatory to report positive HIV test results.

Needle exchange schemes

A 1972 decree on the condition of the sale of needles and syringes was repealed in May 1987 to allow needles and syringes to be purchased without prescription. Needles are not available in prisons, but inmates may request condoms.

Prevention relating to drug use is the responsibility of the Agence de Lutte Contre la Toxicomanie. The AFLS does however implement local initiatives on drug use, as do many of the AIDS and drug NGOs. There are few needle exchange schemes in France and few people are trained in this area; this is partly the result of the strategy of focusing on risk behaviours rather than groups. Those exchange schemes which do exist have been experimental. The Institut de Recherche en Epidemiologie de la Pharmacodépendence (IREP) ran an experimental campaign to promote clean needle and syringe use. Small bottles of water and bleach with instructions for cleaning were distributed, initially in the Paris area, and since in other areas. Such schemes

are being evaluated. L'Association Charonne, an organization for drug users, runs drop-in centres. They see the need to campaign for wider distribution of needles, and to encourage users to return used ones. Médecins du Monde run needle exchange buses in Paris, Strasbourg and Marseille; AIDES do so in Montpellier and Paris. There have been some problems with the police, due mainly to initial poor communication at the outset about the aims of such initiatives.

A Steribox, containing a condom, two syringes, two sterilized cotton pads and one bottle of sterilized water/bleach is also sold at many pharmacies for between five and ten francs. Syringe vending machines have been installed in Paris and Montpellier.

Condoms

Condom advertising was not permitted on television until January 1987, when legislation was changed to permit condom promotion. It is mandatory for packaging to state that condoms protect against STDs.

In 1992 200 condom vending machines were installed in SNCF and Métro stations and in at least 10 per cent (450) of secondary schools. Of the total numbers of condoms sold through pharmacists, in 1991, 1 per cent of their sales were through condom vending machines installed in the walls outside; in 1992 this figure increased to 5.8 per cent.

In June 1992 the Ministry of Education, the Ministry of Health, the Ministry of Women's Rights and the Ministry of Youth and Sports and the AFLS organized a condom promotion campaign – 'Go out covered' – when over 2 million condoms were sold for one franc during August. The campaign was regarded as a success in increasing condom accessibility, as the number of condoms sold increased and the sales of other brands did not decrease, and the visibility of condoms on display increased.

The 1992 sexual behaviour study found a dramatic increase in reported condom use among 18- to 19-year-olds.

Knowledge, attitude and behaviour surveys have shown that condoms are most used by the under 25s and those in unstable relationships, but many do not use them consistently; of those with multiple partners, 42.6 per cent in 1990 and 56.4 per cent in 1992 reported random condom use. In 1990 24.2 per cent and in 1992 35.4 per cent reported systematic condom use. INSERM's 1994 study of 6,500 respondents aged 15–18 found that 78.9 per cent of boys and 74.4 per cent of girls reported using a condom at first intercourse, while 72.5 per cent of boys and 51.1 per cent of girls reported condom use at most recent sexual intercourse, largely because of the use of the contraceptive pill.

Evaluation

Research became more extensive following the establishment of the ANRS in December 1988 to coordinate medical, clinical and sociological AIDS research. The ANRS has ensured that funding is assured for evaluation.

The Minister of Health commissioned an evaluation of French AIDS policy and practice in 1988 and 1993.

Country visit: Claire Gibbons 1990 and 1993

Report preparation: Becky Field and Kaye Wellings

Individuals and organizations contacted:

Nathalie Bajos, Alfred Spira, Jean Paul Moatti
Institut National de la Santé de la Récherche Médicale (INSERM), Paris

Philippe Bocuse
AIDES, Paris

Marie France Casalis
Mouvement Française pour le Planning Familial, Paris

Cedric Claquin
SIDA Info Service, Paris

Christiane Dressen
Comité Français d'Education pour la Santé (CFES), Vanves

Danielle Heed-Le Roux
Conseil National de SIDA (CNS), Paris

Dr Rudolphe Ingold, Susana Cagliero
Institut de Récherche en Epidemiologie de la Pharmacodépendence (IREP), Paris

Jean Louis Missika
Service d'Information et de Diffusion (SID), Paris

Dr Maman Moussa, Hélène Dold
Unité de Refléxion et d'Action des Communautés Africanes (URACA), Paris

Perlette Petit
Directrice de l'Association Charonne, Paris

Yves Souteyrand, Veronique Doré and Michael Pollak
Agence Nationale de Récherches sur le SIDA (ANRS), Paris

Claude Thiaudière, Ariane Revol-Briard, Caroline Serrand, Gwenola Le Troadec
Agence Française de Lutte Contre le SIDA (AFLS), Vanves

Laurent de Villepin, Matthieu Verboud
Journal du SIDA, ARCAT-SIDA, Paris

Bibliography

Actions de communication publique sur l'infection a VIH/SIDA – 1er semestre 95 – Dossier d'information 1995, Ministère des Affaires Sociales de la Santé et de la Ville

AIDS surveillance in Europe, quarterly report no. 44 31 December 1994, European Centre for the Epidemiological Monitoring of AIDS

Bulletin de l'Agence Nationale de Récherches sur le

SIDA (several issues)

Context of sexual behaviour in Europe. Selected indices relating to demographic, social and cultural variables May 1993, Becky Field and Kaye Wellings, EC Concerted Action 'Risks of sexual behaviour and the risk of HIV infection'

Dossier de Presse – Le comportement sexuel des jeunes face au SIDA April 1995, Une enquête nationale auprès de 6,500 adolescents âgés de 15 à 18 ans, ANRS

Evolution de l'épidemie à VIH en France dans la population heterosexuelle December 1994, rapport au Ministre délégué à la Santé Monsieur Phillipe Douste-Blazy, Réseau National de Santé Publique

Free and anonymous HIV testing and counselling sites (T&C) in France: volume and client characteristics (1988–1993) Oliveria, N, A Serfaty, A Rondenet, P Harinck, P Rigaudy, A Laporte, Xth International Conference on AIDS/STDs, Yokohama, Japan, 7–12 August 1994

Guide de Prévention comment conduire des actions en éducation pour la santé sur l'infection par le VIH auprès des jeunes en milieu scolaire Agence Française de Lutte Contre le SIDA

Health Care and AIDS Key Figures June 1994, 3rd edition, Ministère des Affaires Sociales de la Santé et de la Ville

Le marche du préservatif en France 1992, Agence Française de Lutte Contre le SIDA

Multi-city study of drug misuse 1990 update of data Paris report 1992, Cooperation Group to Combat Drug Abuse and Illicit Trafficking in Drugs (Pompidou Group) Strasbourg

Plan à deux ans SIDA 1990–1991 Agence Française de Lutte Contre le SIDA

Le préservatif masculin: dossier de presse 1989 and 1990 editions, Mouvement Française pour le Planning Familial

Programme for the fight against AIDS 3 year prevention plan 1993–1995 Ministère des Affaires Sociales de la Santé et de la Ville, Agence Française de Lutte Contre le SIDA

Programme de Communication sur l'infection à VIH-SIDA 28 November 1994, Ministère des Affaires Sociales de la Santé

Report of the French 'blood scandal' is leaked to press, 1995, A Dorozynski, *British Medical Journal* **310**; (15 April) 959

Sex education in France, 1991, Colette Gallard, *Planned Parenthood in Europe* **20** (1) (May)

Translation of documents: Christina Gonzalez and Lola Martinez

---

GERMANY

Context

Epidemiology

According to the European Centre for the Epidemiological Monitoring of AIDS, by 31 December 1994, the cumulative total of AIDS cases for Germany was 12,379, with an incidence rate (per million population) of 12.9 (n = 1,051). The cumulative total of AIDS cases by transmission group (percentages in parentheses) was as follows: homo/bisexual male 8,433 (68.7); injecting drug user (IDU) 1,634 (13.3); homo/bisexual IDU 111 (0.9); haemophiliac/coagulation disorder 434 (3.5);

transfusion recipient 236 (1.9); heterosexual contact 781 (6.4); other/undetermined 649 (5.3).

The first AIDS case was registered in 1982.

The number of people infected with HIV, estimated on the basis of AIDS cases registered with the Federal Health Office and mandatory reports of cases of discovered HIV infection, is 50,000.

Social and political background

Because of the federal political system in Germany it is difficult to legislate nationally on many issues relating to health and education. Germany has a tra-

Issue	Legislation	Date of legislation	Services provided
Homosexuality	Age of consent 16 (as for heterosexuals)	1994	Yes
Abortion	Unconstitutional but not punishable[1] [2]		Yes
Drug use (non-medicinal)	Illegal. Small amounts of cannabis for personal use is not an offence		Yes
Prostitution	Varies according to Länder; usually 'promotion' of prostitution illegal and restricted areas/'zoning' decided by local authorities;[3] prostitutes under control of local health authorities and STD laws[4]		Yes
Contraception	Free family planning, contraceptive and sexuality advice guaranteed; oral contraceptives medically prescribed	1992	Yes
Contraception for those under age of sexual consent	Legal; oral contraceptives and 'morning-after-pill' free to <21s only	1992	Yes

[1]In May 1993 a law to liberalize abortion was rejected by the Constitutional Court, and the former ruling of a three-month gestational limit was revoked. At the time of writing the issue is not resolved.[2] The operation can no longer be financed through medical insurance. The services that do exist are concentrated in towns. [3]Prostitutes themselves not punishable unless they solicit in prohibited areas and in areas where minors might be affected (e.g. near schools). [4]Only Bavaria requires an HIV test.

dition of organization within small states, or Länder, which have only relatively recently (in most cases post-war) been part of one unified Germany. The Länder have considerable autonomy and any policies made from central government need their agreement and cooperation before they can be enacted. Considerable efforts have been made in relation to policy relating to AIDS/HIV prevention to ensure maximum local participation and harmony with central government policy.

Public attitudes towards homosexuality vary from being tolerant in the large cities, to hostile in country areas, especially in the conservative areas. The National Homosexual Federation has provided the infrastructure for health education among gay men.

Since 1982 a conservative coalition of Christian Democrats/Christian Social Union (CDU/CSU) parties has been in power. What is known as 'Die Wende' (the political-ideological shift from Social Democratic domination to CDU/CSU) heralded a reaffirmation of traditional moral values comparable to a similar shift in Britain.

Health education

The BundesZentrale für gesundheitliche Aufklärung, (Federal Centre for Health Information, BZgA) takes responsibility for health education on behalf of the Ministry of Health. A number of the German Länder have also established their own centres for health education, and at local level the district health authorities also organize health education measures. In the non-statutory sector, the Bundesvereinigung für Gesundheit e.V. – the umbrella organization for non-governmental health education initiatives – coordinates health education.

Sex education

The first legal regulations governing school sex education were produced in 1968 by national government authority, the Permanent Conference of Ministers of Education and Cultural Affairs in 'Recommendations on Sex Education in Schools'. These regulations were highly elaborate, detailed and balanced, especially given that responsibility for education rested at state level. In 1977 the

Constitutional Court widened and extended the power of teachers and schools.

In 1984, new regulations for sex education were published by the Ministry of Education based on the ruling of the federal Constitutional Court that the teaching of sex education should be planned and implemented with the highest possible degree of agreement between parents and schools. The concept of sex education contained within the regulations reflected a broader perspective on the subject, including education in personal relationships as well as biology. A law passed in July 1993 made sex education mandatory in Germany. Responsibility for curriculum in the schools, however, lies with the Länder; some are more supportive of the new law than others.

Other (non-governmental) organizations play a prominent role in sex education provision, notably Pro Familia, the association for sexual education and family planning which has been an innovative force since the 1960s and is the leading non-governmental organization in the field.

The role of the media

Unpaid-for media coverage was, initially, responsible for some scaremongering and hysterical treatment of AIDS issues, notably the newspaper *Der Spiegel*. However, prompt action on the part of health education agencies did much to counter its worst effects. There is evidence that for the most part, the press were responsible for enhancing awareness and increasing information about AIDS in Germany. Time-series evaluation data show a high level of understanding of routes of transmission among the German population in advance of the start of the official campaigns.

AIDS/HIV public education

Aims and objectives

The basis for the federal government's policies concerning AIDS is the coalition agreement made in March 1987, which emphasized three major goals:

- protecting the public from infection;
- giving persons with HIV infection or AIDS optimal counselling and care;
- avoiding isolation and discrimination of people who are afflicted.

Structure and organization

The Federal Ministry for Health (BMG) is the central coordinator for AIDS policy. In March 1987, an interministerial national AIDS committee, the Nationale AIDS-Beirat, was established as an advisory board to the federal government. The Koordinierungsstab AIDS (AIDS Coordination Unit) was established at the BMG in October 1987, to introduce the necessary federal measures in the fight against AIDS as well as coordinating the measures of the federal, Länder, county and community levels. The federal government and the Länder cooperate closely in this area by means of several specially appointed committees.

Responsibility for developing and conducting AIDS public education rests mainly with the BZgA in cooperation with the AIDS centre in Berlin. The AIDS centre in Berlin – an interdisciplinary scientific advisory body within the Bundesgesundheitsamt (Federal Health Office) – was established in January 1988 and is principally responsible for the collection of epidemiological data and coordination of psychosocial and clinical research. It houses the national reference centre for the epidemiology of AIDS and for the diagnosis of HIV infection. Advisory functions have been served by the Nationale AIDS-Beirat and the parliamentary committee, Enquête-Kommission AIDS.

A major assumption of the prevention campaign has thus been that success depends on close cooperation between governmental and non-governmental agencies. AIDS-help organizations and other private organizations have been centrally involved in activities. Principal among these is the Deutsche AIDS-Hilfe. Founded by gay men in 1983 in Berlin as a non-profit-making organization, it is funded by the BZgA to function as a national networking body and coordination agency for 130 regional organizations combatting AIDS.

Development of campaigns

In common with other countries, the Federal Republic of Germany found itself unprepared for the advent of the AIDS epidemic. The public health services, having traditionally attached the highest priority to fighting communicable diseases, had more recently turned their attention towards psychosocial and environmental problems. As in other countries, the earliest preventive efforts were made by NGOs; the first AIDS-help organizations were set up in Berlin and Munich in 1983 and were followed by others in Cologne, Hamburg and Frankfurt the following year. The Deutsche AIDS-Hilfe developed a strategy for HIV prevention as early as 1983. Several Länder, as well as numerous counties and communities, also reacted early with their own comprehensive programmes.

The general population information campaign began in 1985, when the federal government initiated a campaign addressing both the general public and specific target groups. In autumn 1985, the BZgA distributed a letter to every household pointing out the dangers and possibilities of protection. At a special meeting on 27 March 1987, the Conference of Ministers of Health decided on an overall strategy for fighting AIDS, and the AIDS prevention and control programme was officially adopted by the government in 1987.

Campaign chronology

The nature of AIDS public education campaigns in Western Germany do not lend themselves to systematic chronicling in date order. From their inception, the various interventions incorporating different messages have been combined and interchanged to appear repeatedly at regular intervals.

Tone and style

The BZgA has used an approach which attempts to engage people directly and personally by evoking emotions and personal feelings. TV advertisements are more emotive, and posters and press features more informative, but the same images are used in all campaign features. Thus the campaign has incorporated a degree of synergism. For example, 'Don't give AIDS a chance' – the original slogan – has continued throughout the campaign from the beginning.

Fear has rarely been used and the tone of campaigns has become progressively more positive with time. Efforts have been made to motivate young people to talk about sex, and some humour has been used to this end although generally messages have been couched rather seriously. AIDS-Hilfe has been able to be more positive in promoting sexuality than have the statutory bodies.

Messages

The two major goals of AIDS campaigning in Germany are the protection of healthy people, and the avoidance of isolation and stigmatization of those affected. Educational messages have therefore been designed to counter exaggerated fears on the one hand while reducing individual risk behaviour on the other.

In the very early years of the campaign, condom use was very much a subsidiary message, partly because of early resistance on the part of the statutory authorities. Since 1988 the emphasis has shifted more towards motivating condom use. The message to avoid sexual infidelity, although included in early campaign TV spots and advertisements in 1989, for example, is not promoted now. A more recent focus has been on the normalization of condom use and the removal of barriers to use.

Because of a marked tendency at the start of the AIDS epidemic to ostracize and discriminate against people with HIV in Germany, one of the prime aims of the information campaign has been to address irrational fears and avoid stigmatization.

Messages do not contain a general recommendation for HIV testing. The focus of the advice is that those who may have been at risk of HIV infection should seek counselling and possible subsequent testing.

Target groups

In addition to the general popualtion, AIDS information campaigns have been directed towards single people, bisexuals, homosexuals, young people, people having extramarital affairs, workers, clients of prostitutes, and military personnel.

Other measures of prevention and control

HIV testing and surveillance

From the outset there has been a commitment to a prevention campaign based on information leading to voluntary behaviour changes, and adherence to the principle that education and counselling must take precedence over interventions applicable under the law on communicable diseases. Measures provided for in the Communicable Diseases Act are only used where individuals recklessly disregard the value of another person's health. This strategy was re-endorsed in the recommendations of the 59th Standing Conference of the state ministers responsible for health affairs in November 1988.

Testing is not regarded as an important prevention measure. A countrywide programme of voluntary testing centres has been established, and pre- and post-test counselling is strongly recommended. AIDS and HIV infection are notifiable but personal data are subject to confidentiality in coded form, and reporting of results is confidential. Since 1 October 1987, however, all laboratories have been under obligation to report all confirmed positive test results anonymously to the AIDS Centre in Berlin.

A centralized system of registration of laboratory reports from random unlinked anonymous HIV testing, using blood samples taken at hospitals, has been introduced for the purposes of surveillance and health service planning.

All blood which has been donated since 1985 is tested so that infection via transfusion is rare, though there have been instances of contamination; blood and plasma products for use in treating haemophiliacs are heat treated. Regulations laid down by the Länder apply to persons working in the area of tattooing, piercing ears, acupuncture, etc. In all other areas such as schools, kindergartens, sports facilities, swimming pools, etc., normal regulations on hygiene for avoiding transmission of hepatitis B are deemed totally sufficient.

Information and counselling are preferred to epidemiological intervention measures. However, by making use of the Act to Fight Contagious Sexually Transmitted Diseases (Gesetz zur Bekämpfung von Geschlechtskrankheiten) and the Epidemiological Diseases Act (Bundes Sechengesetz), far-reaching measures have been taken in isolated cases.

The situation in Bavaria was, initially, different from that in other Länder. The Bavarian authorities introduced legislation in 1987 which included measures to compel a 'suspected' person to be tested for HIV; to make HIV testing an obligatory part of a medical examination required for employment in the public sector; to remove any guarantee of anonymity in an HIV antibody test; to instruct in appropriate social behaviour those found to be HIV positive; to oblige all foreigners applying for a residence permit to undergo an HIV antibody test (with the exception of certain European countries); and to provide specific authorities for the police in connection with AIDS. However, day-to-day practice in Bavaria does not follow this legislation strictly.

Discussion of the merits of isolating individuals with HIV occasionally resurfaces in Germany but is unlikely to be taken forward.

Needle exchange schemes

Drug use is illegal in Germany and strong actions are taken against both drug consumption and drug trafficking. A twofold AIDS policy has been developed towards IDUs: on the one hand, to persuade them to give up their habit, and on the other, to encourage HIV testing and to use sterile equipment, which is free of charge in many places. Sterile needles and syringes are not available in prisons, though availability of condoms has increased.

Some Länder have not initiated needle exchange programmes. Disposable syringes are easily available in most pharmacies, and there are vending machines for syringes in most cities. There is a greater tolerance among members of the police force for the problem of injecting drug use although possession of syringes and needles may constitute primary suspicion which can trigger police investigation.

Condoms

Pharmacies now display condoms more prominently. They are also advertised in magazines but not on television. The family planning organization, Pro Familia, has actively promoted condoms, and new shops called condomeria have opened geared to the purchase of condoms by young people. Generally there has been an increase in claimed use.

Evaluation

AIDS/HIV prevention programmes in Germany are systematically evaluated. Evaluation studies are categorized as follows:

- general surveys – studies which do not refer to a particular part of the campaign, but investigate knowledge, attitude, behaviour and practice in connection with AIDS;
- programme evaluation – studies of the differential effects of pilot programmes on different levels and in different parts of the target population;
- behaviour studies – research on the causes and effects of the whole campaign in relation to the behavioural changes among different risk groups and the general population.

The evaluation of most public education programmes is initiated and commissioned by the BZgA from different survey agencies and university research institutes. Assesment focuses on the accep-tance and effects of separate measures within the mass media campaign (TV and cinema spots, newspaper advertisements, brochures, etc.), the evaluation of the helpline and the evaluation of the personal communication campaign.

Condom sales trends, STD statistics and HIV prevalence data are used to evaluate the results of the whole prevention campaign, in combination with the above-mentioned surveys.

Country visit: Kaye Wellings 1991 and 1993

Report preparation: Kaye Wellings and Becky Field

Individuals and organizations contacted:

Gerhard Christiansen, Dr Wolfgang Müller, Margarita Nilson Giebel, Dr Elisabeth Pott, Jürgen Töppich
Bundeszentrale für gesundheitliche Aufklärung (Federal Centre for Health Education), Cologne

Dr Wolfgang Heckmann
Federal Ministry for Health, Berlin

Bibliography

AIDS control in the Federal Republic of Germany 1991, Federal Ministry for Health
AIDS im öffentlichen Bewusstsein 1992, Bundeszentrale für gesundheitliche Aufklärung
AIDS surveillance in Europe, quarterly report no. 44 31 December 1994, European Centre for the Epidemiological Monitoring of AIDS
BZgA Untersuchungen zum Themenbereich AIDS in den Jahren von 1986–1993 1994, Auszug der Dokumentation der abgeschlossenen Studien und Untersuchungen
Gerhard Christiansen and Jürgen Töppich, Umfragedaten zum Sexualverhalten. In Wolfgang Heckmann and Meinrad A Koch (eds) *Sexualverhalten in Zeiten von AIDS* 1994, Berlin: Edition Sigma
Context of sexual behaviour in Europe, selected indices

relating to demographic, social and cultural variables May 1993, Becky Field and Kaye Wellings, EC Concerted Action 'Sexual behaviour and the risk of HIV infection'

Damm, C, H Lehmann, G Marsen-Storz, U Sielert and J Töppich *Die personalkommunikative AIDS-Aufklärungskampagne der Bundeszentrale für gesundheitliche Aufklärung* 1990, Prävention; 3/1990: 98-102, BZgA

Jürgen Gerhards and Bernd Schmidt *Intime Kommunikation*, Band 11 der Schriftenreihe des Bundesministeriums für Gesundheit

Niedermeyer, O *Jugendliche und AIDS: Relevanz, Wissen, Einstellungen and Verhalten* no. 39.9. 1988, Institut Universitaire de Médecine Sociale et Préventive, Lausanne

Translation of documents: Jutta King, Ann Snodgrass

GREECE

Context

Epidemiology

According to the European Centre for the Epidemiological Monitoring of AIDS, by 31 December 1994, the cumulative total of AIDS cases was 1,018 with an incidence rate (per million population) of 11 (n = 115). The cumulative total of AIDS cases by transmission group (percentages in parentheses) was as follows: homo/bisexual male 528 (52.9); injecting drug user (IDU) 41 (4.1); homo/bisexual IDU 9 (0.9); haemophiliac/coagulation disorder 67 (6.7); transfusion recipient 45 (4.5); heterosexual contact 106 (10.6); other/undetermined 202 (20.2).

The first AIDS case was registered in Greece in 1983.

The distribution of AIDS cases has not followed the same course as in other southern European countries such as Italy and Spain for instance, where intravenous drug use is a major problem.

Issue	Legislation	Date of legislation	Services provided
Homosexuality	Age of consent 15 (same as for heterosexuals). 'Seduction' (not defined) of 15- to16-year-olds resulting in anal intercourse an offence	1987	In big cities
Abortion	Legal; on request ≤12 weeks, medical/psychological reasons ≤20 weeks, sex crime/eugenic ≤24 weeks. <15s need parental consent. Free if performed in public hospital, but most performed privately	1983, 1986	Yes
Drug use (non-medicinal)	Illegal; no distinction between hard and soft drugs, distinction between dealing (harsh penalties) and using	1989	Yes
Prostitution	If registered with police, legal; mandatory STD check and HIV test every 3 months, health card obligatory	1985	Yes
Contraception	No medical prescription needed for oral contraceptives	1963	Limited in rural and island areas[1]
Contraception for those under age of sexual consent	No legislation, at individual doctor's/GP's discretion		Limited in rural and island areas[1]

[1]Although on the islands condoms are widely available.

Social and political background

Following military rule between 1967 and 1974 the Greek state remains centralized. From 1981 Papandreou led a socialist government until it was defeated in 1990 by a right-wing government but won office again in October 1993. As the new government established itself, public appointments were frozen. Consequently an atmosphere of uncertainty existed in the public health (and other) sectors in relation to job security and financing for projects.

The basis of the national health service is an insurance scheme to which those in employment make contributions. It is generally accepted however that prompt treatment is best achieved through the private sector. The state system compares unfavourably with the private system – conditions are poorer, pay is lower. Most physicians mix private and public work.

In general the Orthodox church is less absolute than the Catholic church in its attitudes towards practices such as birth control, abortion, etc. It allows divorce (up to three times usually) and remarriage in church. Only a vocal minority of the Greek Orthodox church was against the legalization of abortion. Parish priests are usually married; confession is rarely practised among younger generations. The connection between the state and church is long established; although nominally under the state, the church has always exercised considerable power. The Ministry of Education for example, is also the Ministry of Religion. 98 per cent of Greeks declare themselves to be of Orthodox affiliation, though in practice they indicate that they do not consider themselves to be particularly religious. The church has been clear in its support for those with AIDS/HIV.

Taboos surround homosexuality, and many Greek gays may prefer to conceal their homosexuality in order to avoid discrimination, which has in part been reinforced by the association of gay men with AIDS/HIV. There is a strong tendency for those with homosexual inclinations to marry and 'pass' as heterosexuals. According to opinion polls 55–70 per cent of the population disapprove of homosexuality. Homosexuals/bisexuals constitute the majority of declared AIDS cases, of these a considerable number have wives and children (1990). The police are empowered to require people to be tested for STDs – in some cases this has been used to harass the gay community.

Prostitution has for many years been a socially accepted practice, especially for young men. Given the traditional rules of virginity for women and masculine behaviour for men, prostitutes were seen as both an outlet and a schooling for young men. Nowadays, particularly in urban areas, young men are more likely to have a girlfriend with whom they have sex. Registered prostitutes number approximately 270 but there is an estimated ratio of 1:10 of registered to unregistered prostitutes, many of whom are from eastern Europe and the Philippines.

There appears to be an absence of a clear health policy concerning family planning; various governments have had problems separating the demographic problems of Greece (a rapidly aging population and a very low birth rate) from the right to family planning services. Some evidence of the politically sensitive nature of family planning for politicians is their continued avoidance of decision making with respect to the introduction of health and sex education in schools. It is unlikely that a young woman would ask her doctor for contraception, and in rural areas there is little access to contraception. Generally, the pill is regarded negatively and it is rare for a GP to recommend it to under 18s.

Greece has one of the highest abortion rates in Europe with a ratio of abortions to live births of approximately 1:3 in 1988. Abortion is used by women regardless of family and socio-economic status, and is accepted as an established traditional form of birth control. It is not considered a moral issue and there is a general lack of guilt about the subject.

Family life is a core value in Greek society. Unlike many other countries in Europe it is rare for young people to leave home before marrying.

Health education

There is no strong tradition of health education or promotion in Greece, nor any specific agency responsible for health promotion other than the Ministry of Health, Welfare and Social Security. The focus of most state-funded research and projects, for health in general and AIDS in particular, is biomedical.

Sex education

Religious education is taught to all pupils but there is no legislation pertaining to sex education in schools. Consequently provision is scarce. The Ministry of Education is under pressure from those working in AIDS/HIV/sexual health, as well as from the media, to legislate on this matter. The issue is politically contentious, so the *status quo* remains. Some feel that even if legislation were passed, there is no guarantee of quality, given the controversy surrounding the subject and probable lack of teacher training.

The role of the media

At the outset the media treated AIDS/HIV in a sensationalist manner, often portraying it as a gay disease. As elsewhere, a huge epidemic was feared. This soon changed; supportive media coverage of lectures and other educational events has led to significant public education about AIDS/HIV. Much AIDS/HIV information has been disseminated via free media coverage. AIDS/HIV has probably served to create a more open climate in issues relating to sexuality. In general the media have become more liberal, although quite superficial, in their treatment of such issues. This climate has also been encouraged by the growth of satellite TV providing access to American and other European programmes.

AIDS/HIV public education

Aims and objectives

The Public Information Committee (PIC) of the Hellenic Centre for the Control of AIDS and STDs (HCC AIDS and STDs) is the official body responsible for AIDS/HIV public education. Its objectives are:

- prevention through information;
- to shape an appropriate public mentality and attitude towards the disease and those suffering from it, so that nobody panics, yet nobody is indifferent;
- to present the true extent of the problems;
- to make known the actions of the state;
- to facilitate the development of responsibility in individuals, families and social groups.

Structure and organization

The Greek National Committee on AIDS (NCA) was established by and made responsible to the Ministry of Health, Welfare and Social Security (MHWSS) in July 1983 as an advisory committee, with no independent budget. Some problems resulted from the NCA's lack of power and over-bureaucratized procedures. In 1989 it was suggested that an independent body be established for action against AIDS, hence the HCC AIDS and STDs was created in 1992 by a presidential decree. Although this organization has greater autonomy it is still under the authority of the Deputy Minister of Health.

Special committees made up of specialists in the field advise the HCC AIDS and STDs (120 scientists participate), of which the PIC is one. *Ex officio* members of the PIC include representatives of the Greek Orthodox church, the Ministry of Education and Religion, the press and mass media, the Child Health Foundation (CHF), the New Generation Secretariat, the Directorate of Health, the Directorate of Primary Care and the Directorate of Public Health.

The dominance of a biomedical perspective in Greek AIDS policy has resulted in many important decisions being made without open discussion with experts in other fields, even though the government calls AIDS a 'social' problem. The establishment of the HCC AIDS and STDs was intended to remedy this, but some still feel the influence of the biomedical bias.

Development of campaigns

The development of general population campaigns has been erratic. Public education activities began when the National Committee on AIDS was established, and most were initiated through the WHO/National Centre for AIDS of the Athens School of Public Health. A leaflet was distributed to all households with the electricity bill in 1985. Educational efforts were instituted in schools and the armed forces.

The main focus for government public education activities public education has been World AIDS Day (1 December) each year. This highlights the importance of World AIDS Day for Greece and for other countries. Significant contributions to AIDS public education have come from NGOs, including ELPIDA, the Family Planning Association (FPA) and the Hellenic Association for the Study and Control of AIDS (HASCA). HASCA began AIDS public education activities in 1987 and contributed significantly to governmental activities. ELPIDA lobbies the government regarding care, treatment and prevention policy. The FPA has incorporated AIDS education into its general sexual health strategy. Because such independent initiatives lack sufficient resources, however, little preliminary

Campaign chronology

Date and agency	Campaign theme/title	Aims	Media	Main message/endline	Target groups	Tone and style
1985 NCA[1]/ MHWSS	First campaign	Raise awareness	Leaflet drop		General public, armed forces	Informational
1 December 1988 HASCA	World AIDS Day	Raise awareness, improve prevention, encourage solidarity	TV, radio, album, exhibitions of posters all over Greece		General public	
1 December 1990 NCA/MHWSS	World AIDS Day	As above	TV, radio, posters, leaflets, kiosks		General public, women	
1 December 1991 NCA/MHWSS	World AIDS Day	As above	As above	'Sharing the challenge'	General public	
1 December 1992 NCA/MHWSS	World AIDS Day	As above	As above	'AIDS. A community commitment'	General public	
1 December 1993 HCC AIDS and STDs	World AIDS Day	As above	As above	'Time for action'	General public, young people	
1993 HCC AIDS and STDs	Helpline campaign	Provide details of helpline	Leaflet drop (Athens and urban areas)		General public	Informational
1993 HCC AIDS and STDs	Workplace campaign	Correct transmission routes, increase solidarity and inform about precautions	Leaflet, seminars	'Time for action in the workplace'	Workers	Informational
1993 HCC AIDS and STDs/CHF	Schools campaign	Prevention	Leaflet, video	'Time for action'	School children (15–17s)	Informational and moral

[1]National Committee on AIDS

research or evaluation takes place to gauge effectiveness.

Tone and style

Most material produced for the general public has been plainly informative in tone. Leaflets give details about AIDS/HIV in a direct manner, with a focus on correcting misinformation. Booklets for young people are seen by some as paternalistic and didactic.

Messages

Much of the public education material focuses on correcting myths about casual transmission. World AIDS Day themes have been used as the basis for education and prevention activities and materials.

Target groups

In addition to the general population, AIDS information campaigns have been directed towards registered sex workers, women, young people, workers, military personnel and health care professionals.

Other measures of prevention and control

HIV testing and surveillance

It is obligatory for doctors to report an AIDS diagnosis and a positive HIV test result, although the latter is not uniformly adhered to. Since 1993 all newborn babies have been anonymously tested for HIV, otherwise there is no unlinked anonymous testing for surveillance purposes. Free and anonymous voluntary testing is available at four centres in Athens and at clinics attached to hospitals in other urban centres. In theory pre- and post-test counselling is available, but in practice this often, reportedly, fails to take place.

In December 1985 it became mandatory for registered prostitutes to be tested for HIV every three months; the National Centre for AIDS offered counselling, insisting on the use of condoms, and

suggesting avoidance of clients from central Africa. HIV positive prostitutes were advised to abstain from prostitution.

By the end of 1985 all blood banks and transfusion centres were screening blood.

Needle exchange schemes

IDU is a small scale problem in Greece; there is little culture of injecting. There are no needle exchange schemes and their establishment is not foreseen. The sale of needles and syringes by pharmacies is unrestricted and each district has a pharmacy open 24 hours per day on a rota. Methadone is not permitted. Treatment focuses on therapeutic communities financed by government but run independently.

Condoms

A well-established tradition of condom use is said to exist in Greece, although little data exist to demonstrate how widespread use is. The use of condoms is the most common method of contraception, after withdrawal. However, some doubt must be cast on reports of condom use as a contraceptive, given the high abortion rate. Condoms have been advertised on TV and are widely available from the numerous street kiosks, chemists and supermarkets, but it is still difficult to obtain condoms in rural areas. There are no official safety standards for condoms. Incorrect storage in a hot climate can affect quality, and it is not known what proportion of condoms sold are without a kitemark.

Evaluation

Thus far there has been no evaluation of public education campaigns, either under the National Committee on AIDS or the Hellenic Centre for the Control of AIDS and STDs.

The telephone helpline evaluate their service and from this inform policy makers of the gaps in public knowledge of AIDS/HIV.

Country visit: Becky Field 1994

Report preparation: Becky Field

Individuals and organizations contacted:

Mary Antzel, ELPIDA, Athens

Professor D Agrafiotis, George Koulierakis
Department of Sociology, Athens School of Public
Health, Athens

Professor J E Kyriopoulos
Department of Health Economics, Athens School
of Public Health, Athens

Lis Metheneos, Vasso Margaritidou
Family Planning Association of Greece, Athens

Elisa Nicolopoulou, Ralph Hansen
AIDS Helpline and Counselling Centre, Athens

Professor George Papaevangelou
Hellenic Association for the Study and Control of
AIDS, Athens

G Papoutsakis
Director of Public Health, Ministry of Health,
Welfare and Social Security, Athens

Professor Stratigos (President), Maria
Papakonstantinou-Karra (Public Information
Committee)
Hellenic Centre for the Control of AIDS and
STDs, Athens

Bibliography

*Activities of the Information Committee of KEEL for
1 December 1993* M Papakonstantinou, Deputy
Coordinator of Public Information Committee,
Hellenic Centre for the Control of AIDS and
STDs

*AIDS: knowledge, attitudes, beliefs and practices of
young people (pre-test)* 1990, D Agrafiotis *et al.*

Department of Sociology, Athens School of
Public Health

AIDS: research concerning knowledge of the junior
high and senior school students in Thassos,
Greece, 1991, G Apostolides *et al. Primary Health
Care* 3 (9) April–June

AIDS surveillance in Europe, quarterly report no. 44 31
December 1994, European Centre for the
Epidemiological Monitoring of AIDS

*Attitudes to and the use of condoms by the Athenian
population under the threat of AIDS* 1991, E
Metheneous *et al.*, EC Concerted Action 'Sexual
behaviour and the risk of HIV infection'

*Context of sexual behaviour in Europe, selected indices
relating to demographic, social and cultural variables*
May 1993, Becky Field and Kaye Wellings, EC
Concerted Action 'Sexual behaviour and the risk
of HIV infection'

Education in preventing HIV infection in Greek registered prostitutes, 1988, G Papaevangelou *et al.*,
Journal of Acquired Immune Deficiency Syndromes
1; 386–9

Family planning centres in Greece, 1992, V
Margaritidou and E Mestheneos, *International
Journal of Health Sciences*, 3 (1); 25–31

*Hellenic Centre for the Control of AIDS and STDs,
brief description* 1993, J D Stratigos

*Hellenic Centre for the Control of AIDS and STDs,
organogram* 1993

*Knowledge, attitudes, beliefs and practices in relation to
HIV infection and AIDS, the case city of Athens,
Greece* 1990, Department of Sociology, Athens
School of Public Health

*Knowledge, attitudes and practices of Greek health pro-
fessionals, in relation to AIDS* A Roumeliotou *et
al.*, AIDS Reference Centre, Athens School of
Hygiene, Department of Epidemiology and
Medical Statistics

*Report of the Conference of EC Parliamentarians on
HIV/AIDS* 1993, British All-Party Parliamentary
Group on AIDS

Situation in Greece, 1988, A Roumeliotou, paper for
working group B of the EC Concerted Action
'Assessing AIDS preventive strategies', Lucerne,
Switzerland

Sexual behaviour and knowledge about AIDS in a representative sample of Athens area 1991, M Malliori *et al.*, EC Concerted Action, 'Sexual behaviour and the risk of HIV infection'

Sexual behaviour in the years of AIDS in Greece 1991, E Ioannidis *et al.*, EC Concerted Action

'Sexual behaviour and the risk of HIV infection'

Sexuality of Greeks, a bibliographical study 1993, D Agrafiotis and P Mandi, Department of Sociology, Athens School of Public Health

Translation of documents: Vassilis Kontogiannis

ICELAND

Context

Epidemiology

According to the European Centre for the Epidemiological Monitoring of AIDS, by 31 December 1994, the cumulative total of AIDS cases was 35, with an incidence rate (per million population) of 11.3 (n = 3). The cumulative total of AIDS cases by transmission group (percentages in parentheses) was as follows: homo/bisexual male 29 (82.9); injecting drug user (IDU) 2 (5.7); homo/bisexual IDU 0; haemophiliac/coagulation disorder 0; transfusion recipient 2 (5.7); heterosexual contact 2 (5.7); other/undetermined 0.

From 1985 until December 1993, 83 people had been diagnosed as HIV positive.

Health and sex education

Sex education became mandatory in 1975. There is a lack of curriculum materials, development and coordination at secondary school level (for young people age 16–19). Health professionals at primary health care centres are also responsible for providing sex education, counselling and prevention aimed at reducing the spread of AIDs and other STDs. Sex education is now regarded as an important base from which to tackle the spread of AIDS, and AIDS has encouraged more open discussion of sexual issues generally.

Social and political background

Issue	Legislation	Date of legislation	Services provided
Homosexuality	Age of consent 18 (16 for heterosexuals and lesbians)		
Abortion	Legal for ≤16 weeks for reasons of illness, age, too many children, rape, medical. Counselling obligatory. Free of charge	1975	
Drug use (non-medicinal)			
Prostitution	Earning a living from prostitution (heterosexual and homosexual) punishable by 2-year prison sentence; third-party 4 years	1992	
Contraception	Contraceptive advice and provision paid for by client. One clinic in Reykjavik gives free advice and provision	1975	Yes
Contraception for those under age of sexual consent	<16s need parental consent		Yes – one clinic in Reykjavik

Campaign chronology

Date and agency	Campaign theme/title	Aims	Media	Main message/endline	Target groups	Tone and style
1985 GDH		Raise awareness	Leaflet drop		General public	Informational
1987 GDH			TV, posters	Think twice, people die from AIDS	General public	Slightly fearful
1987		Condom normalization	Posters		General public	Famous personalities
1988 GDH			TV, posters	Casual sex can have unforeseen consequences. People die from AIDS	General public, IDUs	Slightly fearful
1989–90 GDH			TV, posters	You alone can protect yourself against AIDS – by being cautious	General public	Erotic
1992 GDH		Increase understanding and tolerance towards people with AIDS/HIV* Change image of the condom† Encourage condom use‡	TV, posters, radio,† posters on buses	*Let's share the challenge against AIDS	General public, †travellers	
1993 GDH		Increase understanding that AIDS is a common problem around the world	Posters, international poster show, theatre in education	Enjoy life ... use the condom. These are good reasons for taking the condom with you on holiday	General public, young people travellers	Positive

AIDS/HIV public education

Structure and organization

The Icelandic National Committee on AIDS was appointed by the Health Minister with responsibility for AIDS public education until January 1994; in 1991 the Icelandic National Committee on AIDS began planning AIDS prevention activities according to a national plan.

Development of campaigns

With a population of 265,000, 100 per cent literacy and a generally high level of education, public health education campaigns are relatively easy to carry out in Iceland.

In 1985 the General Directorate of Health began an AIDS public education campaign with TV and radio spots; brochures were mailed to every home; public lectures were given by health care workers to schools and workplaces throughout the country. Between 1985–88 various educational materials were produced, mainly posters and leaflets aimed at the general population. At the start the tone of such materials was forthright and slightly fear inducing, but it has since become more humorous and positive.

Tone and style

As in some other countries, early campaigns in Iceland relied somewhat on scare tactics. But from 1989–90 onwards, emphasis changed, promoting safe sex in a positive life enhancing way. The 1989 TV spot was markedly different in approach to earlier materials. Set to the pop song 'The power of love' it featured an erotic shower scene filmed in such a way that it is not always clear whether the bodies are male and female together or male and male together.

Target groups

In addition to the general population, AIDS information campaigns have been directed towards travellers, young people and IDUs.

Condoms

Condoms are available in pharmacies, petrol stations, some kiosks, some entertainment clubs and from taxi cabs. Condom advertising is permitted on TV. The Icelandic National Committee on AIDS has tried to make condoms more accessible and available.

Evaluation

The Icelandic National Committee on AIDS has been reponsible for evaluation, which is becoming an integral part of the process of designing campaigns.

No country visit was made to Iceland.

Report preparation: Becky Field

Individuals and organizations contacted:

Jóna Ingibjörg Jonsdóttir
The Icelandic National Committee on AIDS

Bibliography

AIDS surveillance in Europe, quarterly report no. 40 31 December 1993, European Centre for the Epidemiological Monitoring of AIDS

IRELAND

Context

Epidemiology

According to the European Centre for the Epidemiological Monitoring of AIDS, by 31 December 1994, the cumulative total of AIDS cases was 443, with an incidence rate (per million population) of 10.2 (n = 36). The cumulative total of AIDS cases by transmission group (percentages in parentheses) was as follows: homo/bisexual male 149 (34.9); injecting drug user (IDU) 190 (44.5); homo/bisexual IDU 8 (1.9); haemophiliac/coagulation disorder 27 (6.3); transfusion recipient 0; heterosexual contact 48 (11.2); other/undetermined 5 (1.2).

The first AIDS case was registered in Ireland in 1982.

By May 1993, 1,368 people had been found to be HIV positive.

Social and political background

Ireland is a predominantly Catholic country, with 95 per cent of the population being of this religious denomination. There are strong groups in both the Church of Ireland and the Catholic church who would be more liberal and who favour revision, but there are also vociferous factions in each who are staunchly conservative. Among the general public, there exists to some extent a dual morality; many pay lip service to the ideals of the church, but in practice behave differently.

Until 1993 homosexuality was illegal in Ireland; a 1988 European Court of Human Rights ruling overturned this and was translated into actual legislation in 1993. The delay in legally enacting the ruling is an indication of the trepidation with which politicians have viewed the issue of homosexuality. Services are provided for gay men, but overt use of government money for this purpose could, it was felt, create problems for the Ministry of Justice and for this rea-

Issue	Legislation	Date of legislation	Services provided
Homosexuality	Age of consent 17 (same as for heterosexuals)	1993	Yes
Abortion	Illegal	1861, 1983,[1] 1986,[2] 1992[3]	Information only
Drug use (non-medicinal)	Illegal		Yes
Prostitution	Illegal		Yes[4]
Contraception	Legal if for 'bona fide family planning purposes'[5]	1979, 1985, 1992/93[6]	Yes
Contraception for those under age of sexual consent	As above, no legislation concerning age limit for contraception. Condoms available for all	1979, 1985, 1992/93[6]	Yes (few, mainly urban)

[1]Article 40.3.3. of the constitution gave foetuses the 'right to life'. Subsequently women's groups and students were prevented from distributing information on legal abortion services abroad. [2]Offences Against the Person Act: sections 58 and 59 prohibit termination under any circumstances. There are criminal sanctions against anyone assisting this. [3]Following rulings in the European Court of Justice and the European Court of Human Rights, article 40.3.3 was amended to permit abortion information and freedom of travel. [4]In STD clinics and by a voluntary religious organization. [5]The enforceability of this is questionable. [6]Legislation concerning condom availability (see 'Condoms' section, below)

son is channelled through more general networks, such as the Irish Gay and Lesbian Associations. The general Irish attitude to homosexuality is perhaps more tolerant than it was, in spite of the teachings of the church.

There is little legislation or regulation pertaining to AIDS. Anti-discriminatory regulations and guidelines on correct practice have been issued by the trade unions and employers' associations. There have been complaints by gay organizations of discrimination against homosexuals and people with HIV, but these have proved difficult to substantiate.

Health education

The main statutory agency dealing with health promotion and education is now the Health Promotion Unit (HPU) of the Department of Health (DoH), which received funds of approximately IR£1.5 million from the state in 1993. Many voluntary agencies also contribute to health promotion such as the Irish Cancer Society and the Irish Heart Foundation.

Health education was, until 1988, the responsibil-ity of the Health Education Bureau (HEB), a quango (quasi non-governmental organization) which enjoyed a considerable degree of independence despite being funded by the DoH. After 1988, however, the HEB was superseded by the HPU, which has a closer relationship with government, being responsible to the Minister for Health and thus subject to a greater degree of political control.

Sex education

Nearly all schools in Ireland are Roman Catholic. There are also a small number of 'multidenominational' schools. Sex education is not mandatory and no programme is laid down at secondary level by the government, though the Department of Education has issued guidelines for post-primary schools on the subject. The approach suggested by the Department of Health is that sex education takes place in the context of a broader health education curriculum, allowing for a full discussion of human relationships in addition to facts relating to physical aspects of reproduction. The climate surrounding the teaching of sex education is more facilitating than it was a decade ago yet it remains a contentious issue.

The role of the media

In general, issues relating to sexuality and sexual health are dealt with in a non-sensationalist manner. Over time it has become more acceptable for matters of sexuality to be portrayed in the media. Initially, AIDS/HIV issues were treated in a fairly emotional fashion by the media, which tended to reinforce prejudice with scare stories and a sometimes hysterical approach. More recently, the attitude of the media has generally been more responsible. As an information source, the press has been quite helpful, and has shown a willingness to be corrected when errors have been made.

Generally, the media have been sympathetic towards people with AIDS, though there has been a tendency to single out individual cases for overemotional treatment rather than focus on the broad issues.

AIDS/HIV public education

Aims and objectives

The National AIDS Strategy Committee's integrated AIDS/HIV strategy for public education aims to take measures to avoid discrimination, and to implement more direct and intensive education and information programmes.

Structure and organization

Responsibility for national implementation and coordination of AIDS policy rests with the National AIDS Strategy Committee, representative of the voluntary and statutory services, under the auspices of the Department of Health (DoH). The DoH works closely with the eight regional health boards, most of which have established AIDS coordinating committees to which NGO AIDS organizations apply for funding.

Each regional health board is divided into community care areas (CCAs). It is not mandatory for a CCA to run an AIDS education programme for schools in the area nor for those working with AIDS/HIV; provision of this tends to depend on the policy adopted by the director of the CCA.

No statutory body exists to oversee and coordinate NGO activities. The AIDS Liaison Forum, however, performs a networking function, bringing together NGO and statutory AIDS/HIV organizations from all over Ireland, (including care and treatment organizations). The NGO sector is responsible for a very significant proportion of AIDS/HIV service provision and prevention.

Development of campaigns

An early AIDS information leaflet was produced by the Gay Men's Health Project in 1985, after receiving a grant of IR£15,000 from the government.

The first attempt at AIDS public education was made in 1986. In 1986-87 the government produced its first AIDS information leaflet. Initially campaigns were carried out by the HEB. By that time a number of measures to combat AIDS had already been employed.

The NGO Dublin AIDS Alliance produced the first AIDS prevention cinema spot which ran for two weeks nationwide and four weeks in Dublin in September 1993, and again in February 1994 to coincide with the opening of the film *Philadelphia*. An AIDS/HIV factpack, which it also helped to compile was mailed out to schools/colleges for special screenings of the film. The cinema spot was sponsored by Durex for IR£3,000 but cost IR£50,000 to make; crew, actors and space were all donated. Rank Screen Advertising donated the cinema spots free of charge.

Tone and style

Although in general the tone and style of campaigns have been informative and educational in nature, there have been some exceptions. The 1988 'Shooting AIDS' posters could be viewed by some as stigmatizing and fear inducing. Similarly, the 1992 TV

Campaign chronology

Date and agency	Campaign theme/title	Aims	Media	Main message/endline	Target groups	Tone and style
1986 HEB		Raise awareness	TV, posters	Casual sex spreads AIDS; sharing needles spreads AIDS	General public, IDUs	Low key, informative
1987 HEB		Reinforce message to IDUs	Posters	Sharing needles spreads AIDS; information hotline available	IDUs	Low key, informative
1988 HEB	Shooting AIDS	Reinforce message to IDUs	Bus shelter posters, billboards	'Sharing needles can be the death of *YOU*. Don't shoot yourself with AIDS'	IDUs	Frightening
1988/89 AIDS Alliances		Advertise helplines		Confidential phonelines available	General public	Low key, informative
November 1989 HPU and DoE	AIDS resource materials for schools	Raise awareness and inform	Video, teaching pack		14–18s, teachers	Informative
January 1990 HPU	AIDS. The facts	Raise awareness and inform	Leaflet		General public	Informative, moral[1]
March 1991 HPU	Convenience advertising strategy	Correct misinformation, inform of risk-reduction strategies for HIV, STDs, unwanted pregnancy	Posters in toilets	'Be safe. Be sure'	General public third-level colleges, women, entertainment venues	Informative
May 1991 HPU and IASW[2]	Ciara's story	Help parents raise HIV issue with children	Booklet		Parents, children	Story book
May 1992– May 1993 HPU	'Domino' campaign	Sustain awareness	TV, radio	'Education can stop the spread'	General public	Sombre
May 1993 to date HPU	Condom campaign	Encourage condom use/ safe sex	TV, radio, posters	'Protect yourself. Use a condom'	General public, young people	'Straight talking'
September 1993– February 1994 DAA	Cinema campaign	Encourage condom use	Cinema		Young people	Stylish, modern

[1]'It cannot be too strongly stressed that to avoid sexual transmission of HIV, the most effective way of all is to: • Stay with one faithful partner • Remain faithful to that one partner.' [2]Irish Association of Social Workers

campaign featured a chain of dominos falling with a sombre voice-over, associated by some with the UK tombstone/'Don't die of ignorance' campaign.

Messages

The first campaign concentrated on disseminating messages concerned with modes of transmission and the need to avoid discrimination against people with AIDS/HIV. The message of condom use was subsidiary but has now increased in prominence. An additional message was to adopt responsible behaviour, which in essence meant one *safe* partner. This led to some discussion, since medical experts maintained that such a definition was neither realistic nor achievable. In general, messages of the campaign have veered towards the moralistic rather than the pragmatic, in order to appease the church.

AIDS/HIV appears to have contributed to the development of a more down-to-earth atmosphere surrounding sex and sexuality in general, which in turn has led to changes in legislation increasing condom availability. This perhaps has made a more pragmatic approach more feasible.

Target groups

In addition to the general population, AIDS information campaigns have been directed towards IDUs, young people, university students and homosexual men.

Other measures of prevention and control

HIV testing and surveillance

AIDS cases but not HIV diagnoses are reported, on a voluntary basis, to the Ministry of Health. Testing is available on a voluntary basis with guarantees of confidentiality; counselling services are available.

On the National AIDS Strategy Committee's recommendation, the surveillance programme has been extended to include anonymous, unlinked surveillance of HIV from blood taken for routine clinical

purposes at antenatal clinics (which is surplus to requirements). From May 1993 testing of unlinked surplus blood taken at STD clinics and outpatients departments was to be phased in.

Since 1985 all blood has been tested for HIV, and blood products treated. The Blood Transfusion Services Board does not accept blood from men who have had same-sex relations at any time since 1978.

Needle exchange schemes

Since injecting drug use is the principal mode of transmission of HIV in Ireland, efforts at developing effective preventive programmes focusing on injecting drug users have been accorded a high priority. The huge majority of IDUs live in and around Dublin.

The first needle exchange scheme was piloted in 1989; AIDS/HIV had led those working with IDUs to favour a less didactic treatment and prevention strategy. There was some public controversy surrounding the idea, but avoidance of publicity eased the situation. There are now eight such schemes in Dublin, which also offer cleaning equipment, one-to-one addiction counselling, condoms, advice on safer sex, anonymous testing and counselling.

AIDS/HIV has served to open up the debate surrounding drug use. Until 1992 the Drug Treatment Centre was the only agency offering actual *treatment* for IDUs, based on a rigid programme of methadone maintenance with emphasis on a drug-free lifestyle, in contrast to the harm-minimization approach of Eastern Health Board (EHB) clinics. Since then the EHB clinics have been able to offer treatment as well as preventive measures. Outreach work is important – making contact with users locally, providing information services, educating about HIV prevention.

Condoms

Ireland has seen major advances recently, possibly AIDS-linked, in relation to condom availability. Condoms have been legally available for sale in pharmacies since 1980 with a doctor's prescription. From

1985, condoms and other non-medically prescribed contraceptives became available from pharmacies, family planning centres, doctors' surgeries and health clinics for those over the age of 18 without a medical prescription. The same Act was amended in 1992 and 1993. The 1992 amendment allowed the sale of condoms and spermicide to persons over 17 years of age and removed the anomaly whereby pharmacies (which were limited companies) were legally prohibited from selling contraceptives. The 1993 amendment removed controls over the supply of condoms, allowing distribution through unrestricted outlets including vending machines. Chemist shops in even the smallest towns now have condoms on open display, clubs and pubs have vending machines in toilets. Supermarkets do not stock condoms and commercial TV condom advertising is not permitted.

Evaluation

Three knowledge, attitude, behaviour and practice (KABP) surveys have been carried out in Ireland to date, by Irish Marketing Surveys under the direction and scientific guidance of the Health Promotion Unit (HPU) at the Department of Health (DoH). The first was conducted in February 1987, prior to the national public education campaign which began in May 1987, with the dual aims of providing information which would guide the design and execution of the campaign and the form it should take, and providing baseline information on knowledge, attitudes and behaviour against which the effectiveness of the campaign could be measured. A post-campaign survey using the same protocol was carried out in September 1987, and a further survey was carried out two years later in September 1989.

At the time of writing, the HPU plans to carry out another KABP survey using comparable questionnaire design, although they hope to include questions on sexual behaviour for the first time. While evaluation is acknowledged to be vital to effective prevention campaigns, in practice lack of resources prevents evaluation from being built into the prevention strategy.

In 1992 an evaluation of the Convenience Advertising strategy was completed for the DoH. The use of and reactions to the HPU AIDS education resource materials were evaluated by the Educational Research Centre, St Patrick's College, Dublin in September 1992, on behalf of the HPU.

Country visit: Becky Field and Carol Morgan 1993

Report preparation: Becky Field and Kaye Wellings

Individuals and organizations contacted:

Shauneen Armstrong
Union of Students in Ireland, Dublin

Mags Gerhaghty
Dublin AIDS Alliance, Dublin

Irish Gay Alliance, Dublin

David Nowlan, *Irish Times*

Mick Quinlan
Gay Men's Health Project/AIDS Liaison Forum/National AIDS Strategy Committee, Dublin

Ruth Riddick (Development Consultant)
Irish Family Planning Association, Dublin

Dr Mary Scully
Eastern Health Board, Dublin

Noel Usher, Owen Metcalfe, Mary Jackson, Anna May Harkin
Health Promotion Unit, Department of Health, Dublin

Dr James H Walsh
Irish AIDS Coordinator, Department of Health, Dublin

Bibliography

Address by Mr Brendan Howlin TD, Minister for Health, at the launch of the New AIDS Media Campaign and on the occasion of the publication of the Health (Family Planning) (Amendment) Bill 1993, May 1993

AIDS education resource materials: survey of their use in post-primary schools 1993, M O Martin and A Mythen, Educational Research Centre, St Patrick's College, Dublin

AIDS surveillance in Europe, quarterly report no. 44 31 December 1994, European Centre for the Epidemiological Monitoring of AIDS

Irish women who seek abortions in England, 1992, Colin Francome, *Family Planning Perspectives* **24** (6); 265–8

National survey of public knowledge of, and attitudes to, AIDS 1989, A M Harkin, summary based on IMS tabular report, Health Promotion Unit/Irish Marketing Surveys

National survey on public knowledge of AIDS in Ireland, 1988, A M Harkin and M Hurley, *Health Education Research* **3** (1); 25–9

Public knowledge of, and attitudes to, AIDS in Ireland 1989 1989, A M Harkin, based on survey conducted by Irish Marketing Surveys for DoH 1989, Health Promotion Unit, Department of Health

ITALY

Context

Epidemiology

According to the European Centre for the Epidemiological Monitoring of AIDS, by 31 December 1994, the cumulative total of AIDS cases was 25,783, with an incidence rate (per million population) of 73.9 (n = 4,222). The cumulative total of AIDS cases by transmission group (percentages in parentheses) was as follows: homo/bisexual male 3,676 (14.5); injecting drug user (IDU) 16,565 (65.4); homo/bisexual IDU 566 (2.2); haemophiliac/coagulation disorder 224 (0.9); transfusion recipient 292 (1.2); heterosexual contact 2,822 (11.1); other/undetermined 1,184 (4.7).

The first AIDS case was registered in Italy in 1982. The Ministry of Health anticipates 4,500 new cases per year.

In December 1993, Italy had the third highest number of AIDS cases in Europe, after France and Spain. Italy has between 150,000 and 200,000 IDUs, with an estimated 50,000 to 60,000 of them (80 per cent males) HIV infected. HIV prevalence among IDUs in northern cities is high, for example, approximately 50–60 per cent in Milan and Genoa, but only around 5 per cent in Naples.

Social and political background

Although Italy is a Catholic country, for the past twenty years Catholic culture has not been the dominant influence on social behaviour, especially in urban areas and among young people. In southern and rural areas, though, the influence of the church remains strong. The Vatican does however influence political decisions and social policy via the Christian Democrat party, for example in its policy on condom promotion and the shape of school sex education.

In many respects the Italian family exerts more influence over actual behaviour than the church. Free sexual contact for young people, (especially for gay men) is difficult. Although homosexuality is legal, it remains covert and stigmatized; public demonstrations are rarely held. Fear of discovery is

Issue	Legislation	Date of legislation	Services provided
Homosexuality	Age of consent 14 (same as for heterosexuals). Legal, although 'public decency' law has been used against gays	1930 (penal code)	Yes
Abortion	Legal <90 days for social, socio-medico, socio-economic grounds, >90 days if eugenic, medical or sex crime grounds. Doctor's certificate required, minimum 7-day wait and counselling obligatory. <18s need parental consent	1978	Yes but limited
Drug use (non-medicinal)	Illegal. Possession for other than personal use punished	1993[1]	Yes
Prostitution	Legal to work as a prostitute. Soliciting and third-party involvement illegal	1958	Yes but limited
Contraception	Legal: public family planning clinics established	1975	Yes[2]
Contraception for those under age of sexual consent	Legal		Yes but limited[2]

[1]In 1990, prison sentences of not less than twenty years were introduced for drug trafficking. This was repealed in 1993. [2]Clinics and counselling are concentrated in north and central Italy.

great, and this inhibits people from being tested. There is some evidence of gay men travelling to other countries to be tested. AIDS has certainly increased the visibility of gay men. Gay organizations like FUORI and Arcigay pioneered AIDS information and have worked increasingly with the government.

Abortion was legalized in 1978 after heated debate. Two subsequent referendums have not succeeded in recriminalizing it.

In July 1990 a repressive drug law regarding punishment for possession of drugs for personal use was passed; heavy penalties and prison sentences of not less than twenty years for trafficking were introduced. Critics condemned it as an emotive reaction to AIDS. In 1992 the Minister of Social Affairs introduced a risk-reduction programme and a complete reversal of the former policy. In 1993 the law was repealed following a referendum proposed by the Radical Party. Critics suggest that the 1990 law did more than anything else to increase HIV transmission in Italy by effectively preventing the establishment of needle exchange schemes.

A law passed in 1990 (No. 135/90) provided for funding of HIV prevention and care of AIDS patients and explicitly states that 'HIV infection may in no way constitute a reason for discrimination, in particular concerning environment in schools, participation in sports, access and maintenance of employment.'

Health education

Conceived as a decentralized system, services remain heterogeneous. Before the first national AIDS campaign in 1988, there had been no national health education campaigns, although local campaigns, for example on smoking, had been mounted. A positive effect of AIDS campaigns has been the impetus for collaborative efforts between national and local levels. Social factors influencing disease are increasingly being considered. The reduction in syphilis and hepatitis A and B, since the AIDS campaigns, has also persuaded people of the potential effectiveness of health promotion.

Sex education

School sex education is not mandatory and provision of sex education is rare. Many teachers lack confidence in tackling sexual issues, and discussion of condoms is difficult. The Ministry of Education has to take the Catholic point of view into account.

In March 1992 the Ministries of Health and Education collaborated to produce joint guidelines for a school health education/HIV prevention programme. Prior to this, there had been little contact between the two.

The role of the media

Media coverage of AIDS was often alarmist in the four years prior to the first national campaign, the existing vacuum being filled by media misinformation. Epidemiologists also argue that the media attention given to possibilities of a cure or vaccine has generated false optimism and undermined AIDS public education campaigns, reducing the incentive for preventive action.

Since the inception of national campaigns, prominent TV personalities have been enlisted to include AIDS education material in their shows. Independent scientists, members of the National Committee and NGOs cooperate with the media to promote AIDS awareness.

AIDS/HIV public education

Aims and objectives

- To raise awareness of AIDS as a problem;
- to dispel unfounded fears;
- to provide accurate information about the means of transmission and methods of prevention;
- to focus permanent attention on the need for solidarity towards the infected.

Structure and organization

The Ministry of Health (MoH) is responsible for AIDS policy and public education campaigns. Changes in the administration over the last decade have militated against continuity.

The Commissione Nazionale per la Lotta Contro l'AIDS (National Commission for the Fight against AIDS) was established in 1987 – a year before the first national campaign began – to advise the Minister of Health, its president. The creation of this body at national level acknowledges that a national strategy was called for in a country where regionalism prevails. A consultative committee of the Commission allows formal consultation with NGOs.

The Istituto Superiore di Sanita (ISS), staffed by doctors, epidemiologists and psychologists, is part of the MoH, and provides technical assistance. The Centro Operativo AIDS (COA) is a subsection of the ISS specializing in AIDS and is responsible for surveillance and training. The Centro Informazione AIDS was established by the MoH in the course of the third and fourth national education campaigns (1991–93) in order to mail materials connected with the campaigns (leaflets, videos, books, stickers, kits, etc.). The COA houses the Telefono Verde – a free national AIDS helpline, staffed by doctors, psychologists and social workers – established by the MoH in 1987.

Although Italy lacks a strong tradition of NGOs, FUORI and Arcigay – the national gay organizations – were the first to attempt AIDS public education, before the government had recognized AIDS as a problem for Italy. LILA and other national associations providing services and support for people with AIDS/HIV have also been active in prevention, and were involved in the 1992–93 national campaign, although they have also been outspoken critics of government AIDS policy. Since 1985 ANLAIDS (Associazione Nazionale per la Lotta Contro l'AIDS) has disseminated information, leaflets and run training courses.

Development of campaigns

Arcigay began distributing condoms to gay men in 1985 and launched a low budget campaign. Soon their remit widened to include non-gay activities.

National government AIDS public education campaigns began in 1988. By the end of 1993 four had been conducted. Some regional health authorities had conducted their own campaigns earlier, but the slow response of many regions prompted

Campaign chronology

Date and agency	Campaign theme/title	Aims	Media	Main message/endline	Target groups	Tone and style
1988–89 MoH and AT[1]	First national campaign	Raise awareness, dispel unfounded fears	TV, posters, press ads, videos, brochure mailed to all families	AIDS. If you know it, you can avoid it. If you know it, it won't kill you.	General public, gays/bisexuals, IDUs, health professionals	Stark
1990–91 MoH and AT	Second national campaign	Sustain awareness, increase solidarity, draw attention to risk behaviours, reach specific sectors of population	TV, posters, press ads, leaflets	As above	General public, gays/bisexuals, IDUs, young people, travellers, women, armed forces, prisoners, health professionals	Near-silent black and white TV ads
1991–92 MoH and SCR[2]	Third national campaign	Create greater awareness, increase sense of personal responsibility and solidarity, focus on high risk population; promote testing for certain groups	TV, posters, press ads, leaflets, posters on buses and trains	As above	General public, gays/bisexuals, IDUs, young people, women, armed forces, prisoners, health professionals, blood donors	Informative, microstories, cartoons
1992–93 MoH and MoE, AT, SCR Publicis FCB-Mac	Fourth national campaign	Encourage school AIDS education, increase solidarity, sustain awareness, especially among target populations	TV, posters, leaflets, press and magazine ads, educational pack	As above	General public, gays/bisexuals, IDUs, young people, health professionals, sports people, workplace colleagues, immigrants, blood donors	Informational

[1]Armando Testa [2]SCR Associates

national action. Donat-Cattin's proposal for a national policy met some resistance from the regions, who were concerned about autonomy. Donat-Cattin insisted it was a national emergency, and although money was given to the regions, emphasis was placed on the national programme.

From 1988–91 Arcigay worked with central government and became members of the NGOs' consultative committee, the National Commission; Arcigay conducted specific campaigns for gay men, supervised by the Ministry of Health. Funding difficulties have hindered further interventions.

Following the allegations of corruption against former Minister of Health De Lorenzo, government AIDS campaign strategy appeared to have reached a standstill.

Tone and style

The campaigns have to some extent been evolutionary, attempting to sustain public awareness. Each has addressed different themes while using different techniques to achieve continuity: a yellow and blue colour scheme, the Commission logo and the same typography for the names of the National Commission and the Ministry of Health, the repetition throughout the different campaigns of the solidarity message and the endline, 'AIDS: if you know about it you can avoid it. If you know about it, it won't kill you.' Campaigns have tended to be concentrated in three or four months of the year.

A somewhat controversial aspect of the 1991–92 campaign was the comic book-style leaflet 'How I Cheat the Virus!' featuring the cartoon character *Lupo Alberto* (Albert Wolf) in an adaptation of a popular comic. The comic book was targeted at young people and the text used their argot. Its distribution was impeded by the Ministry of Education (MoE). The MoH noted that young people preferred this to other official leaflets because it was funny, which also made it popular with teachers. The MoH distributed it on request. Independent distribution was subsequently organized by some NGOs, and by young people themselves through discos and a music magazine. 1,375,559 copies were sent out between 1991–93 by the Centro Informazioni AIDS alone.

Messages

The letter sent by the Health Minister to each household on 1 December 1988 was criticized, especially for its judgemental line on condoms. The leaflet reads 'Anyone who says that contraception offers total safety is, according to all the experts, lying. Informed American opinion is that "the contraceptive is far from safe". We write: "It isn't completely safe". The condom today is the only barrier against dangerous sexual relations, but it's a limited barrier.' The letter urged normality in sexual relations and chastity for HIV positive people, and ended by castigating lack of solidarity, asserting that AIDS was not the plague.

First used in 1988, the endline 'AIDS: if you know about it, you can avoid it. If you know about it, it won't kill you' has been often repeated in subsequent campaigns. However some confusion over the wording (in Italian this can also mean 'If you know *him*, you can avoid *him*') led to criticism that the message was too oblique, and may have been

counterproductive to achieving solidarity.

The 1991–92 TV and radio spot aimed at young people gave the more didactic message 'Don't be afraid of saving your life. Say no to drugs, say no to AIDS.'

The second, third and fourth campaigns all attempted to encourage solidarity and anti-discrimination, with messages such as 'One of these people is seropositive. Their colleagues can rest easy' (1990–91); 'Those who aren't ill with AIDS are often ill with indifference', 'The desire to stop AIDS is contagious' (1991–92); and 'You can fight AIDS by word of mouth too' (1992–93).

Target groups

In addition to the general population, AIDS information campaigns have been directed towards homosexuals and bisexuals, health care professionals and pharmacists, military personnel, prisoners, women, travellers, blood donors, teachers and young people.

Other measures of prevention and control

HIV testing and surveillance

In 1990 the Ministry of Health established a surveillance system to gather demographic information and monitor HIV trends, offering free HIV testing – on a voluntary basis – to all who attended. Reporting of all positive test results, anonymously, to the regional surveillance system for HIV infection is mandatory only in some regions. The 1990 law (No. 135/90) explicitly forbids testing for HIV without consent.

National health service counselling and testing centres were established in 1985 in many regions by the regional health departments and offer confidential testing and counselling free of charge. Pre-test visits are required if the client has not been referred by their GP; prior to 1989 pre-test visits were required for all.

Needle exchange schemes

The concept of harm reduction has only recently been accepted. Needle exchange was hitherto equated with encouraging drug use. Critics argue that had an outreach harm-reduction programme with free condoms and a needle exchange scheme been established in 1987–88, lives could have been saved. Even now, there are few needle exchange schemes in Italy although syringes are freely available without prescription and at low cost. A number of vending machines (automatic exchanges or syringe distributors) have been recently placed in different sites in several cities.

Condoms

Condoms are available in chemists without prescription. There are few vending machines in public places. Opposition from the Catholic church has hindered national family planning campaigns. Condom advertising on private and public TV is permitted after 10 p.m. Condoms have featured in TV spots, but condom use has not been one of the primary messages of the campaigns, and the Ministry of Health has not felt able to advocate overtly condom use. Although AIDS has certainly increased discussion about condoms, they are not widely used. Condom use among IDUs is also low; it has proved easier to change drug-related behaviour (i.e. not sharing syringes) than sexual behaviour. Voluntary groups have failed to gain permission from the Ministry of Education to place condom vending machines in schools.

Between 1988 and 1991 1.5 million free condoms were distributed, purchased free or at cost price from a manufacturer thankful for free publicity.

Evaluation

The first campaign was evaluated before and after the campaign in July and November 1988, and another evaluation was conducted at the end of the third campaign. Since then, specific campaign evaluations have been commissioned from market research companies (Abacus, Telecontatto, Unicab) by the advertising agencies who conduct campaigns. More recently, the Ministry of Health directly commissioned a campaign evaluation.

Country visit: Anne Karpf 1994

Report preparation: Anne Karpf and Becky Field

Individuals and organizations contacted:

Dr Luigi Bertinato
Istituto Superiore di Sanita, Rome

Professor Gaetano Maria Fara
Istituto di Igiene, 'G Sanarelli', Universita di Roma 'La Sapienza', Rome

Dr Annarosa Frati
Ministry of Health, Rome

Professor Elio Guzzanti
National Commission for the Fight Against Aids

Dr Giuseppe Ippolito
Centro di Rifercimento AIDS,
Ospedale L Spallanzani, Rome

Gilberto Lucca
LILA, Milan

Maurizio De Martino
Arcigay, Bologna

Dr Carlo Perucci
Director, Osservatorio Epidemiologico Regionale, Rome

Dr Giovanni Rezza
Director, Centro Operativo AIDS, Istituto Superiore di Sanita, Ministry of Health, Rome

Enrica Rosa
Ministry of Health, Rome

Doriana Torriero
ANLAIDS, Rome

Bibliography

AIDS surveillance in Europe, quarterly report no. 44 31 December 1994, European Centre for the Epidemiological Monitoring of AIDS

Context of sexual behaviour in Europe, selected indices relating to demographic, social and cultural variables May 1993, Becky Field and Kaye Wellings, EC Concerted Action 'Sexual behaviour and the risk of HIV infection'

Informative campaigns for AIDS prevention from 1988 to 1992 1992, Ministry of Health, National Commission for the Fight Against AIDS

IV Campagna informativa per la prevenzione dell'AIDS 1992–1993 Ministry of Health, National Commission for the Fight Against AIDS

LUXEMBOURG

Context

Epidemiology

By 31 December 1994 the cumulative total of AIDS cases in Luxembourg was 90, with an incidence rate (per million population) of 32.4 (n = 13). The cumulative total of AIDS cases by transmission group (percentages in parentheses) was as follows: homo/bisexual males 46 (51.7); injecting drug users (IDUs) 16 (18.0); homo/bisexual IDUs 0; haemophiliacs/coagulation disorder 3 (3.4); transfusion recipients 3 (3.4); heterosexual contact 13 (14.6); other/undetermined 8 (9.0).

The first AIDS case was registered in Luxembourg in January 1985.

It is estimated that there are 400 HIV positive people, (including 55 who have died from AIDS) in a population of 400,000. Transmission via homosexual sex has been and remains the largest transmission group.

Social and political background

Luxembourg is a Catholic country, although in practice most people do not strictly adhere to the Catholic doctrine. The church exerts influence through the daily newspaper *Luxembourger Wort*, and via the governing Christian Democratic Party (which governs in coalition with the Social Democrats). The church was against the legalization of abortion in the 1970s.

Some doctors may conscientiously object to performing abortions and prescribing contraception to those under 18 without parental consent. Social and medical insurance does not cover the cost of oral contraceptives. Patients must pay towards the cost of medical care at the time of use; medical insurance is mandatory.

The gay community in Luxembourg is not formally organized; socially, homosexuality remains taboo. A dedicated 'support group', the Family Planning Association and the NGO AIDS-Berodung provide advice and support to gay men and lesbians. Legislation passed in 1994 prohibits HIV tests and discrimination of any kind for employment purposes.

Prostitution, which takes place in the railway station area, is tolerated in practice.

Legislation controlling drugs is among the toughest in Europe. If a user refuses to be medically examined, s/he can be sent to prison. Treatment is voluntary, although if refused it can be made mandatory. Sentences for possession (personal use) can be between one and five years, with the same for

Issue	Legislation	Date of legislation	Services provided
Homosexuality	Age of consent 16 (as for heterosexuals)[1]	1993	Limited
Abortion	Legal <12 weeks with certain indications (medical, foetal abnormality, rape, social)		Yes[2]
Drug use (non-medicinal)	Illegal. No distinction between hard and soft drugs		
Prostitution	Third-party involvement illegal, prostitution itself legal		
Contraception	Legal		Yes
Contraception for those under the age of consent	Legal		Yes but some doctors do not prescribe pill to <18s without parental consent

[1]Previously 18 for homosexuals and 15 for heterosexuals. [2]Catholic doctors can and do refuse to perform abortions.

dealing, although a previous conviction can mean a life sentence. A working group is currently debating the decriminalization of cannabis.

Health education

The Ministry of Health Division of Preventive and Social Medicine (DPSM) is responsible for health education. It runs campaigns promoting healthy lifestyles, prevention of cancer, smoking, alcohol and medication abuse, and vaccination campaigns. These campaigns combine outreach work, work in schools, printed materials – distributed to schools, health professionals, places of work and other relevant associations – and mass media information campaigns.

Sex education

In 1992 sex eduction became mandatory for 10- and 11-year-olds. For the past twenty years it has been mandatory for 13- and 19-year-olds. However, in practice it is often not taught, and where it is, it is generally included in the biology syllabus. Teachers are not specifically trained and feel uncomfortable with the subject. The lack of uniform provision of more general sex education makes it difficult to incorporate AIDS education into the school curriculum.

The role of the media

The media have been responsible in their presentation of AIDS – there has been little scaremongering or blaming. Interest in the AIDS issue has waned and it is often necessary to persuade the media to sustain coverage. Nevertheless a good relationship generally exists between radio and TV and those working in AIDS public education. The Catholic newspaper *Luxembourger Wort*, however, is reluctant to print references to condoms, sex outside marriage or homosexuality.

The DPSM is charged the same to air AIDS public education TV spots as commercial advertisers. At the time of writing it is currently trying to persuade the Minister of Health to institute at least a reduced rate for public health messages.

AIDS/HIV public education

Aims and objectives

The stated aims of the AIDS Surveillance Committee are to prevent the spread of the AIDS epidemic through voluntary measures and the responsibility of the individual; to reduce the personal and social consequences of infection; and to encourage an atmosphere of solidarity.

Structure and organization

Following the recommendation of the World Health Organization, the Director of Health recommended that a national AIDS committee be established. In January 1984, the AIDS Surveillance Committee was created, before the first AIDS case had been reported in Luxembourg. Formally an advisory body, the government and the Ministry of Health rely heavily on it for advice on AIDS issues. Originally made up of medical personnel, it soon became a multisectoral committee. The president is head of Infectious Diseases at the Central Hospital, and other members are director of health; head of the DPSM; head of the Health Inspectorate; director of the National Health Laboratory; a psychologist; a prison doctor; a lawyer; an educationalist (from the Jugend-an Drogenhëllef); director of the Red Cross transfusion centre; and a clinician. The Ministry of Health develops AIDS policy according to five-year plans. Between 1988–94 AIDS and drugs were both incorporated in one plan.

The DPSM is responsible for AIDS public education and conducts mass media campaigns aimed at the general population. Targeted and outreach prevention (non-mass media) are implemented by NGOs, notably AIDS-Berodung and Jugend-an Drogenhëllef, with whom the DPSM has formal agreements and partly funds. Close cooperation exists between the DPSM and the NGOs in regard to development and implementation of interventions. AIDS-Berodung runs various events to maintain AIDS awareness in the general population but its 2.5 paid staff are employed to do psychosocial work, and there is not enough money to pay staff specifically to do prevention work.

Since Luxembourg is a small country, coordination between the different AIDS NGOs, the AIDS Surveillance Committee and the DPSM works well.

Development of campaigns

The initial aim of the first national campaign (1987–89) was to provide information and raise awareness. It began with a leaflet drop of a fourteen-page booklet entitled *AIDS. What Everyone Should Know* to all households (150,000) in Luxembourg. In 1988 and 1989 leaflets about testing were distributed via large specific mailings.

In 1991 a new head was appointed to the DPSM; in 1993 a new three-year national campaign was launched. A leaflet entitled 'Me? AIDS?', with the aim of encouraging recognition of personal susceptibility, was distributed to all households. Billboard posters were produced for bus stops. TV and cinema spots also ran. Press advertisements, posters and leaflets featuring older people and a baby were produced to encourage solidarity.

There is no free AIDS telephone helpline. The AIDS-Berodung phone number is given on materials as the number from which to obtain advice and information.

The 1993 TV spots were developed by a commercial advertising agency.

In addition AIDS-Berodung runs campaigns and awareness events for World AIDS Day each year and at other times.

Tone and style

The 1993–94 posters and leaflets featured photographs of a young woman, an old couple, a baby and a gay couple. The text follows a 'testimonial' approach, where the characters featured talk about their lives, possible infection, safer sex and solidarity. The TV spot is sombre in tone, showing ink dripping into clear water. The cinema spot, in contrast, is more light-hearted: in a supermarket a young man woos a young woman with a heart of condoms, loud blues music plays and the couple happily run off into the distance together.

Campaign chronology

Date and agency	Campaign theme/title	Aims	Media	Main message/endline	Target groups	Tone and style
1987* 1988[†] 1989[‡] DPSM	First 3-year national campaign	Provide information, raise awareness and encourage condom use [‡]Inform about testing	*Leaflet drops to all households [†]Specific mailings, posters, press ads, conferences, TV, radio, cinema	*'AIDS. What everyone should know' [‡]'To be or not to be … there is only one answer: the AIDS test is anonymous, free of charge'	General public, young people	
1992 1993 1994 DPSM	Second 3-year national campaign	Increase information available, improve solidarity, correct condom use and increase recognition of personal risk	Leaflet drop (every household), posters, brochure, press ads, TV, radio, cinema	'AIDS? Me?' 'AIDS? Us?'	General public, young people, gays, IDUs	TV: sombre Cinema: positive

For 1 December 1994 a new leaflet in the same style as the 1993 materials (a photograph and the endline 'AIDS? Me?') was produced.

Messages

The 1987 booklet explained how the disease was and was not transmitted, and gave information about testing and symptoms. Reducing sex with strangers and partner change were mentioned before the regular and proper use of condoms.

The AIDS Surveillance Committee states that prevention messages must be based on science; that as it is scientifically proven that condoms protect against HIV, this must be clearly stated. Messages to people who are sexually active must be unambiguous; the choice is either non-penetrative sex, mutual monogamy or condom use. In practice this message has not been promoted as openly as some would like, because of fear of Catholic objections. Some feel this results in partial self-censorship by those producing AIDS public education materials. The emphasis placed on condoms in the 1987 campaign was criticized by the Catholic church. However, opposition to the condom message has since lessened, and there has been little adverse reaction to the 1993 campaign materials. In 1989 AIDS-Berodung produced a poster with a picture of a condom and received a shocked reaction.

Target groups

In addition to the general population, AIDS information campaigns have been directed towards IDUs, gay men, sex workers, young people and immigrants (all materials are produced in French and German and Luxembourgisch; with 25 per cent of the population foreign to Luxembourg, it is hoped that most people can read one of these languages).

Other measures of prevention and control

HIV testing and surveillance

HIV tests are confidential, free, and if desired, anonymous. The two laboratories involved give an accurate picture of HIV infection in Luxembourg; there are 300 positive test results recorded, and estimates are of 100 more. Testing is not regarded as a preventive strategy. There is no formal provision for pre- and post-test counselling, although the AIDS Surveillance Committee has produced a leaflet to be given to those having a test. Screening of blood and blood products began in July 1985. AIDS is a notifiable disease.

The issue of mandatory HIV testing continues to be raised from time to time, as in the 1994 elections, when the Christian Democrats included this in their manifesto, but has not been implemented.

Needle exchange schemes

Needle exchange schemes operate in Luxembourg. There are 24-hour automatic machines in Luxembourg City, Esch and Ettelbruch dispensing low cost syringes and needles. Syringes and needles are also selectively available from chemists without prescription, at a slightly higher price; there are some hospitals where needles can be exchanged.

Condoms

Condoms are easily available from chemists and supermarkets, although some think they are too expensive. They are sold at a subsidized price at the Family Planning Association and other outlets targetting young people. There has been no commercial advertising of condoms on TV. Condom machines have been installed in a few secondary schools.

Evaluation

There has been no systematic evaluation of campaigns and no part of the budget is allocated to evaluation.

Country visit: Becky Field 1994

Report preparation: Becky Field

Individuals and organizations contacted:

Dietmar Denzel
Jugend-an Drogenhëllef, Esch/Alzette

Dr Henri Goedertz
AIDS-Berodung Croix Rouge, Luxembourg

Dr Robert Hemmer
Chief of Infectious Diseases Department, Chairman of the AIDS Surveillance Committee, Central Hospital, Luxembourg

Claudiene Mardaga
Family Planning Association, Luxembourg
Dr Simone Steil
Médecine Chef de Division, Division de la Médecine Préventive et Sociale, Ministry of Health, Luxembourg

Bibliography

AIDS surveillance in Europe, quarterly report no. 44 31 December 1994, European Centre for the Epidemiological Monitoring of AIDS

Comité de Surveillance du SIDA Rapport d'activité 1993, Dr Robert Hemmer *et al.*

Context of sexual behaviour in Europe, selected indices relating to demographic, social and cultural variables May 1993, Becky Field and Kaye Wellings, EC Concerted Action 'Sexual behaviour and the risk of HIV infection'

Santé pour tous 1994, Ministry of Health, Luxembourg

Translation of documents: Lola Martinez

THE NETHERLANDS

Context

Epidemiology

According to the European Centre for the Epidemiological Monitoring of AIDS, by the 31 December 1994, the cumulative total of AIDS cases was 3,372, with an incidence rate (per million population) of 21.9 (n = 337). The cumulative total of AIDS cases, by transmission group (percentages in parentheses) was as follows: homo/bisexual male 2,507 (75.0); injecting drug user (IDU) 331 (9.9); homo/bisexual IDU 35 (1.0); haemophiliac/coagulation disorder 54 (1.6); transfusion recipient 36 (1.1); heterosexual contact 332 (9.9); other/undetermined 46 (1.4).

The first AIDS case was registered in the Netherlands in 1981.

Of patients found to have AIDS, approximately 50 per cent are resident in Amsterdam.

There are few data on which an accurate estimation of HIV prevalence in the Dutch population can be based since there is no central registration of seropositive individuals. Based on research, it is estimated that in 1991 there were between 9,000 and 12,000 people with HIV.

Social and political background

Human rights and liberties play a predominant part in Dutch society. The government has subscribed to international human rights conventions such as the Council of Europe's European Convention on the Protection of Human Rights and Fundamental Freedoms (1950). The principles of non-discrimination, the right to bodily integrity and the right to privacy are also enshrined in the Dutch constitution.

Dutch society is relatively harmonious. It has a long tradition of tolerance and acceptance of different political, ideological and religious positions. The influence of religion does not generally have negative consequences; where efforts are made fully to inform and involve representatives of religious groups, their cooperation can usually be depended

Issue	Legislation	Date of legislation	Services provided
Homosexuality	Age of consent 16* (same as for heterosexuals); discrimination on grounds of homosexuality forbidden and punishable by law;† civil marriage acknowledged by some local governments; legal contract can give partnership rights	*1971, †1983	Yes
Abortion	Legal when 'intolerable situation' defined jointly by woman and doctor <24 weeks; <18s need parental consent; compulsory 5-day waiting period; cost is reimbursed	1981, 1987	Yes
Drug use (non-medicinal)	Officially illegal, in practice tolerated; soft drugs legal for personal use	1976	Yes
Prostitution	Soliciting illegal, in practice prostitution and brothels tolerated	1854	Yes
Contraception	Legal, oral contraceptives on prescription		Yes
Contraception for those under age of sexual consent	There is no legislation concerning age; confidentiality is guaranteed. In practice, easily available (generally and for <16s)	1969 onwards	Yes

upon. Where there has been opposition to AIDS/HIV interventions (as in the case of AIDS educational materials for schools produced by the Dutch School TV, for example), it has generally been the result of an inadequate consultation process, which has since been redressed. The STD Foundation has subsequently produced two educational packages on AIDS/STDs with the blessing of both Catholics and Protestants. The National Committee for AIDS Control regards the churches as valuable intermediaries.

In the context of health care, individual human rights find expression in the principle of informed consent prior to any medical action, in the right to confidentiality in the doctor–patient relationship, and in the right to privacy and the protection of professional security.

In addition, there is a strong belief that society should be self-regulating without widespread recourse to legislative means of control. Laws tend to be enforced flexibly. Although prostitution and drug use are officially prohibited, in practice a 'blind eye' is turned; authorities are conscious of the need to avoid driving those at risk underground, where surveillance would be more difficult. Legislation to legalize brothels was debated in 1993 but not enacted. Homosexuality is legal and has for a long time been openly tolerated. Gay parades and other events are common in the Netherlands. Gay organizations contend that although homosexuality is now generally accepted at societal level, it is not always so at the personal level.

Health education

In the past two decades there have been public information campaigns relating to heart disease, contraception, dental health, smoking, abortion, road accidents, STDs, infant health, pregnancy, as well as to AIDS/HIV.

Two STD campaigns have previously been run in the Netherlands, so the AIDS campaign was by no means the first safe-sex campaign although it was the first to be directed towards *primary prevention*. The previous campaigns concentrated on familiarizing the public with the symptoms of STDs and advising medical attention if symptoms were suspected.

Sex education

It is mandatory for schools to cover the biological aspects of sex education. There is no legislation relating to wider aspects of sex education. There is, however, a 15- to 20-year tradition of sex education in schools in the Netherlands; a recent study showed that more than 85 per cent of all secondary schools have some kind of sex education. From August 1993 health education became a legislated part of both the biology and care curriculum for the first three years of secondary school (12- to 15-year-olds).

By prioritizing sex on the public agenda, AIDS may have contributed to the advancement of sex education; in 1987 the National Committee on AIDS Control gave the Dutch Centre for Health Promotion and Health Education responsibility for coordinating AIDS education policy in schools on a national and regional level, receiving funding from the Ministry of Health, Welfare, and Culture. Since 1988 projects have been directed towards the integration of sex and health education in schools.

The role of the media

From the beginning of the AIDS epidemic, the media have been supportive and informative in the Netherlands. There has been little hysterical reporting, misinformation or attempts to stimulate fear, as there was in Germany and the UK for example, nor any labelling of this disease as a 'gay plague'. As a result, AIDS educators have been able to make good use of the media. Their responsible behaviour is indicated by the fact that in 1987, before the Netherlands had ever had a general population education campaign, accurate knowledge relating to AIDS/HIV was already high.

Campaigns have had their message reinforced by the press, television and radio.

AIDS/HIV public education

Aims and objectives

The general aims of prevention policy are to prevent the further spread of HIV (to inform the general public about AIDS/HIV, how HIV can and cannot be transmitted, and on how infection can be avoided; and to limit undesirable social consequences of the AIDS epidemic on society and individuals). Recently more attention has been given to the information programme for people with HIV and AIDS.

Dutch AIDS public education has been characterized by an emphasis on freedom of choice backed up by good information. The approach has been pragmatic rather than moralistic, aiming for what is feasible and achievable, in the belief that the most effective approach will be one which stimulates lifestyle adaptations rather than drastic changes, taking reality as a starting point. It has been explicitly stated that the campaigns should aim to adopt a positive, supportive approach to sexuality, avoid coercive measures, prevent stigmatization of certain groups and avoid fear.

Structure and organization

Officially, the Ministry of Health, Welfare and Culture (MHWC) is responsible for AIDS policy. The National Committee on AIDS Control (NCAC), established in October 1987 to coordinate and advise on AIDS prevention activities, plays the central advisory role. There are three main sections of the NCAC's work: prevention and public education; care and treatment; ethical and legal issues. The sub-committee for HIV prevention (NCACEP) deals with prevention of all kinds, both targeted and general population. Its function is to advise and coordinate the different interests in prevention programmes.

The AIDS Fund is an NGO which raises funds privately and is responsible for distributing government funds to other NGOs, but does not actually run public education campaigns itself.

NGOs involved include the STD Foundation, the Rutgers Foundation (contraception), organizations providing services for prostitutes (Red Thread, De Graaf Foundation), gay men (coordinated by the SFD Schorer Foundation), drug users (Junky League and National Institute on Alcohol and Drugs), etc.

The advantages of this structure – the expertise of NGOs being coordinated by the NCAC, which is loosely attached to government – are seen by the NCAC as threefold. Firstly, the AIDS problem is seen to be on the political agenda, but at the same time remains unpoliticized. Secondly, campaigns can be properly synchronized so that they are not competing for public attention at the same time. Thirdly, there was no necessity to set up a new organization, with the inevitable attendant difficulties and disruption; only a coordinating body with a networking function was needed, so that existing skills and experience could be directly harnessed to the problem. The MHWC, for example, funded the STDF (between 1987–91) to conduct safer-sex campaigns, thereby relieving the government-linked NCAC of the need to be associated with more controversial national advertising. In 1991 the NCAC and the STDF combined to form a working group for all mass media campaigns. A hotline, set up in 1985, is now coordinated and funded by the NCAC.

Development of campaigns

From the start, campaigns have been guided by the idea that efforts to inform are most effective when developed and carried out in close cooperation with representative bodies and individuals from affected groups. Thus campaigns have been devolved from the centre; hardly any prevention activities are carried out directly by the NCAC. AIDS intervention activities were already at an advanced stage when the NCAC was set up, previously having been developed and executed in specialist NGO groups. In 1982, under the auspices of the Amsterdam Municipal Health Service, a small group of gay men and haemophiliacs formed the basis of what was to become Dutch prevention policy: information and prevention of discrimination. Coordination of spe-

Campaign chronology

Date and agency	Campaign theme/title	Aims	Media	Main message/endline	Target groups	Tone and style
April 1987 NCAC	First information campaign	Increase knowledge about transmission and prevention of HIV	TV, press, brochures, billboards	'Please inform yourselves. Stop AIDS'	General public	Gentle and informational (bees and flowers)
October 1987 STDF	Condom campaign	Change attitudes towards condoms	Press, posters	Use condoms	Young people, general public	Humorous
Spring 1988 NCAC	AIDS and the workplace	Relieve anxiety, promote necessary prevention at work	TV, press, leaflets	'AIDS, take blood bloody seriously. Stop AIDS'	Health care and other workers at possible risk	Informational
Summer 1988 STDF	Safe sex on holiday	Protect young travellers from HIV	Multi-media (no TV)	Practise safe sex on holiday	Young people 15–25	Romantic
October–December 1988 NCAC	AIDS and youth	Stimulate sex/HIV education programmes	TV, press, brochures	'AIDS education at school, not easy, but necessary. Stop AIDS'	Teachers, parents, governors, children, social workers	Pragmatic
June–September 1989 May 1990 STDF	Excuses campaign	Remove barriers to action	Posters, brochure, press, cinema, radio	Adopt safe-sex practices	Young people 18–25	Emotive
October 1989–October 1990 NCAC	Second information campaign	Maintain public involvement with AIDS issues	TV, radio, local and national press, brochures	'Think twice. Stop AIDS'	General public and high risk groups	Awe-inspiring (candles)
1990–92 NCAC	Solidarity campaign	Encourage solidarity/compassion for people with AIDS/HIV	TV, radio, billboards	'A little bit of understanding never gave anybody AIDS'	General public	Gentle and story-like
1991–92 STDF	Cupido campaign	Promote safe sex	Posters, brochures. Focus on discos – no mass media	'Think about it, play safe'	Young people, general public	Humorous (cartoon)
February–June 1993 MHWC Working Group	Safe-sex campaign	Promote safe sex	TV, posters, brochures, press, billboards, cinema	'I have safe sex or nothing'	Young people, general public (including gay men and ethnic minorities)	Soft and romantic

cific interest groups from the centre continues to form the framework of Dutch prevention policy. Government money is provided for projects and the NCAC advises the government on how it should be allocated. Thus campaigns have always been primarily directed towards special target groups. The pre-existing structure of NGOs, with expertise in particular areas and with specific groups, were responsible for all preventive activities between 1983 and 1987. For the general public, information was available on request, but was not actively promoted.

In the early years a nationwide campaign was

deliberately avoided for fear of generating an emotional response to AIDS and because there was felt to be insufficient need. The public were already receiving the requisite information, partly because of the good cooperation between the press and the authorities, so that there was no need to correct disinformation, and partly because the STD Foundation (STDF) had already mounted information initiatives on safer sex. At the time, it seemed that the epidemiological data also supported such a strategy. As a result, a series of planned and targeted national initiatives were implemented focusing on particular groups thought to be at risk from, or practising, behaviours thought to be implicated in the spread of HIV – a 'step-by-step' approach. Only in 1987 did the government mount a nationwide mass media campaign directed at the general population.

Between 1987 and 1991 the mass media were used for two separate campaigns: the Safe-sex campaign for young people, run by the STDF, and the National information campaign (knowledge of HIV and solidarity), run by the sub-committee for HIV prevention, in close collaboration with the MHWC.

In 1991 the dual campaign strategy of the sub-committee for HIV prevention and the STDF was combined into one working group responsible for safer-sex, solidarity and general information campaigns, for reasons of economy and efficiency. The working group is responsible to the MHWC and consists of representatives from the NCAC, the MHWC, the STDF, the Dutch Information Service and the AIDS Fund, and has considerable autonomy.

Tone and style

An important principle from the campaign's inception has been the need to avoid frightening people. The tone has therefore been life rather than death orientated. The campaign has been deliberately positive and pragmatic in tone about sexuality. In the safer-sex campaigns of the STDF, humour was used to lighten the initiatives with all groups except the youngest, who were found in research to prefer a more romantic approach. Informational initiatives have been soft and down to earth, rather than didactic and hard-hitting.

Messages

The starting point of messages relating to the Dutch campaign was that people should take responsibility for themselves. The message is generally that sex is pleasurable but has some adverse side effects which can be avoided by practising safer sex by using condoms. AIDS prevention messages are now being integrated into other sexual health issues.

Target groups

In addition to the general population, AIDS information campaigns have been directed towards men with homosexual contacts, IDUs, sex workers (female, male, migrant and drug users) and their clients, young people (over 12) and young travellers, women, workers and immigrants. Information for immigrants has been further specifically directed to males and females, and refugees; for the 64 nationalities resident in Amsterdam, an own-language education programme is available in which people from Surinam, Turkey and Morocco are trained to train people of their own language group.

Other measures of control and prevention

HIV testing and surveillance

AIDS is not a notifiable disease within the framework of the Communicable Diseases Act of 1928; patients with AIDS are reported anonymously and voluntarily to the Medical Officer of Health for Infectious Diseases. Mandatory testing has not been introduced, nor has anonymous testing for purposes of surveillance. The belief is that testing can play only a minor part in prevention. The only justification for AIDS testing is as a protection for third parties.

The Communicable Diseases Act of 1928 makes possible compulsory notification of certain diseases and temporary quarantine of persons infected, but HIV is *not* classified as a notifiable disease. In Amsterdam there is cooperation between the municipal health service and the hospitals; an AIDS diagnosis is reported anonymously to the Amsterdam AIDS Coordination Centre.

All blood donated has been tested for the presence of antibodies to HIV since 1985, as has routine screening of sperm, tissue and donated organs. Anonymous voluntary HIV testing with counselling is easily accessible to those who want it.

Needle exchange schemes

Some needle exchange schemes existed in the Netherlands before the onset of AIDS as a way of combating the hepatitis B problem. Since AIDS/HIV, a supervised system of distributing sterile syringes and needles to drug users has been well established. This is in line with the Dutch policy of pragmatism.

Needle exchange schemes for AIDS/HIV began in summer 1984. There are currently projects in 40 municipalities of the Netherlands, funded by the MHWC. The highly favourable evaluation of the early Amsterdam project helped pave the way for later initiatives, though introduction of the schemes has not been without controversy; critics claim that it encourages drug use and discourages people from giving up the habit. Now the schemes are generally very much accepted, needle distribution is being further developed, as exchange is regarded as only one form of prevention. Various schemes involve chemists and local organizations which can make a contribution to needle distribution.

The number of IDUs who are HIV positive in Amsterdam is high (30 per cent). Numbers in other cities and rural areas are small (0.1–3 per cent).

Condoms

Condom advertising on television is permitted, though in practice they have been mentioned but not advertised. The London Rubber Company (which produces Durex condoms) has a monopoly of about 95 per cent of the market, and so does not advertise on TV. The number of vending machines for condoms is reported to have doubled in recent years.

In April 1987 the University of Utrecht knowledge, attitudes, behaviour and practice (KABP) study found that 11 per cent of respondents claimed always to use a condom; 9 per cent claimed sometimes to use a condom; 23 per cent expressed an intention to use condoms in the future. By May 1992, figures had increased to 13, 23 and 41 per cent respectively, indicating reported condom use has increased but that behaviour still falls short of intention.

About 25 million condoms are sold each year, which is low compared to other countries. This may be due to the high proportion of women who use the pill. After the first condom campaign in 1987, condom sales increased by approximately 20 per cent but now remain stable, increasing maybe 2 per cent each year.

Evaluation

Between 1987 and 1991, the STDF established a research programme aimed at informing their campaigns, for example, to investigate the perceived advantages and disadvantages of condom use. Pre- and post-testing was carried out by the University of Utrecht, with whom the STDF has close contact. In 1986–87 two evaluative studies to monitor the effects of AIDS public education began. One is a KABP-style survey funded by the MHWC and run by the University of Utrecht, relating to safe-sex practices, including condom use and STDs. The second is more general, relating to AIDS/HIV knowledge and attitudes, run by the Dutch Information Service (a government research agency). Both help to inform the development of new campaigns. Both surveys take place once a year, with samples of around 1,000. In addition, smaller surveys take place every three months regarding 'involvement' (defined as knowledge, interest, emotional/affectional feelings and practices) of the general public with AIDS. The University of Utrecht study is currently facing financial problems; the government has been advised by the Scientific Research Council to discontinue funding for the survey, given financial constraints on scientific and financial grounds – though this is not the view of the NCAC. KABP surveys by commercial agencies have also been conducted for the NCAC.

Country visit: Dominic McVey (Health Education Authority, London), Becky Field and Carol Morgan, 1991 and 1993

Report preparation: Kaye Wellings and Becky Field

Individuals and organizations contacted:

Professor Roel Coutinho
Municipal Health Service, Amsterdam

Lilian Kolker, Katinka Vries, Maria Paalman
STD Foundation, Utrecht

Dr Cees van der Meer
AIDS Coordination Amsterdam, Amsterdam

Jo Reinders
School Health Unit, Dutch Centre for Health Education and Health Promotion, Utrecht

Rutgers Stichting
The Hague

Theo Sandfort
University of Utrecht

Cees Van Eijk, Dr Carla van der Wijden,
Dr Fred J Lijdsman
National Committee on AIDS Control, Amsterdam

Gertjan van Zessen
Programme Leader AIDS Research, NISSO, Utrecht

Bibliography

AIDS information and education in the Netherlands HIV prevention policy 1983–1992, summary of the national programme 1993 1993, National Committee on AIDS Control

AIDS Policy in the Netherlands 1988, Ministry of Health, Welfare and Cultural Affairs

AIDS policy in the Netherlands 1992, factsheet (V-3-E), Ministry of Health, Welfare and Cultural Affairs

AIDS policy in the Netherlands 1992, progress report, Ministry of Health, Welfare and Cultural Affairs

AIDS surveillance in Europe, quarterly report no. 44 31 December 1994, European Centre for the Epidemiological Monitoring of AIDS

AIDS Werkplan Voorlichting en Preventie: 1990 en verder 1989, National Committee on AIDS Control

AIDS Werkplan Voorlichting en Preventie: 1994–1995 1993, National Committee on AIDS Control

The Dutch approach to AIDS 1992, City of Amsterdam

Education and contraceptive provision in the Netherlands: lessons to be learned? 1993, Adrianne Earnshaw (funded by NBS)

The effectiveness of the 1989 multi-media safe sex campaign in the Netherlands, 1989, Katinka de Vries *et al.*, paper presented at the First European Conference on Effectiveness of Health Education, Rotterdam

Mass media campaigns, the Netherlands 1987–1992 1992, Cees van Eijk, staff member education and prevention, National Committee on AIDS Control

Safe sex and condom use in the general population. Results of 11 time-points April 1987–May 1992 1992, Dr A A M Dingelstad, Dr E M M de Vroome and Dr T G M Sandfort, University of Utrecht

Translation of documents: Greet Peersman

NORWAY

Context

Epidemiology

According to the European Centre for the Epidemiological Monitoring of AIDS, by 31 December 1994, the cumulative total of AIDS cases in Norway was 442, with an incidence rate (per million population) of 15.7 (n = 68). The cumulative total of AIDS cases, by transmission group (percentages in parentheses) was as follows: homo/bisexual male 258 (59.3); injecting drug user (IDU) 68 (15.6); homo/bisexual IDU 6 (1.4); haemophiliac/coagulation disorder 7 (1.6); transfusion recipient 15 (3.4); heterosexual contact 70 (16.1); other/undetermined 11 (2.5).

The first AIDS case was registered in Norway in January 1983. Later, it was established that three persons in a single family had died of AIDS in 1976. These are among the earliest documented cases of AIDS in Europe. In December 1993 the registered number of HIV-infected persons was 1,337; the cumulative total of reported HIV positive persons was between 1,500 and 2,000.

Social and political background

Norway finds itself somewhere between Sweden and Denmark with regard to the liberality of the social and moral climate. As one of the first countries to pass a law (1981/82) criminalizing discrimination on sexual grounds, it has provided an environment in which an excellent relationship exists between gay associations and health agencies.

The influence of the church is generally stronger at municipal than at the national level, although this varies across the country. Periodically the church together with some Christian Democrats in Parliament have opposed openness relating to sexuality and acceptance of homosexuality. There has also been occasional government pressure to amend STD legislation to be harsher.

In general, however, AIDS prevention campaigns have been conducted unimpeded by political or moral pressure. Despite the influence of the church, Parliament has taken a pragmatic as opposed to a moralistic stance, and generally deferred to the professional authority of the Directorate of Health.

Anti-discrimination legislation protects HIV positive persons, especially in terms of housing and

Issue	Legislation	Date of legislation	Services provided
Homosexuality	Age of consent 16 (same as for heterosexuals).* Anti-discrimination law concerning religion, cultural background, sexual orientation, etc.† Partnership recognition‡	*1972, †1981/82, ‡1993	Yes
Abortion	Legal and free of charge <12 weeks on request; >3 months for medical, eugenic, sex crime grounds. Two doctors must be consulted	1975, 1978	Yes
Drug use (non-medicinal)	Illegal		Yes
Prostitution	Prostitution not a criminal offence 'but illegal to "encourage"' (brothels, pimping, advertising, clubs)		Yes (mainly in Oslo)
Contraception	Legal. Oral contraceptives on prescription from pharmacies; there are no regulations about others		Yes
Contraception for those under age of sexual consent	Legal		Yes

employment. The dismissal of a bartender because of his HIV status was established by the Supreme Court to be incompatible with Norwegian law. Efforts to ensure HIV positive persons their legal rights are founded on rules applying to society in general, rather than because of statutory rights for HIV positives as a group, since defining HIV positives as a special group is seen as potentially reinforcing negative attitudes.

HIV is included in the list of dangerous communicable and easily transmitted diseases such as tuberculosis and cholera. The existing legislation provides general regulations about intervention in epidemics, for example contact tracing and quarantine. It is generally accepted that a person entering Norway with active cholera who refuses to be quarantined can be obliged by law to be so. HIV-infected people and those working with them are concerned that this law could result in more restrictive practices for people with HIV than to date, and fear that some forces in Parliament may attempt to create a separate law for HIV. The Directorate of Health and the Ministry of Health and Social Affairs see this as unlikely, and have made clear their commitment to continue dealing with the epidemic through consent and collaboration.

Health education

At state level responsibility for health education rests with the Directorate of Health, at community level with the municipal and local authorities' offices, while services are administered at county and local level. NGOs work closely with the official authorities. Health education campaigns are popular in Norway: in the past twenty years there have been public education campaigns about heart disease, contraception, dental health, smoking, abortion, road accidents, STDs, infant health and pregnancy.

Sex education

Sex education is formally integrated into the curriculum in upper primary school (13- to 16-year-olds). Officially AIDS education is included in sex education classes, but quality of provision varies with the teacher. Only a small group within the church are opposed to this.

The role of the media

The Norwegian press has not been above occasional sensationalist treatment of sexual issues in order to sell papers, and AIDS has been no exception. In 1982–83 the disease was described as a gay plague; in 1984–85 similarly sensationalist headlines described the epidemic among IDUs. In general, however, the media have made a positive contribution to AIDS education. The national tabloids are read more for titillation, but Norway is characterized by a proliferation of local newspapers to which people turn for reliable information and in which there has been a more sober treatment of the issues.

AIDS/HIV public education

Aims and objectives

The government's action plan to counter the AIDS epidemic focuses on measures which will help to chart the distribution and current spread of infection. The objective, as stated in 1989, was to promote changes in behaviour and attitudes by teaching each individual to protect him/herself and others against infection by avoiding risk behaviour and risk situations, and to adopt a rational attitude towards risk groups and persons with AIDS/HIV in order to prevent stigmatization and segregation.

In 1990 the Ministry of Health declared two further goals for AIDS prevention work, in addition to the above: to prevent discrimination and marginalization of people with AIDS/HIV and persons at risk, and to increase the competence of health workers and social workers.

Structure and organization

To a large extent the structure and organization for AIDS prevention was already in existence in Norway, and needed only some modification to carry out the work. Close cooperation exists between NGOs and the Directorate of Health.

Until January 1994 the Directorate of Health was the professional coordinating body for AIDS prevention policy, at central level. It was accountable to the Ministry of Health and Social Affairs, but had considerable autonomy, authority and self-regulation in the field of health promotion/disease prevention.

From January 1994 the Directorate of Health became the Norwegian Board of Health. Funded by the national government, it retains responsibility for implementation of the AIDS/HIV National Action Plan and for AIDS policy, funding, information campaigns, targeted activities and monitoring. It reports to and gives technical advice to the Ministry of Health and Social Affairs, as do other national health bodies. This has led to the Ministry taking a more active coordinating role and placing responsibility for implementation with appropriate agencies.

A professional advisory group was appointed jointly by the Ministry of Health and Social Affairs and the Directorate of Health to ensure access to experience from different disciplines and social environments and as a forum for discussion of new measures against the epidemic. In the mid-1980s the Minister for Health and Social Affairs also appointed her own national advisory council with broad political as well as professional membership. This committee was active in laying the foundations for what has since been a collaborative effort. For clinical advice on preventive measures, the Directorate of Health consults the Director General of Health Services' advisory committee on infectious disease control, the National Institute of Public Health and the WHO. In 1987 the AIDS Information and Awareness Centre was established at the National Institute of Public Health as a documentation and information centre for AIDS public education.

Norway's chief county medical officers plan, initiate and coordinate county-specific preventive measures; at a local level these functions are taken care of by the chief municipal medical officer. Centrally, the Ministry of Justice is responsible for the efforts of the police and prison service, the Ministry of Church and Education for those in schools, and the Ministry for Cultural and Scientific Affairs for disseminating information to youth groups. Other important collaborating partners include the Gay Health Committee, the Norwegian AIDS Association and PLUSS, the organization for people with HIV and AIDS.

Development of campaigns

In 1983, following the first report of an AIDS case in Norway, the Gay Health Committee wrote to all members of gay organizations and asked them to stop donating blood. The Directorate of Health circulated all hospitals with AIDS information, and all blood banks were advised to distribute written information to potential donors. This prompt response was largely the result of close and easy collaboration between health authorities and the Gay Health Committee, such that the extensive and active efforts of the latter could be utilized and harnessed without disharmony.

Another key factor explaining the ease with which the Norwegian programme began was the role played by key personnel; strategies depended very much on the people who mobilized support in the gay community and among medical staff. As a measure of their effectiveness the budget allocated to the Gay Health Committee increased from NKr35,000 in 1984, to NKr625,000 in 1986 and to NKr1,900,000 in 1987. By 1985, when the Directorate of Health appointed the first official with special responsibility for AIDS prevention (Sven Erik Ekeid), a firm foundation had already been laid for the cooperation that has marked the combat of the epidemic. When the Gay Health Committee travelled to the USA to learn from 'Gay Men's Health Crisis', Ekeid accompanied the group, and this tour became the starting point of his efforts. Thus the early framework was built on two extremely important supportive planks: a pre-existing and established close collaboration between the gay organizations and the Directorate of Health, characterized by an unusually high level of mutual trust.

Campaign chronology

Date and agency	Campaign theme/title	Aims	Media	Main message/endline	Target groups	Tone and style
1985 DoH[1]	First AIDS/HIV public health education film strip	Raise awareness	Video, TV	Focus on condoms	General public	Informative, serious
1986 DoH	First national campaign	Encourage condom use	TV, billboards, press, posters (still used), face-to-face communication	'AIDS is transmitted by sexual contact – use a condom!'	General public	Light, humorous, non-didactic
1987 DoH	Second national campaign	Encourage condom use	National press ads	'Use a condom if you have sex'	Young people, gay men, travellers, prostitutes and clients, adult couples	
1987 MoCE[2] MoH[3]	Schools information campaign	Provide facts about AIDS	Leaflets, face-to-face communication	Information and guidelines for protection	Teachers, pupils (13–18s)	Frank, open
1988 DoH	Travellers' campaign	Provide risk-reduction guidelines	Posters, TV, music cassettes	Interrail as common theme	Travellers, young people	Light, humorous
1988 NAA[4]	Anti-discrimination campaign	Promote anti-discriminatory attitudes to those affected	Posters	'Human care is not contagious'	General public	Empathetic, emotional, sentimental
1989 and 1991 DoH	Third national campaign	Encourage responsibility	Posters on trains and trams	'Take AIDS seriously!'	General public, gay men, IDUs	B/w photos, light
1989 DoH	Testing campaign	Encourage testing	Posters		Those at risk	
1990–91 DoH	Fourth national campaign	Encourage responsible sex	Posters, national press	Safer sex	General public, gay men, adult couples	Stark, simple
1992 DoH		Provide accurate information	Brochure distributed to clinics, doctors' surgeries, pharmacies		General public, health workers	Informative
1992–93 DoH	Fifth national campaign	Encourage condom use	Posters	'Be the first to say it. Condoms protect you against HIV infection'; 'Let's talk about it. Man to Man'; 'Do more than 10 people really have to be HIV-infected each month? You know how to avoid it'; 'Do you think that the pill protects you against HIV and other STDs? The condom is the only contraceptive which gives you such protection'	General public, gay men, adult couples	Erotic, stylish

[1]Directorate of Health [2]Ministry of Church and Education [3]Ministry of Health [4]Norwegian AIDS Association

In 1986 Norway had no commercial television stations, Norwegian public service television being state-run, licence-funded and non-commercial. It shows public information spots (messages from the government, fire hazards, Red Cross, etc.) without charge as part of their public duty, and thus showed the first AIDS prevention spots.

Tone and style

The Directorate of Health has taken the view that it is acceptable to use emotions to raise awareness. From the campaign's inception, no one believed in the use of fear to initiate appropriate behaviour. Instead, the emotive use of humour has permeated the advertisements. For health education personnel this was already regarded as established knowledge in 1985, having worked on drug use issues. Advertisements have been relatively low key, no attempt has been made to compete with glossy, slick advertising in magazines.

Messages

A clear philosophy in relation to the messages of the Norwegian campaign was stated in the official booklet, *AIDS prevention in Norway* (May 1989); when choosing illustrations and text, the Directorate of Health has tried to ensure that the message is specific and unambiguous, that it does not lead to increased discrimination of individuals or groups and that the message does not cause anxiety, over and above the objective and factual information that exists about the disease.

The most important single message, and the earliest to be featured has been 'use a condom'. Reduction of the number of sexual partners has been a subsidiary message. In 1989, for the first time, testing was promoted as a campaign message.

The aim of messages has been to tell people what action to take themselves; emphasis has not been 'don't transmit to others' but 'don't become infected yourself'. An important principle has been to show what people *can* do, avoiding where possible negative instructions, the tone being one of guidance rather than imperatives. The rationale for all messages was that the smaller the modification required, the more easily the goal would be achieved.

Drug users and gay men are regarded as part of the general public and so it has been seen as important to include messages to them as part of public campaigns.

Early attempts were made to prevent stigmatization of infected persons by explaining clearly the ways in which HIV could not be transmitted. Later, in 1988, these efforts were strengthened in an anti-discrimination campaign with solidarity as the main theme run by the Norwegian AIDS Association (an NGO).

Target groups

In addition to the campaigns, AIDS information campaigns have been directed towards gay men, sex workers, drug users, travellers (business and holiday), young people, teachers, social workers and health care professionals.

Other measures of prevention and control

HIV testing and surveillance

All testing in Norway takes place on a voluntary basis, with informed consent. The national surveillance system is based on various schemes. Some of these are intended to reach persons at special risk, men with homosexual experience for example; others are aimed at segments of the general population, e.g. pregnant women. Tests are also available on a bus used to distribute clean needles and syringes, as well as in STD clinics and special AIDS/HIV centres. HIV patients are registered anonymously. Details of the patient's risk factor, age, etc. are recorded. Norway is one of the few countries in the world which registers HIV as well as AIDS cases. There is a higher test rate for Norway than for most other countries. Consequently epidemiological surveillance data are of high validity and reliability.

All pregnant women are offered an HIV test as

part of the general antenatal screening programme. In addition, the test is offered to first-time military recruits, immigrants and those receiving a hepatitis B vaccine.

A system in place before the AIDS/HIV epidemic provides for contact tracing to be carried out. Existing legislation provides for coercive measures to be used to detain people with HIV who do not act responsibly, although this has been used in only one instance to date.

Needle exchange schemes

There are approximately 6,000 IDUs in Norway, mostly in the Oslo area. Of drug users, 80–90 per cent have taken an HIV test, 50 per cent more than once. A full and comprehensive programme of HIV preventive work has been developed in relation to drug use. Large scale residential facilities are available for treatment and rehabilitation, street visits have been set up to provide field work support, and health care personnel have been regularly informed on different aspects of AIDS/HIV. Information (brochures and leaflets) developed for IDUs deal with safer sex, syringe sharing, disinfection and disposal of syringes and needles. In two towns needle exchange schemes have been established. Vending machines for the sale of needles have been installed in a number of towns, the first one in 1988. Needles and syringes are sold in pharmacies, and are also an unrestricted commodity, and as such may be sold by anyone.

Methadone treatment is not widely used.

Condoms

Condoms, though expensive, are widely available in Norway, in petrol stations, supermarkets, etc. RFSU, the largest condom importer in Norway, has been influential in increasing availability. A diploma signed by the Directorate of Health is offered for display to every shop selling condoms.

In 1994 the Board of Health subsidized the distribution of condoms in night clubs, bars, youth clubs and places where sex is thought about or planned. The Gay Health Committee distributes condoms in parks, discos, bars and cruising areas; people who work with IDUs distribute condoms all the time. According to figures from the Board of Health condom sales decreased in 1993.

Evaluation

Little systematic evaluation took place at the early stage of the campaign. Knowledge, attitude and behaviour surveys are carried out by the National Institute of Public Health. Although these surveys are not intended specifically to evaluate campaigns, efforts have been made to interpret results in the light of future interventions.

The first overall evaluation of the Directorate of Health's HIV prevention activities from 1985 has been undertaken and was to begin in 1994. The Board of Health has assigned this evaluation to the Norwegian Research Council and is the main source of funding. There are three parts to this evaluation: further analysis of all of the quantitative survey data, e.g. researching persistent misconceptions about transmission; examining the Board's own choices relating to resourcing – the level, distribution and responsibilities; and a qualitative study of practices and attitudes among female sex workers, IDUs and men who have sex with men. The respondents are asked to comment on campaigns which have targeted them specifically or the general population. The aim is to identify changes by comparing earlier studies of these populations, thus identifying areas of need for further preventive efforts.

Country visit: Kaye Wellings and Carol Morgan, 1991 and 1994

Report preparation: Kaye Wellings and Becky Field

Individuals and organizations contacted:

Sjur Hansen
Norwegian Gay and Lesbian Organization, Oslo

Odd Johannsen, Dr Pål Kraft, Hilde Pape, Dr

Bente Traeen
National Institute of Public Health, Oslo

Jo Kittelsen
Head of Section, National Board of Health, Oslo
Dr J Kristofferson, Dr Sven Erik Eiked, Anna Lise
Middlethon
AIDS Directorate of Health, Oslo

Dr Annick Prieur
Research Fellow, Department of Sociology, Faculty
of Social Sciences, University of Oslo, Oslo

Kari Rvang
Norsk Forening for Familieplanlegging (Family
Planning Association), Oslo

Per Kristian Svendsen
AIDS-Informatsjonsenheten (AIDS Information
and Awareness Centre), Oslo

Bibliography

AIDS Prevention in Norway May 1989, Ministry of
Health, Directorate of Health, National Institute
of Health
AIDS surveillance in Europe, quarterly report no. 44 31
December 1994, European Centre for the
Epidemiological Monitoring of AIDS

PORTUGAL

Context

Epidemiology

According to the European Centre for the Epidemiological Monitoring of AIDS, by 31 December 1994, the cumulative total of AIDS cases was 2,221, with an incidence rate (per million population) of 36.8 (n = 362). The cumulative total of AIDS cases, by transmission group (percentages in parentheses) was as follows: homo/bisexual male 707 (32.5); injecting drug user (IDU) 641 (29.4); homo/bisexual IDU 31 (1.4); haemophiliac/coagulation disorder 41 (1.9); transfusion recipient 70 (3.2); heterosexual contact 598 (27.5); other/undetermined 90 (4.1).

The first AIDS case was registered in Portugal in 1983.

The number of cases reported as having been heterosexually transmitted has increased, as has the number of IDU transmissions; the rate of homosexual transmission has declined, although the stigmatization of homo/bisexuality and inclusion of IDU transmission may well swell rates of reported heterosexual transmission. There are an estimated 10,000 to 20,000 people infected with HIV, most of whom are concentrated in Lisbon.

Social and political background

The last two decades have seen a relaxation of much legislation relating to personal behaviour. An example of this is the change in attitude shown by the government towards drug users. Users are treated less repressively than previously, more as victims, while dealers are criminalized. A multiministerial project was established to coordinate action against drugs. Special services include a helpline for users. There is generally, however, a strong reaction against drug users from the general public.

The Catholic church still has a strong influence in Portugal, though less so at governmental level than at local level. The church was initially quiet in its response to AIDS. There was little obstruction of public health campaigns, except for local opposition to condom use from individual priests. Recently the church has become slightly more liberal; generally priests in rural areas are less liberal than their urban counterparts.

Issue	Legislation	Date of legislation	Services provided
Homosexuality	Age of consent 16 (same as for heterosexuals). 3 years gaol for >18s who have sex with person of same sex <16 (no equivalent for heterosexuals)	1982	No
Abortion	Legal <12 weeks on grounds of sex crime, risk to woman's life/physical/mental health, or for eugenic reasons. 2 medical opinions needed, <18s need parental consent	1984	Yes, but limited
Drug use (non-medicinal)	No legal sanction		Yes
Prostitution	Abolitionist, prostitution not punished; exploitation/facilitation illegal	1983	Yes
Contraception	Legal, state provides family planning services and information	1984	Yes
Contraception for those under age of sexual consent	Legal	1985	Yes

Abortion is generally accepted, except by practising Catholics, and there is active anti-abortion agitation, especially from conservative groups allied to the church. The cost, lack of information, procedural difficulties, legal barriers and the negative attitude of some health workers make access difficult.

While prostitution is generally disapproved of, attitudes have become more tolerant recently. There is no registration of sex workers but STD clinics cater largely for their needs and are free of charge. Condoms are not generally used by sex workers – clients often refuse to use them.

Portuguese society is macho orientated and homosexuality is not well tolerated, although AIDS has brought about a greater tolerance. Gay interests are not articulated through a 'gay organization' or well organized.

There have been cases of discrimination against people with HIV.

Health education

Some NGOs are concerned with health promotion. Each of the eighteen provinces and two autonomous regions has its own district health administration within which there is a health education group. The NGO AIEPS (Association of Information,

Education and Promotion of Health) was established in 1991 and runs projects on public health issues such as hepatitis and drug use as well as AIDS, which is a priority at the moment. AIEPS is one of a limited number of organizations that the Ministry of Education (MoE) allows into schools. In January 1994 the MoE began a national programme of health education in 250 schools, focusing on AIDS but also covering other aspects of sex education and drug use.

Sex education

Since educational reforms began in 1990, sex education has in theory been introduced into the curriculum. In practice, provision has remained limited and often poor. School programmes refer primarily to human reproduction in natural science classes, contraception and the prevention of STDs in biology. In 1991 the MoE announced programmes for a new discipline, 'Personal and social development', intended for the first nine years of schooling. In January 1993 the MoE sent 'AIDS packs' out to all teachers in secondary schools. There is some conservative resistance among educational reformers themselves but it is regarded as an achievement that sex education of some kind has now been incorporated into the school curriculum. This is in large part due to AIDS since the lack of sex education in schools presented major problems for AIDS education in Portugal.

The role of the media

In general, sex is still a taboo area in Portugal and there are few programmes on radio or television on the subject. Sections of the press have treated AIDS in a sensationalist way, creating an atmosphere of fear by overstating the numbers of those affected but generally media treatment of AIDS has been responsible and anti-discriminatory. Television treatment of the subject in particular has been helpful and well balanced. Representatives of the Ministry of Health have been invited to speak. In an effort to discourage sensationalism, the National Commission for the Fight Against AIDS (CNLCS) inaugurated a prize for the best AIDS-related coverage or individual article each year in the press, TV or radio.

AIDS/HIV public education

Aims and objectives

In 1985 a national programme on AIDS was established. Specific objectives relating to public education are to monitor the spread of the epidemic, minimize spread of infection, care for the sick and HIV infected, and encourage non-discrimination.

Structure and organization

In June 1985, the CNLCS was established and made responsible for national AIDS policy and public education, directly linked to and coordinated by the Ministry of Health (MoH). The idea was to establish a body which could coordinate and oversee work carried out in other sectors. CNLCS is made up of representatives from the National Blood Institute, the MoH and its department of primary health care, health education, hospitals, primary care and social security. Individuals from the Ministries of Health, Education, Employment, Justice and NGOs advise on specific topics such as education, psychosocial

issues, law, ethics, the workplace, drug use, biostatistics, epidemiology, youth, public health, sexual behaviour and social security.

Conflict relating to the biomedical and epidemiological bias of CNLCS membership has led to changes in senior personnel. In 1992 a new director in favour of a stronger focus on prevention was appointed. At the same time, the MoH's budget was being reduced, and consequently CNLCS's funding decreased. Many felt that changes that had been made under the new director were attempted too suddenly and without adequate finance; for example, the CNLCS telephone line closed due to lack of funds. In addition, this director (an immunologist) had been advocating a hepatitis B vaccine for the whole population, which proved politically unacceptable. Consequently, tension developed with the MoH and members of CNLCS, and the director resigned. In early 1993 a new director was appointed (a virologist), whose relationship to the government is reportedly closer.

Initially the Portuguese Red Cross was important to AIDS public education, providing its own projects and information network. A substantial amount of AIDS public education work is done by NGOs, of which there are several. The most visible is Abraço, which was established in 1992 with the aims of solidarity and support for people with HIV. It raises funds (e.g. for hospital facilities) and trains volunteers to work with AIDS/HIV patients and run prevention campaigns.

The Liga Portuguesa Contra a SIDA (Liga) was established in 1991 by a group of doctors and psychologists. Liga's main objective is to support people with AIDS/HIV and those affected. Liga also gives informative talks in schools, cultural and leisure centres and to companies, produces teaching material for distribution, and provides pre- and post-test counselling and legal advice. In 1991 Liga began a free and anonymous helpline.

Development of campaigns

In 1985 information about AIDS was placed in all newspapers, but the first major intervention was in

1987, when the CNLCS produced the pamphlet *AIDS – what everyone must know*. This was posted to every household, 3.6 million in total, and to special groups.

In 1987–88, CNLCS directed campaigns to travellers. The mass media and newspapers were used extensively. Courses were organized for physicians, teachers, rehabilitated drug users and priests so as to

Campaign chronology

Date and agency	Campaign theme/title	Aims	Media	Main message/endline	Target groups	Tone and style
1987 CNLCS	Leaflet drop	Awareness, provide basic information	Leaflet, TV debate	What AIDS is, transmission facts, prevention strategies	General public	Informative
Summer 1987 CNLCS	First TV campaign	As above and condom use	TV	As above	General public	Informative
Summer 1988 CNLCS	'Travel without risk'	Protect travellers	Leaflets at train stations, airports, motorway toll booths	Avoid risks which could spoil your trip	General public, travellers	
Summer 1989 CNLCS	SIDA or VIDA		TV, posters	'AIDS: don't trust it with your life'	General public	Dramatic
Summer 1990 CNLCS		Motivate risk-reduction behaviour	TV, radio	'Don't fall victim – protect yourself'	Young people	Fast, snappy
1991–93 CNLCS	Information campaign		TV, radio, posters, leaflets	Transmission facts		Informative
1991–93 CNLCS	Solidarity campaign	Encourage solidarity with people with AIDS/HIV	TV, posters, leaflets	'Against AIDS. Against discrimination'	General public	Dramatic
1991 onwards AIEPS	Schools campaign	Raise awareness, inform schoolchildren, teachers	TV, radio, posters, teaching pack	'AIDS…depends on your personal behaviour'	Young people 14–20s	
1992 Abraço	Condom campaign	Encourage condom use	TV, leaflets, posters, press ads	'Because AIDS exists. Use a condom'	General public	
1992 Abraço	Information campaign	Information about Abraço, AIDS	Newspapers		General public	Informative
April 1993 Abraço	Solidarity campaign	Encourage solidarity with people with AIDS/HIV	Leaflets, posters, billboards	'Make the first move. AIDS can't be caught by friendship'	General public	Soft
June 1993 Abraço	Condom campaign	Encourage condom use	Posters, postcards, *Cosmo* features	'Condom use obligatory. Because AIDS exists'	General public	Humorous
October–December 1993 CNLCS NAP[1]	Needle exchange	Safe IUD use	Kit, leaflet, billboards, TV	'Say no to a second-hand syringe'; 'If you need a syringe we have some here'	IDUs	

[1]National Association of Pharmacists

prepare them for education and counselling activities. In 1989 activities were directed towards health professionals, schoolchildren, homosexuals, drug abusers, workers, Africans, journalists, and parents and teachers of infected children. In 1991–93 CNLCS ran campaigns to combat discrimination and provide more factual information on AIDS/HIV (e.g. transmission facts).

The various NGOs and CNLCS produce information leaflets for World AIDS Day each year (e.g. in 1989, the Institute of Social Affairs and Education sent a document to all schools). During World AIDS Day 1993, Abraço and other NGOs in Lisbon provided information to the general public by distributing leaflets, stickers and condoms.

Tone and style

CNLCS's 1992 solidarity campaign used quite hard-hitting moody black and white images, and was felt to be well received. Other earlier CNLCS campaigns had been more informative in tone and style. 'Life or death, the decision is yours' played on words and the gambling message to bring the message home. There was a negative reaction from people with AIDS/HIV to the 1991-onwards AIEPS schools campaign, 'Messages of death'.

Messages

The messages of the CNLCS's 1987 leaflet campaign were:
- avoid more than one partner;
- use condoms if you have sex with a casual partner;
- don't share syringes or needles;
- don't share toothbrushes;
- make sure equipment for tattooing and ear piercing is sterile;
- there is no danger in social contact.

CNLCS's 1992 solidarity campaign aimed to encourage empathy, hoping especially to appeal to Catholics in this way.

Between the different NGOs and CNLCS, messages covered have included transmission routes, mutual fidelity, condom use, solidarity, and non-

drug use as well as promotion of clean works for users. The term 'safer sex' or 'non-penetrative sex' has not been used by CNLCS, except in material specifically for gay men and IDUs. Abraço's main message is solidarity, followed by prevention through condom use, although this is not specified in terms of anal, vaginal, non-penetrative sex, or number of partners. An underlying aim of their campaigns is to facilitate talking about safe sex and encourage negotiation of condom use.

Target groups

In addition to the general population, AIDS information campaigns have been directed towards IDUs, sex workers, health care professionals, young people (high school and university students) and travellers.

Other measures of prevention and control

HIV testing and surveillance

In 1985, the Centre for Epidemiological Surveillance of Communicable Diseases established a programme of surveillance for AIDS. In addition, HIV surveillance studies are carried out at the National Institute of Health.

Theoretically tests for HIV and AIDS are confidential and consent is obtained, but involuntary testing does occur. Pregnant women are tested and in practice are not given counselling or the option to refuse. All new prison inmates are systematically tested. Testing also takes place to confirm suspected diagnosis and sometimes for surveillance purposes. Since 1986, all seropositive cases have been notified to the National Blood Institute in Lisbon. Pre- and post-test counselling exists, but with inadequate professional training. Despite efforts to ensure confidentiality and make possible the detection of double notifications, there have been problems with confidentiality.

In April 1986 it became mandatory for all blood used for treatment to be screened for HIV-1 and HIV-2 (Portugal has a higher than average prevalence of HIV-2). Members of high risk groups (including Africans and Portuguese citizens who have stayed in Africa during the last three years) are requested not to donate blood. Except for blood donations, HIV testing is neither compulsory nor advised except for some high risk groups.

Needle exchange schemes

Needles and syringes can be sold in chemists without any restrictions, but in practice, chemists often only sell them selectively.

Controversy has long surrounded the notion and cost of needle exchange schemes. The first programme introduced by the Red Cross met with serious opposition. However, a national needle exchange scheme ran from 1 October until 31 December 1993, following an agreement reached between CNLCS and the National Association of Pharmacists. A kit containing a syringe, a disinfectant towel, a condom and an advice leaflet was given free by chemists in exchange for used syringes.

Condoms

Until 1986 condoms were only available through pharmacists. The law has since been changed and they are now more widely available in supermarkets, chemists and some bars; they are distributed free of charge in the army and navy and in health centres (family planning out-patient consultancies). The sale of condoms is authorized in prisons but inmates explicitly have to ask for them. Television advertising is permitted. A decrease in price is due to come into force following an agreement reached between CNLCS, chemists and manufacturers. Approximately 20 million condoms are sold each year and this remains stable.

Evaluation

Systematic evaluation of CNLCS's campaigns began in 1993 and there is financial commitment to evaluate all campaigns. Evaluations were carried out previously but not consistently. Research has also been used to inform campaign development.

Liga produces a quarterly evaluation report of

calls to their helpline. Abraço has not evaluated its campaigns. Evaluation of the 1993 AIEPS schools programme was planned before, immediately after and six months following the intervention.

Country visit: Helen Ward (St Mary's Hospital Medical School, London) and Claire Gibbons (London), 1990 and 1993

Report preparation: Becky Field

Individuals and organizations contacted:

Fausto Amaro
National Commission for the Fight Against AIDS (CNLCS)/Bom Sucesso Foundation, Lisbon

Francisca Avillez
Instituto Nacional de Saúde, Lisbon

Dr Laura Ayres (National AIDS Coordinator)
Dr Teresa Avillez Paixao
Instituto Nacional de Saúde, Lisbon

Maria Barros
Liga Portuguesa Contra a SIDA, Lisbon

Maria Jose Campos, Margarida Martins (Director)
Abraço, Lisbon

Luis Goncales (Coordinator of National School Campaign on AIDS), Filipa Lance Rodrigues (Coordinator of 'Students teaching about AIDS in school')
Associaço de Informaçao, Educaçao e Promoçao de Saúde (AIEPS), Lisbon

Professor Odette Santos Ferreira
President of the National Commission for the Fight Against AIDS, Ministry of Health, Lisbon

Dr Joao Santos Lucas
Human and Social Sciences Department, Escola Nacional de Saúde Publica, Lisbon

Bibliography

AIDS surveillance in Europe, quarterly report no. 44 31 December 1994, European Centre for the Epidemiological Monitoring of AIDS

Context of sexual behaviour in Europe, selected indices relating to demographic, social and cultural variables May 1993, Becky Field and Kaye Wellings, EC Concerted Action 'Sexual behaviour and the risk of HIV infection'

Diz no a uma seringa em segunda mo (Dossier) Comisso Nacional Luta Contra a SIDA, Associaço Nacional das Farmácias

Perguntas e respostas sobre a SIDA 1988, Divisao de educaçao para a saúde direcçao-geral dos cuidados de saúde primários + Grupo de trabalho da SIDA

Plano Nacional de Luta Contra a SIDA 1993–1994 Ministéro da Saúde, Comisso Nacional de Luta Contra a SIDA

Public awareness of AIDS and sexual behaviour change in Portugal, 1987, L J Santos, paper presented at Xth Conference on Social Science and Medicine

Report of Abraço's activities from April 1992 to June 1993

Sexual behaviour in the city of Lisbon, 1991, F Amaro, L Teles, A Dantas, paper for VIIth International Conference on AIDS, Florence 16–21 June 1991

Sexual behaviour in the city of Lisbon, 1995, F Amaro, A Dantas and L da Cunha Teles, *International Journal of STD and AIDS* 6; 35–41

Spartacus International Gay Guide 1990/1991, B Gmunder and J D Stamford (eds)

Translation of documents: Melissa Herman, Lola Martinez, Maria de Pereira, Edvaldo da Silva Souza

---

SPAIN

Context

Epidemiology

According to the European Centre for the Epidemiological Monitoring of AIDS, by 31 December 1994, the cumulative total of AIDS cases was 29,520, with an incidence rate (per million population) of 117.5 (n = 4,650). The cumulative total of AIDS cases, by transmission group (percentages in parentheses) was as follows: homo/bisexual male 4,324 (15); injecting drug user (IDU) 19,012 (66); homo/bisexual IDU 592 (2.1); haemophiliac/coagulation disorder 514 (1.8); transfusion recipient 246 (0.9); heterosexual contact 2,531 (8.8); other/undetermined 1,601 (5.6).

The first AIDS case was registered in Spain in 1981. There is little reliable information on the number of people infected with HIV; several studies are now trying to establish more realistic data about HIV prevalence in Spain through the use of sentinel surveillance.

Social and political background

Spain is a country of strong regional differences in both culture and geography. Since the restoration of democracy in 1975, there has been a gradual increase in decentralization with regional authorities enjoying a considerable degree of autonomy. 1978 saw the establishment of seventeen constitutionally autonomous communities. Thus regional administrations collaborate with central government in the administration of their respective territories.

Since its privileged position during the Franco era, the power of the Catholic church has been declining recently. Its role in terms of AIDS public education has been mixed; most of its leaders have been critical of AIDS prevention campaigns which promote condom use or other 'safer-sex' practices. In contrast to the relatively liberal attitudes to the campaigns in Catalonia and Madrid, strong resistance from the church and the Right in Galicia at the end of 1989 led to withdrawal of posters and other publicity materials. However, many priests

Issue	Legislation	Date of legislation	Services provided
Homosexuality	Age of sexual consent 12 (same as for heterosexuals)	1978	Yes
Abortion	Legal if resulting from sex crime, risk to woman's life/ physical/mental health, eugenic reasons	1985	Yes[1]
Drug use (non-medicinal)	Possession of small amounts legal, use in public subject to fines. Manufacture and trade are criminal offences	1992[2]	Yes
Prostitution	Abolitionist: no offence committed by sale/purchase of sexual services by consenting adults; assisting/ persuading <23s illegal; pimping/providing accommodation illegal	1963	Yes
Contraception	Contraceptive information legal.* Information free of charge, provision of method not free[†]	*1978, [†]1980	Yes, but limited
Contraception for those under age of sexual consent	Not regulated		Yes

[1]Free in theory but the majority are performed privately. [2]1984–92 cannabis legal for personal use (to buy or sell illegal). Since 1988, the police have taken tougher action against drug dealers.

care for AIDS patients or work with groups particularly affected (e.g. IDUs, prostitutes). The credibility they have gained among these populations allows them to promote AIDS prevention education and interventions.

Generally, there has been less controversy surrounding interventions which aim to prevent IDU transmission through safe drug use than for programmes which aim to prevent sexual transmission of HIV by promoting safer sex.

The rights of those infected with HIV and AIDS should, theoretically, be protected by the constitution, many articles of which more than adequately cover contingencies raised by AIDS. Article 14, for example, asserts the individual's fundamental right to equality and protects against discrimination; article 18 upholds the right to privacy and intimacy; article 27 safeguards the right to be educated; article 35, the right to work; article 47, the right to a roof over one's head; and article 60 dictates that sick people should not be kept in jail if in need of treatment which cannot be provided there. However, cases of discrimination have occurred in some schools, hospitals and workplaces.

In prisons, there is a high prevalence of AIDS (50 per cent in certain prisons). AIDS education and

prevention programmes for prisons began in 1989, involving health education, methadone, condoms and bleach. Article 60 prescribes that seriously ill inmates with a terminal disease can be released from imprisonment. Yet there are no special services and few centres prepared to accept released prisoners with AIDS/HIV. Some NGOs, often in collaboration with priests, are trying to remedy this situation, as far as resources allow.

Homelessness is a common problem for people with AIDS. Recently hospices for AIDS patients without family support have opened in several of the regions, the majority of which are managed by priests (from different religious denominations).

Health education

Since Spain is virtually a federal country, legally health promotion and public health are the responsibility of regional governments. The task of central government is one of basic legislation and coordination. Traditionally, the Ministry of Health has had overall responsibility for the organization and coordination of regional and national health campaigns. With the advent of AIDS/HIV, a need was recognized for greater liaison between relevant ministries to ensure that information on the disease and means of preventing transmission reached all sections of the population. Much prevention, however, takes place at local level and it is hard to generalize on the provision of health education and prevention projects across Spain. In the past few years, the role of the autonomous communities and local government councils (through programmes like 'Healthy cities') has been important in the implementation of health education interventions to prevent AIDS/HIV.

Sex education

AIDS has been largely responsible for progress in sex education. Provision of sex education became mandatory in 1990–91 but inclusion into school curricula has been gradual, the number of schools actually teaching sex education remains low. Sex education and AIDS/HIV education for young people has caused controversy, for example, during the '*Póntelo, pónselo*' campaign, parental response stopped the planned distribution of one million condoms to young people in colleges (*El Independiente* 25 October 1990).

The role of the media

At the beginning of the epidemic, the tone of media presentations of AIDS issues was sensationalist. It has since become more informational. AIDS/HIV has been frequently misrepresented as a problem of marginal groups, though again, more recently, the focus has shifted to heterosexual transmission. Sex is not a taboo subject for Spanish television; a TV programme on sex problems and adult sex education, for example, was broadcast at peak viewing time in 1990. This change in media treatment of AIDS is in part due to the work of the NGO Fundación Anti-SIDA España (FASE), which organized workshops designed for mass media professionals with the aim of achieving news treatment which would help to prevent both AIDS/HIV and discrimination.

AIDS/HIV public education

Aims and objectives

The Spanish programmes of public education are intended to prevent further transmission of HIV in the population ('biological AIDS') and to quell unfounded fears and prevent discrimination ('social AIDS').

Structure and organization

In May 1983, a National AIDS Committee was established under the Ministry of Health and Consumers Affairs. Spain has had a National Plan on AIDS since 1987, defining all AIDS activities. Responsibility for AIDS programmes is shared between central government and the seventeen autonomous regional communities, which have established regional anti-AIDS committees. While the task of the Ministry has been to attract the attention of the broad mass of the general population, activities more closely tailored to the needs and characteristics of regional populations have been undertaken by the autonomous communities, with a special budget from the government for this purpose. Although the Ministry of Health is nationally responsible for HIV health education, each region has autonomy in deciding the content and style of local campaigns which are tailored specifically to particular local problems.

Between 1992–94 the National Plan on AIDS was without a general secretary, which represented a substantial setback to the national campaign strategy. Although a general secretary was appointed in 1993, administrative problems provoked his hasty departure. A new general secretary was appointed in the first half of 1994 and created four sub-committees intended to advise on prevention, research, epidemiology and assistance projects.

NGOs have been important for AIDS public education in Spain, providing drop-in centres, hotlines, self-help groups, psychological support and documentation centres, as well as implementing interventions for IDUs and prostitutes. Many of the NGOs cooperate as a federation of NGOs at regional

Campaign chronology

Date and agency	Campaign theme/title	Aims	Media	Main message/endline	Target groups	Tone and style
1985 MoH[1]	National information campaign	Provide prevention information to those at risk	Leaflets, booklets		General public, gay men, IDUs, prisoners	Direct, factual
1987 1988 1989 1990 MoH	'SiDa, NoDa'	Inform about the ways HIV is and is not transmitted	TV, posters, packs of cards, badges, T-shirts	'This transmits, this doesn't. Don't change your life for AIDS' (play on words to illustrate transmission routes)	General public	Humorous, informational
1987 1988 1989 1990 MoH	'SIDA, VIDA' (AIDS, life)	Prevention of HIV, STDs and unwanted pregnancy	TV	'If you don't have a stable partner, use a condom'	Young people	Down to earth, friendly
1988 1989 1990 MoH	'No piques' ('Don't get hooked')	Persuade IDUs to protect themselves and others	TV, billboards	'Use disposable syringes and dispose of them carefully'	Young people	Serious
1988 (MoH and MoE)	Schools campaign	Reinforce information on modes of transmission; Prevent discrimination	Booklets	What's AIDS? How to prevent AIDS in school	Teachers, parents, educationalists	Informational, clear
1988 MoH and trade unions	Workplace	Quell unfounded fears	Booklets	'Don't change your life because of AIDS'	People in the workplace	Reassuring
1989 NGOs	Solidarity	Prevent discrimination	TV, booklets	'Don't underestimate'; 'Don't isolate yourself'	HIV positive people, general public	Direct, clear
1990 1991 MoH and MoSA[3]	Condom campaign 'Póntelo, pónselo' ('Put it on, put it on him [your partner]').	Correct condom use	Posters, TV, radio spots	'We can share AIDS prevention, condom use protects against many diseases'	Young people	Explicit, familiar
1993 MoH	'Deja vivir y vive' ('Let live and live')	Promote solidarity and condom use	Billboards, posters, leaflets, TV, press	Let live (red ribbon) and live (condom)	General public, HIV positive people	Positive
1993 1994 FASE[4]	'Los pájaritos' ('The birdies')* 'Las 7 respuestas al SIDA' ('The 7 key answers to AIDS')†	Provide prevention information and promote hotline, encourage solidarity	TV, billboards, leaflet	*AIDS is a question for everyone. If you have sex, take precautions	*General public †General public, young people	*Humorous †Direct, clear

[1]Ministry of Health and Consumer Affairs [2]Ministry of Education [3]Ministry of Social Affairs [4]Fundación Anti-SIDA España (Spanish Anti-AIDS Foundation)

and national level. Collaboration between the regional administrations and NGOs is increasing and consolidating; NGOs are consulted for their experience and have become key participants in the identification of priorities and design of programmes.

Development of campaigns

As in many other countries, the first response to the need for intervention in the fight against AIDS came from the gay movement. The existence of a network, more or less organized, allowed information to move quickly among the most aware members of this population (located in the big cities of Spain: Madrid, Barcelona, Bilbao and Valencia).

The regional anti-AIDS committees have run their own campaigns with financial support from the national government. The NGOs from each autonomous community have frequently collaborated in these campaigns. It is common for both the regional administrations and the NGOs to mount informational and awareness raising events on World AIDS Day, as well as during local festivals and celebrations.

A national information campaign on AIDS began in 1985 using brochures, posters, leaflets, etc., but efforts were intensified following the establishment of the National Plan. Since June 1987, health promotion and education programmes have been coordinated by the National Health Secretariat. Also since 1987, television has become a major medium for the provision of information, particularly that which is aimed at young people. TV campaigns have focused on the ways in which HIV is and is not transmitted and on the means of prevention. In addition there is a permanent and continuous campaign aimed at IDUs in recognition of their importance with respect to AIDS. Other central government institutions have also developed information campaigns. The Marine Institute, for example, has prepared brochures and posters for sailors, and the Ministry of Justice has produced information for prisoners.

Tone and style

A distinct contrast can be seen between interventions designed and executed by the national government and by the regional authorities. A more careful and cautious use of language characterizes the former, while those responsible for the latter have been freer to use the language of the people and to employ more down-to-earth imagery. The language used in the official leaflet for prisoners was almost crude, employing prisoners' slang. In contrast, TV advertisements, by the skilful use of cartoons, have deflected possible criticisms that they are too frank. This strategy has allowed the use of material which might otherwise have been considered too explicit. The tone of the campaign directed towards IDUs, while sombre, avoided the use of fear, concentrating instead on a clear and factual presentation aiming to lead to practical action. Generally a positive approach has been used, as the choice of endlines demonstrates e.g. '*SIDA, VIDA*' ('AIDS, life'), '*Que tu vida no cambie por el SIDA*' ('Don't change your life because of AIDS') and '*Deja vivir y vive*', where the red ribbon of solidarity is shown with the words 'Let live' and the condom with the word 'Live'. This latter campaign used real people for the TV spots, rather than actors, using everyday language. The '*Póntelo, ponselo*' campaign was perhaps the most controversial of the Spanish campaigns. In 1993 a court ruled in favour of CONCAPA (National Catholic Confederation of Parents of Pupils), which argued that the campaign encouraged promiscuity. The magistrates passing the sentence called the campaign invalid and biased because among the messages publicized it failed to state that abstinence or fidelity among non-infected partners would completely eliminate the risk of infection (see also 'Condoms' below).

Messages

The first messages to be transmitted in Spain focused on the ways in which HIV is and is not transmitted. These were initially described in brochures distributed through pharmacies, health centres and NGOs throughout the country. The *'SiDa NoDa'* campaign on TV continued this message using cartoon figures to illustrate situations and behaviours which do and do not involve risk of infection. In terms of preventive strategies, the main message of the Spanish campaigns has been to use a condom. No attempt has been made to tell people to keep to one exclusive partner. Spain is one of the few countries to have featured messages in the mass media aimed at high risk groups. The television campaign aimed at IDUs advised them to use disposable needles to protect themselves, and to dispose of them safely to protect others. Anti-discrimination messages first concentrated on quelling panic by telling people that it is not necessary to isolate themselves in order to avoid infection. Later solidarity messages have been more positive, promoting solidarity ('Let live').

Target groups

In addition to the general population, AIDS information campaigns have been directed towards men who have sex with men, IDUs, female prostitutes and their clients, prisoners, travellers, young people, military personnel, teachers, social workers, health care professionals and pharmacists.

Other measures of prevention and control

HIV testing and surveillance

AIDS case reporting varies in quality across the country. In Andalusia, Aragon, the Basque Autonomous Region and Catalonia, AIDS is included in the list of notifiable diseases. Only two of these regions, Aragon and the Basque Autonomous Region, have enacted regulations guaranteeing the confidentiality of the results of the tests and the persons tested.

HIV antibody testing is voluntary in Spain. Counselling services for seropositives and their contacts are becoming more widespread, supported by the work of the NGOs. In many regions there are hotlines providing additional support. Confidentiality in general is guaranteed by order of the central health authorities. Testing for HIV infection is also voluntary in Spanish prisons.

In Spain, 81 per cent of blood for blood transfusions and blood products is imported. For a long period there was no possibility for screening or heat treatment to eliminate the risk of infection. All blood for transfusion is now screened and all blood products treated. Before giving blood, donors are issued a leaflet on AIDS, which urges all those who have been involved in high risk behaviour to withdraw themselves voluntarily.

Needle exchange schemes

The major thrust of preventive efforts in Spain is towards drug users. A campaign has been developed encouraging injecting drug users to bleach injecting equipment. Bleach is provided in prisons to enable prisoners to clean needles.

Needle exchange schemes have been established in major cities in Spain. Methadone programmes and drug abuse education is available and methadone is prescribed in some prisons. Syringes and needles are available, at low cost, from some pharmacies, most of which sell direct to the public.

The policy on heroin abuse treatment varies widely throughout Spain. Methadone maintenance programmes have served to increase contact between the social and health care systems and IDUs, providing further opportunities for prevention messages to be directed to IDUs. In some areas, like Barcelona, these programmes are thought to reach 20 per cent of heroin users; in other areas, such programmes are non-existent. Other harm-reduction strategies are also being implemented in the autonomous communities.

Condoms

Condoms are actively promoted, and television advertising of condoms has been permitted since 1985. The Spanish Ministry of Health and Consumer Affairs and the Department of Prisons have authorized the distribution of condoms in prisons. Group meetings have been set up to make prostitutes aware of the facilities, and drop-in centres have been established in areas of prostitution. Efforts have been made by NGOs to promote – through education materials and workshops – a more erotic approach to safer sex in general and to the condom in particular.

Evaluation

National prevention campaigns generally undergo some form of evaluation. This may be carried out by the ministries responsible or commercial survey agencies.

Knowledge, attitude, behaviour and practice surveys have been carried out on behalf of the AIDS Unit at the Institute of Health Carlos III, and their results published in report form.

Country visit: Marina Barnard (Glasgow University) and Pilar Estebanez (London School of Hygiene and Tropical Medicine), 1991 and 1993

Report preparation: José-Luis Bimbela (Escuela Andaluza de Salud Pública, Granada, Spain) and Becky Field

Individuals and organizations contacted:

Dr Rafael de Andres Medina
Ministry of Health and Consumer Affairs, Madrid

Enrique Garcia-Huete
Fundación Anti-SIDA España (FASE), Madrid

Dr José Antonio Nieto
Universidad Nacional de Educación a Distancia, Madrid

Francisco Parras, Carmen Martinez Ten
National Plan on Aids, Ministry of Health and Consumer Affairs, Madrid

José Torres
Fundación Anti-SIDA España (FASE), Madrid

Joan Ramon Villalbi
Institut Municipal de la Salut, Barcelona City Health Department

Bibliography

Actitudes sociales ante el SIDA 1990, Ministry of Health and Consumer Affairs
AIDS surveillance in Europe, quarterly report no. 44 31 December 1994, European Centre for the Epidemiological Monitoring of AIDS
La sentencia del 'Póntelo pónselo' califica la campaña de 'inveraz y parcial', *El País*, 17 March 1993
National plan on AIDS: activities of penitentiary institutions 1993, Ministry of Health and Consumer Affairs
National plan on AIDS: memories of activities from autonomous communities 1993, Ministry of Health and Consumer Affairs
National plan on AIDS: national register of cases of AIDS 1994, Ministry of Health and Consumer Affairs
National plan on AIDS: organisational plan and structure December 1988–January 1989 investigation of publicity campaign Ministry of Health and Consumer Affairs
Notebook on AIDS information spring 1988, Federation of Citizens Commissions against AIDS in Spain
Sanidad insiste en el condón para prevenir, *El País*, 17 March 1993
Second survey of public opinion about AIDS February 1988, Sigma
Spanish Anti-AIDS Foundation (FASE): memory of activities 1993–1994 FASE

SWEDEN

Context

Epidemiology

According to the European Centre for the Epidemiological Monitoring of AIDS, by 31 December 1994, the cumulative total of AIDS cases was 1,128, with an incidence rate (per million population) of 17.2 (n = 150). The cumulative total of AIDS cases, by transmission group (percentages in parentheses) was as follows: homo/bisexual male 727 (64.9); injecting drug user (IDU) 114 (10.2); haemophiliac/coagulation disorder 34 (3); transfusion recipient 39 (3.5); heterosexual contact 110 (9.8); other/undetermined 89 (7.9).

The first AIDS cases in Sweden were diagnosed in Stockholm in December 1982 and reported in the following year. There are approximately 4,000 HIV positive people diagnosed in Sweden, 60 per cent of whom live in the Stockholm area.

Social and political background

According to the National Institute of Public Health a number of factors facilitate the implementation of preventive measures in Sweden: comprehensive health and medical care services; a system for reporting and registering communicable diseases; a well-established system of partner notification; a strict drug policy combined with highly developed services for the care of drug users; a relatively open attitude to sexual matters and social relations; a tradition of sex education in schools based on over 40 years experience; an early start with preventive measures; and free and anonymous testing at a wide variety of health and medical care centres and clinics throughout the country.

Sweden is a country in which the state assumes a major responsibility for social issues, and in which social responsibility is accorded high priority. Social tasks and bureaucracy have grown rapidly, as has the professionalization of social work and health care.

Issue	Legislation	Date of legislation	Services provided
Homosexuality	Age of consent 15 (same as for heterosexuals).* Anti-discrimination act for public service (not labour market).[†] Homosexual cohabitees have the same rights as heterosexual cohabitees concerning inheritance, tax, property.[‡] Partnership law[§]	*1978, [†]1987, [‡]1988, [§]1995	Yes
Abortion	Legally permitted;* Socio-medical causes introduced as grounds;[†] Available on request: <18 weeks after consultation with doctor and >18 weeks with approval from the National Board of Health and Welfare[‡]	*1938, [†]1946, [‡]1974	Yes
Drug use (non-medicinal)	Illegal, 6 months maximum for use. Convicted drug users can be forced to undergo treatment for addiction as an alternative to prison	1980s, 1993	Yes
Prostitution	Prostitution legal; profit making from others' 'immoral life', working in groups, renting flats, supporting family by prostitution forbidden	1950s, revised 1980s	Yes
Contraception	Law which prohibited information on contraceptives repealed;* Consultation and advice free of charge, oral contraceptives subsidized[†]	*1938, [†]1974	Yes
Contraception for those under age of sexual consent	Contraceptive advice and provision available to <15s. Approximately 190 youth clinics	1974–75	Yes

The absence of war since 1814 has facilitated social reform.

Sweden has the reputation of being a country relatively free from sexual repression (Meredith 1984). Nevertheless state response to sexual issues contains some apparent contradictions: a Bill passed by Parliament in 1987 included far-reaching proposals to give gay and lesbian couples cohabitation status, and government grants were given to enable city centre gay centres with restaurants, pubs and meeting rooms to be opened; yet in the same year bath houses and gay saunas were closed down by a law passed in haste by Parliament.

Attitudes towards drugs have hardened since the advent of AIDS. There is, for example, no recognition of the term 'recreational drugs', and in the 1980s a new law was introduced criminalizing the use of drugs, before which only possession was illegal.

Treatment of some people with HIV is one aspect of Sweden's AIDS/HIV prevention approach which initially caused some consternation internationally, and indeed nationally among some AIDS workers and physicians. Under the Communicable Diseases Act of 1989, 'the county administrative court, on petition from the county medical officer, can order the compulsory isolation of a person carrying infection from a serious infectious disease if that person does not voluntarily comply with the measures needed to prevent the infection spreading.' An order of this kind is also to be made when there is good reason to suppose that the infected person is not complying with practical instructions issued and this omission entails a manifest risk of the infection spreading (see below, 'HIV testing and surveillance').

Health education

Sweden has a well-established tradition of public information on health and social problems. Traditionally health promotion has been the responsibility of the National Board of Health and Welfare, and some counties have their own information campaigns. In the early 1970s a radical locally based drug prevention programme was designed by the government. It addressed structural as well as individual and lifestyle factors in drug use (how society itself, rather than the individual, could be changed to prevent drug misuse). This approach departed from the paternalistic and moralistic advice which had characterized previous campaigns. Also in the early 1970s, the Swedish Association for Sex Education – an organization with a great deal of expertise in the area of sex education and contraception – launched a campaign to reduce the incidence of gonorrhoea. Combined with the Communicable Diseases Act and partner notification, it was notably successful.

In July 1992 the National Institute of Public Health (Folkhälsoinstitutet, FHI) was created to develop preventive health strategies. The FHI comprises three sections: the Health and Environment Unit runs programmes for allergic complaints, diet and exercise, physical injury, tobacco use and associated disease, and matters relating to mental illness, old age, etc.; the Health and Dependence Unit runs programmes for alcohol and drug misuse and dependence, gambling addiction, etc.; the Sex, Gender and Health Unit is responsible for programmes concerning AIDS/HIV, sex and social relationships, STDs, unwanted pregnancies and women's health. There is also a special programme for children and young people.

Sex education

Sweden has a long history of sex education. It was the first European country to establish compulsory sex education, in 1956. Much earlier, in 1933, the Swedish Association for Sex Education (RFSU) was established; the subject was officially recognized in 1942 when the government recommended its introduction into the school system. The introduction and implementation of sex education in Sweden has been a slow, careful and thoughtful process. A highly elaborate national curriculum was developed by successive national commissions. An official manual for use in all schools was produced in 1946, and revised in 1956 and 1977. Large scale surveys of sexual behaviour (such as that conducted by Zetterberg in 1967, for example) and evaluations of sex education programmes were conducted. Nevertheless, according to some, provision is still uneven.

The role of the media

Issues relating to sexuality are treated relatively sensibly. The Swedish public is familiar with free discussion of sexual matters on TV, discussion is open-minded and free of prejudice. As a result television and the more serious morning papers treat these issues seriously.

At the start of the AIDS epidemic, the media helped fuel much of the moral panic around the disease, for example the name of one man with HIV was disclosed by the press in violation of existing press rules. In recent years, however, the press has been supportive of public education about AIDS/HIV. On the issue of heterosexual spread of HIV, there has been no suggestion in the media that AIDS will not affect the general population.

AIDS/HIV public education

Aims and objectives

The FHI states that the principal objectives of its prevention strategy are to:
- minimize the spread of infection;
- alleviate public anxiety and fear;
- provide support for sufferers, families and relatives;
- reduce discrimination against people with AIDS/HIV.

The intention of the FHI has been to achieve these aims without resorting to scaremongering.

Structure and organization

Parliament is responsible for health care decision making and the Ministry of Health and Social Affairs takes responsibility for putting the measures into effect. The task of practical implementation then falls to relatively independent administrative agencies, primarily the National Board of Health and Welfare and the FHI, to whose remit health information programmes fall.

County councils and local authorities have their own programmes with direct links with the health care system, the social services, schools, youth counselling centres, armed forces unit, local branches of NGOs, organized sports bodies, refugee accommodation centres, etc.

Several voluntary associations make an invaluable contribution to public education, such as RFSU, the Noah's Ark-Red Cross Foundation, the Swedish Federation for Gay and Lesbian Rights (RFSL), the Swedish Association for Help and Assistance to Drug Abusers (RFHL), the National Swedish Parents' Anti-Narcotics Association, Save the Children, etc.

In 1985, Parliament created a special commission to deal with AIDS – the state AIDS Delegation – which represented the five main political parties, with the Minister of Health as chairperson. The intention was to provide strong leadership for the national AIDS prevention campaign. The location of control within the Ministry reflected the spirit of a national emergency since normally, and on past precedent, health educational initiatives would have been mounted by the National Board of Health and Welfare, which has the expertise to deal with preventive health issues.

It had been planned that responsibility for the campaign would pass from the state AIDS Delegation to the National Board of Health and Health and Welfare in summer 1990. Instead, in 1992 responsibility for AIDS public education campaigns was taken under the direct control of the Ministry of Health and operational control lodged with the newly created National Institute of Public Health (FHI). In July 1992, a special AIDS/HIV programme – incorporating the tasks formally undertaken by the state AIDS Delegation – was established within the FHI. Attached to the FHI is a consultative AIDS council with an advisory role, consisting of twelve government-appointed members (later to be appointed by the FHI) representing the parliamentary political parties, the National

Board of Health and Welfare, the Institute for Infectious Diseases Control, Noah's Ark, RFSU, RFSL and the respective associations of county councils and local authorities. A good working relationship with constructive collaboration between FHI, RFSL and RFSU has developed, exemplified by the development and implementation of the 'Love power' (1991 onwards) and 'Man + man' (1993) campaigns.

Development of campaigns

As in many other countries, important initiatives were taken by NGOs before the start of the official campaign. Noah's Ark, (later subsidized by the Swedish Red Cross) set up a number of activities including the AIDS hotline. The Swedish Federation for Gay and Lesbian Rights (RFSL) worked intensively with the problem and issued early (1983) safer-sex advice.

In 1986 the government set up a contract with the Ted Bates commercial advertising agency and large scale, national campaigns began in autumn 1986, directed from the centre. Campaigns have continued mostly at six-monthly intervals. The FHI provides funding for campaigns, given to the FHI by the government on an annual basis, which makes forward planning and continuity a problem.

Tone and style

A major preoccupation from the outset was to find an appropriate level of information to raise awareness without generating anxiety. According to the AIDS Delegation's documented strategy, the information of the campaign was to be matter-of-fact, clear and truthful, avoiding didactic or moralistic overtones, thereby counteracting prejudices. Despite this, early campaigns were criticized on several fronts, and in 1988 the National Audit Bureau (Riksrevisionsverket, RRV) was commissioned by the AIDS Delegation itself to evaluate the public education campaign. This government agency was openly critical of the campaigns. In the opinion of the RRV, the Delegation had succeeded in avoiding causing offence or anxiety, and materials were well presented, but had neglected to communicate delicate and difficult issues in a more concrete and open way without provoking negative emotions. The Delegation was also criticized by the RRV for conveying a tradition-

Campaign chronology

Date and agency	Campaign theme/title	Aims	Media	Main message/endline	Target groups	Tone and style
Winter 1986 AD[1]/TB[2]	The alarm clock	Raise awareness, alert people to danger	Press, posters	Take action before it's too late	General public	Alarming
Winter 1986 AD/TB	Information campaign	Raise awareness, encourage people to obtain information and protect themselves	Posters, TV, cinema	Ring AIDS-Jouren ... 'read the leaflet you will get through the letterbox. Knowledge is the best protection against AIDS'	General public, young people, parents	Questioning, serious, discursive
Spring 1987 AD/TB	Risky situations		Posters	'Ring AIDS-Jouren if you have questions'	General public young people, gay people, IDUs	Alarming, grave
Autumn 1987 AD/TB	Information campaign	As above	Posters, TV	'Take a test. Ring AIDS-Jouren' (You must take love seriously)	General public	Serious, long text

238

Spring 1988 AD/TB	Risk groups	Warn of transmission through prostitutes and multiple partnerships	Posters (strategic sites), press, cinema, TV	'Ring AIDS-Jouren' (AIDS is spreading. You can't see it. Keep to one partner Use protection)	Prostitutes and clients, 'swingers', general public	Ominous, questioning
Spring–autumn 1988 AD/TB	Solidarity	Give accurate information to counter discrimination	Posters, TV	'Ring AIDS-Jouren' (Live with it; Togetherness is vital)	General public	Factual
Spring 1989 AD/TB	'Long live lust'	To remind that AIDS is still a serious threat but we can enjoy love and sex if we take responsibility	Posters, TV	'Long live lust!'	General public	Sex positive
Spring 1990 AD/Garbergs[2]	Personal responsibility	To address flaws in risk-reduction strategies, encourage responsibility	Posters, TV	'Ring AIDS-Jouren' (AIDS will influence you for the rest of your life...We cannot protect you but *you* can)	General public, young people	
Spring/ summer 1990 AD/BRO[2]	Condom normalization	Encourage condom use	Posters	E.g. 'Have a nice trip; Head over heels'	General public	Minimalist, humorous
December 1991 AD/ Garbergs	World AIDS Day 'A sunny story'; 'A bedtime story'	Illuminate risk situations rather than risk groups	Brochure, posters, cinema, story-book	Encourage individual responsibility and awareness	General public	Humorous
1991–92 onwards FHI/RFSU/ RFSL	Love power campaign	To decrease number of unsafe sexual contacts by increasing number of safer sexual contacts	Posters, brochure, TV, cinema	Make love not AIDS	Young people	Metaphorical, sensual
1992 FHI/Nikita[3]	Love without fear	Promote condoms, encourage condom use	Poster, leaflets	'Some of the fun is to put it on', Where to go for information (posters placed in restaurants)	Gay people, heterosexuals	Humorous
September/ October 1993 FHI/RFSU	Man + man campaign	Make safer sex the norm	TV, cinema, press, gay media, brochure, posters	'Condom + water-based lubricant = safer sex'	Gay people, general public	Warm, personal

[1]Aids Delegation; counties, boroughs, RFSU, RFSL and RFHL were involved in their own campaigns. [2]TB (Ted Bates), Garbergs and BRO are all advertising agencies. [3]Nikita is a famous Swedish cartoonist.

ally moralistic attitude to sex, recommending monogamy and sexual restraint (Information-skampanjen om HIV/AIDS, RRV 1988).

The AIDS Delegation's immediate response was to change advertising agencies, and a marked change towards a more positive approach became evident. The subsequent condom normalization campaign (1990) used condom 'collages', for example, a heart, with the endline 'head over heels', a palm tree with the endline 'have a nice trip'. Since the creation of the National Institute of Public Health in 1992, collaboration with the Swedish Association for Sex Education and the Swedish Federation for Gay and Lesbian Rights has resulted in the further development of more sex-positive initiatives, pragmatic in tone and style, as illustrated by the 'Love power' and 'Man + man' campaigns.

Messages

The National Institute of Public Health (1992) states that AIDS public education should address such questions as cohabitation, sex and sexual expectations, and attitudes to those infected or at risk. Key concepts are an open and positive approach to sexual matters and the various ways of preventing HIV infection, as well as sympathy and respect for those afflicted by or exposed to the disease.

The RRV criticized early messages for not offering enough in the way of practical risk reduction and safer-sex advice: 'Messages have often been unspecifically and cautiously worded. Descriptions of how the virus spreads have been rare. RRV believes that the message would have been better with a clearer wording. Information giving practical advice about behaviour would have been more effective. The campaign recommends monogamy and urges restraint as to the number of sexual contacts... but well-balanced descriptions of safe ways for expressing affection and satisfying each other are very rare' (RRV 1988).

Later campaign messages have encouraged safer-sex practices; the condom normalization campaign and 'Love power' campaigns used images and associations rather than direct messages to signify safer-sex practice. For example, some slogans from the 'Love power' campaign were 'Make love not AIDS', 'Rubber revolution', 'Wake up happy'.

Target groups

In addition to the general population, AIDS information campaigns have been directed towards men who have sex with men, IDUs, people from countries where the infection is common, people who have or have had unprotected (i.e. without a condom) sex abroad in high prevalence countries, donors or recipients of untested blood or blood product components abroad, people injected with unsterile hypodermic needles, sex workers and their clients, sexual partners of such people, children of HIV positive mothers, young people, social workers and the media.

Other measures of prevention and control

HIV testing and surveillance

More tests for HIV have been carried out per million population than in any other European country. At present about 1,000,000 tests are carried out annually in Sweden, but this figure does not represent the total number of people tested – for example blood donors account for more than half of all tests as they are tested each time they give blood.

HIV testing is voluntary. As a general rule, HIV testing is offered liberally and at no charge to the patient. Grounds for testing include a patient's suspicion of being infected or the presence of HIV-related symptoms. Testing is offered on a routine basis to those attending prenatal or venereal clinics, and certain groups such as IDUs, migrants and pregnant women are encouraged to have HIV tests. Non-voluntary tests may also be performed in the course of contact tracing.

HIV infection is a notifiable disease in Sweden; under the Communicable Diseases Act of 1989 an HIV-infected person can be detained in hospital if he/she poses a threat of spreading the infection to others. Physicians are obliged to report cases of HIV infection to the county council's medical officer. The report of cases of HIV infection include a coded (anonymous) case number as well as sex, year and country of birth, risk category, and if possible, time and place of transmission. The doctor is obliged to inform the patient of the binding regulations, which are:

* to inform sexual partners of his/her HIV infection before intercourse;
* to practise safe sex;
* not to share needles or injecting equipment; and
* not to engage in prostitution.

HIV-infected people must inform medical personnel before receiving treatment that could involve blood contact. Any patient not adhering to these rules can be reported to the medical officer by the doctor. Since 1989 40 people (1 per cent of the 4,000 HIV-infected population) have been detained for up to three months through the action of an administrative court. These compulsory measures are the last resort when counselling and referral have failed. Cases of these more extreme measures tend to receive extensive media coverage.

Blood and blood products/components used within the health and medical care system have been tested since 1985.

Needle exchange schemes

Sweden has a restrictive drug policy, yet it also has one of the best voluntary drug prevention and treatment programmes. Many of the hardline compulsory regulations which were abandoned in the 1970s have been revived in the 1980s because of AIDS. An official report recommending the widespread adoption of syringe exchange schemes was rejected after considerable debate in the press, at public meetings, in Parliament and government. The medical consensus in favour of syringe schemes was rejected by a wider consensus of drug agency workers, militant pressure groups and the political establishment. It was felt that syringe exchange schemes would not only condone drug use but encourage it. A clean needle exchange programme is, however, in operation in the cities of Malmö and Lund.

Condoms

There has been some commercial advertising of condoms on television. Condoms are widely available in supermarkets, grocery shops, petrol stations and are generally well accepted.

Evaluation

Little systematic evaluation has been undertaken, either before or since the transfer of operational responsibility from the AIDS Delegation to the National Institute of Public Health.

The 1988 National Audit Bureau (RRV) report was commissioned by the government to evaluate the AIDS Delegation's campaigns, for which RRV studied the results of a number of independent surveys. One example is the knowledge, attitude, and behaviour (KAB) surveys conducted by the Department of Social Medicine at Uppsala University. The objective of these surveys is to study the effects on the population of the actual prevalence of HIV, as well as the effects of measures taken as to prevention, diagnosis and treatment. A series of reports of KAB surveys among young people, health care workers and sixth-form college students were commissioned by the AIDS Delegation between 1986 and 1989.

The work of Noah's Ark, the Swedish Federation of Sex Education and the Swedish Federation of Gay and Lesbian Rights was to be evaluated in 1995.

Country visit: Kaye Wellings and Julian Heddy, 1990 and 1993

Report preparation: Kaye Wellings and Becky Field

Individuals and organizations contacted:

Luis Abascal, Bodil Långberg
National Board of Health and Welfare, Stockholm

Anna-Karin Asp
Stockholm County Programme, Gröndal

Anders Bolin
Stockholm

Benny Henriksson
Institute for Social Studies, Stockholm

Bo Lewin
Uppsala University

Torsten Malmqvist, Gudrun Winfridsson
Folkhälsoinstitut (FHI, National Institute of Public Health), Stockholm

Jan-Olof Morfeldt
Noah's Ark-Red Cross Foundation, Stockholm

Kerstin Strid, Joakim Johansson, Margó
Ingvardsson
RFSU (Swedish Association for Sex Education),
Stockholm

Tobias Wikström, Anna Mohr
RFSL (Swedish Federation for Gay and Lesbian
Rights), Stockholm

Bibliography

AIDS Newsletter 1994 9 (9); 2

AIDS surveillance in Europe, quarterly report no. 44 31 December 1994, European Centre for the Epidemiological Monitoring of AIDS

The Communicable Diseases Act and other legislation on control of communicable diseases October 1989, Ministry of Health and Social Affairs International Secretariat

Context of sexual behaviour in Europe, selected indices relating to demographic social and cultural variables May 1993, Becky Field and Kaye Wellings, EC Concerted Action 'Sexual behaviour and the risk of HIV infection'

HIV and AIDS in care 1988, 1992, National Swedish Board of Health and Welfare

HIV/AIDS in Sweden, an analytical survey for the health and medical care services 1992, H Malmqvist and O Ramgren (eds) National Swedish Board of Health and Welfare (Socialstyrelsen), Stockholm

Information about HIV/AIDS – goals and strategy for public policy measures; further measures proposed September 1986, Ministry of Health and Social Affairs, National Commission on AIDS

Informationskampanjen om HIV/AIDS – samhällsinformation som styrmedel (The Information Campaign about HIV/AIDS – national information as a means of direction) 1988, Riksrevisionsverket, Regeringsuppdrag, Stockholm

Informativa styrmedel – ett sätt att lösa samhällsproblem 1989, Riksrevisionsverket

Managing HIV/AIDS in Sweden, 1993, Dagmar Von Walden Laing and Victor A Pestoff, paper presented at the Managing AIDS project meeting in Reichenau, Austria, 10–13 October

Sex education: political issues in Britain and Europe 1994, P Meredith, London: Routledge

Social democracy or societal control – a critical analysis of Swedish AIDS policy 1988, B Henriksson, Stockholm: Glacio Bokforlag

Sweden's syringe exchange debate: moral panic in a rational society, 1994, A Gould, *Journal of Social Policy* 23 (2); 195–217

Working with HIV and AIDS May 1993, National Institute of Public Health in Sweden (Folkhälsoinstitutet), The HIV/AIDS Programme, Stockholm

Translation of documents: Tulla Hacking and Julia Hacking

SWITZERLAND

Context

Epidemiology

According to the European Centre for the Epidemiological Monitoring of AIDS, by 31 December 1994, the cumulative total of AIDS cases was 4,268, with an incidence rate (per million population) of 43.5 (n = 310). The cumulative total of AIDS cases by transmission group (percentages in parentheses) was as follows: homo/bisexual male 1,690 (40.1); injecting drug user (IDU) 1,647 (39.1); homo/bisexual IDU 52 (1.2); haemophiliac/coagulation disorder 27 (0.6); transfusion recipient 53 (1.3); heterosexual contact 666 (15.8); other/undetermined 78 (1.9).

The first case of AIDS was reported in Switzerland in 1982.

It is estimated that between 20,000 and 30,000 people with HIV are living in Switzerland. Whereas at the start of the epidemic the group most affected by HIV was homosexual and bisexual men, the virus is currently spreading most rapidly among injecting drug users.

Social and political background

Switzerland is a federal country with a population of almost 7 million. Three main languages are used in the country according to region: French, German and Italian. Over 1.18 million people living permanently in Switzerland are foreign nationals, including close to 400,000 Italians, 100,000 Spaniards, 100,000 former Yugoslavs and 56,000 Turks.

In general homosexuality is relatively well tolerated by the general population. A variety of gay NGOs provide support and services to homosexuals in Switzerland. The existence of a well-organized gay community enabled a swift response to the AIDS epidemic. As early as 1983, the organization known as Homosexual Working Group began discussing some of the issues raised by AIDS and started to disseminate information about the disease to its members.

There are approximately 4,000 female prostitutes working in Switzerland, and roughly 250,000 to 300,000 clients of prostitutes. The enforcement

Issue	Legislation	Date of legislation	Services provided
Homosexuality	Age of consent 16 (same as for heterosexuals). Legal in all cantons	1937–42, according to canton	Yes
Abortion	Legal where there is risk to woman's life/physical/ mental health	1942	Yes
Drug use (non-medicinal)	Trafficking and possession prohibited in all cantons	1975	Yes
Prostitution	Prostitution legal, exploitation illegal		Yes (some cantons)
Contraception	Legislation and provision differs according to canton; available on prescription		Yes
Contraception for those under age of sexual consent	As above, on prescription		Yes

laws relating to prostitution vary considerably from one canton to another, as does the provision of health and welfare services for prostitutes.

The country is divided into cantons, each of which has considerable powers to determine policy on a variety of social and political issues. Possession of drugs is illegal but some cantonal authorities exercise a degree of discretionary leniency in cases of possession of soft drugs.

Over 90 per cent of the population in Switzerland are Christian, half of which are Catholic and the other half Protestant. Both the Catholic and Protestant authorities have officially approved the AIDS campaign. From early on in the campaign church representatives have met twice each year with those responsible for the campaign in order to exchange information and views.

Health education

Cantonal health departments are responsible for most health promotion and disease prevention activities. Several NGOs are also involved in health promotion. A number of local campaigns have been carried out over the past decade, including prevention of heart disease, anti-smoking and dental health. In addition, there have been nationwide campaigns to prevent road accidents.

Prior to the AIDS epidemic, health promotion activities were carried out through leaflets and television spots. Posters were rarely used, other than in relation to the road accidents campaign. In general, health promotion campaigns preceding the AIDS campaign were didactic in tone.

Sex education

At present there are no national regulations requiring schools to provide sex education. While some cantonal education departments have historically encouraged the provision of sex education in schools, others have not, leading to a distinctly variable situation across the country. However, in recent years even those cantons which previously did not provide sex education have begun to introduce it in conjunction with the AIDS education which is provided at classroom level.

There has been a broad shift away from an exclusive emphasis on medical, physiological and reproductive aspects of sex towards issues concerning personal relationships.

The role of the media

Prior to 1986–87, contradictory messages were put across by the press and television. The introduction of the 'Stop AIDS' campaign in 1987 was generally well received, however, and journalists and editors have been largely supportive of the campaign over the years.

The cooperation of the media has been vital to the implementation of the Swiss campaign. The cost of the campaign would have been considerably higher than the 4 million Swiss francs allocated, except for the fact that all television broadcasts were free of charge until 1991 and billboard posters were charged at half price. One reason for the concession was that, as a state monopoly, the broadcasting companies recognized their public duties to assist in the AIDS prevention campaign. However, in response to market pressures, the television companies began in 1991 to charge for the broadcast of AIDS spots, albeit at a reduced rate. In 1991 the campaign qualified for charitable status which meant a 75 per cent discount. This dropped to 65 per cent in 1992, and further still in 1993. The concessions granted to the campaign were crucial to the financing of the campaign activities, but they carried certain disadvantages. In particular, campaign organizers were unable to control the scheduling of the television spots, and could not reverse the ruling that spots be broadcast only after 9 p.m.

There are three television channels, one for each of the three languages spoken in the country. In 1992 the campaign bought 42 minutes of air time per language area, for a net reach of 72.6 per cent of the overall population.

AIDS/HIV public education

Aims and objectives

The objectives of the Swiss AIDS prevention campaign have been clearly defined. They are to prevent new infections, reduce the negative impact of the epidemic and to promote and reinforce solidarity with those affected by the epidemic.

Structure and organization

In the absence of a Ministry of Health in Switzerland, issues relating to public health fall under the auspices of the Ministry of the Interior. The Federal Office of Public Health (FOPH) is responsible for the whole AIDS prevention strategy.

Much of the earliest work in response to AIDS/HIV in Switzerland was carried out by AIDS-Hilfe Schweiz (AHS, Swiss AIDS Help). AHS is an NGO which was established in 1985 by a group of gay men who recognized the need for a rapid response to AIDS/HIV. AHS now obtains most of its funding from the federal government. It is independent of all political parties, the FOPH and religious denominations.

Since 1986 AHS and the FOPH have joined forces to cooperate in the design and implementation of the 'Stop AIDS' campaign. The FOPH provides scientific and professional expertise and financial resources while the AHS contributes its considerable experience of, and direct contact with, people affected by AIDS/HIV. A creative team is responsible for the 'Stop AIDS' campaigns.

Other organizations which have been active in AIDS public education include Pro Familia, which has a long tradition in sex education, family planning and marriage guidance; and the Swiss Red Cross which has played a major role in professional training. In addition there are twenty regional AIDS relief centres in Switzerland which provide telephone counselling and advice.

Development of campaigns

Between 1983–86 virtually all of the information on AIDS which was disseminated in Switzerland was provided by gay organizations, many of which were staffed in large part by volunteers.

Recognizing that HIV was spreading rapidly, the FOPH took action in 1986. In March of that year the FOPH issued a leaflet presenting the basic facts about AIDS/HIV which was delivered to every Swiss household. The impact of the leaflet was evaluated immediately after the leaflet was distributed, and again three months later. The evaluation indicated the need for a long-term, sustained information campaign about AIDS prevention which would address specific risk behaviours.

The continuous information campaign which was subsequently developed by the FOPH and AHS came to be known as the 'Stop AIDS' campaign. The campaign logo itself – 'Stop AIDS' – was not only verbal but also visual, as the O was replaced by a picture of a pink, rolled up condom. Over time the image of the condom came to symbolize the campaign and its message of HIV prevention.

Tone and style

The continuity of the agencies and personnel involved in the design and execution of the campaign has allowed for consistency in tone and style. The creative team worked collaboratively in determining the direction of the campaign. From the beginning members of the team unanimously rejected the use of fear in AIDS/HIV messages. In relation to sexuality, the tone has been generally permissive and positive. The creative team was clear from the start that its aim was to prevent the spread of HIV rather than to pass moral judgements on specific forms of behaviour.

Those responsible for designing and executing the campaign have endeavoured to ensure a steady rhythm of output. Publicity has been generated at regular and evenly spaced intervals, with each wave of publicity having similar direction and force, thus avoiding 'bursts' of publicity which are difficult to sustain. A common symbol – the circular condom

Campaign chronology

Date and agency	Campaign theme/title	Aims	Media	Main message/endline	Target groups	Tone and style
1986	AIDS leaflet	Provide and clarify basic facts about AIDS	Leaflet	Routes of transmission and means of prevention	General public	Informational
February 1987	Stop AIDS phase I	Encourage risk-reduction behaviour	TV, posters	Condoms protect	General public	Incremental, prominent logo
June 1987	Stop AIDS phase II	As above	TV, posters	Condoms protect; fidelity protects; don't share needles	General public, young people, IDUs	As above
December 1987	Stop AIDS phase III	As above	TV, posters	Use a condom, or stay faithful; don't share needles; ways in which HIV is not transmitted	General public, young people, IDUs	As above
September 1988	Stop AIDS phase IV	As above, and to combat stigmatization and discrimination	TV, posters, cinema	As above and solidarity with people with AIDS/HIV	General public, young people, IDUs	As above
1989	Stop AIDS	As above	As above	As above	As above	
January 1990* July 1990† September 1990‡	*Excuses campaign; †Holiday campaign; ‡Solidarity campaign	*Address barriers to risk-reduction practices; †Highlight risks to travellers; ‡Encourage positive attitudes towards the sick	*Posters; †posters; ‡posters	*Highlight excuses for avoiding safer sex; †Practise safer sex when abroad	General public, young people	*Informational, motivational; ‡Empathetic
1991	Without a condom? Without me!	Promote condom use	Posters	Condoms protect	General public, young people	Motivational
1992	Without a condom? Not me! Correcting misinformation	Promote condom use, explain how HIV is not transmitted	Posters, TV	Condoms protect; HIV is only spread in limited ways	General public, young people	Humorous, informational
1993	Unfaithful to partner, faithful to condom	Promote condom use	Posters	Condoms protect	General public	Broad-minded

All campaigns have been run by the Federal Office of Public Health and AIDS-Hilfe Schweiz/Swiss AIDS Help.

rim, variously depicted as a moon and a slogan, 'Stop AIDS' in which the O is replaced by a condom – has unified the campaign and created a strong visual and verbal image. Evaluation has shown that people have a very high recognition of the campaign's central symbol.

Messages

The message most strongly associated with the campaign is that condoms protect against HIV infection. Opposition from some sectors of the community to overreliance on the single message of 'use a condom' – on the grounds that this emphasized a practical rather than moral solution to HIV prevention – prompted the introduction of a message which stressed fidelity. In June 1987, the second wave of the campaign featured the additional message 'Faithfulness protects'. This ad featured a wedding ring, rather than a condom, replacing the O of 'Stop AIDS', which was less well understood.

Having made this concession to the groups which had lobbied for moral messages, the 'Stop AIDS' campaign returned to its primary theme of condom promotion as a means of HIV prevention. In 1993, for instance, five new posters were produced with the theme 'Unfaithful to partners – faithful to condoms'. These posters – including one focusing for the first time on unfaithfulness between male lovers – conveyed the message that HIV infection could be avoided even if individuals were not faithful to their partners, provided they used a condom.

In 1987 the campaign organizers recognized that the sharing of needles among intravenous drug users was becoming an increasingly important HIV transmission route. The main drug-related message of the campaign was not to start using drugs at all.

Messages about the need for solidarity with people affected by AIDS/HIV have been transmitted regularly in the campaign since 1989. Swiss personalities and celebrities from the world of sport and entertainment have spoken on television about the need for compassion and acceptance. In 1990 a billboard campaign was introduced to promote solidarity. The solidarity messages were reinforced by messages which underlined how HIV is and is not transmitted. These messages were put across in print and billboard ads, as well as radio, television and cinemas.

A unique feature of the Swiss campaign has been the way in which messages have been introduced cumulatively in each wave of advertising, each adding to, rather than replacing, the earlier one(s). While the first wave of the 'Stop AIDS' campaign concentrated on the basic condom message, the second broadened attention to injecting drug use and the need for fidelity. In the third phase of the campaign, messages relating to the ways in which HIV is not transmitted and about the need for solidarity were added to the three permanent basic messages.

Target groups

In addition to the general population, AIDS information campaigns have been directed towards young people, women, homosexuals, IDUs, sex workers and their clients, foreign nationals (materials in German, French, Italian, English, Spanish, Portuguese, Serbo-Croatian, Albanian and Turkish) spending extended periods of time in Switzerland, tourists, workers, health care professionals, blood donors/recipients, military personnel and prisoners.

Other measures of prevention and control

HIV testing and surveillance

HIV testing is carried out in Switzerland on the basis of voluntary informed consent. In September 1987 a special ordinance was introduced making the reporting of both AIDS and HIV compulsory. The ordinance includes special provisions to ensure the confidentiality of all notifications and of any other information relating to cases of AIDS/HIV.

The Swiss campaign has supported voluntary – as against compulsory – testing, but has never explicitly recommended that individuals be tested.

Needle exchange schemes

There are an estimated 20,000 to 30,000 injecting drug users in Switzerland. Several of the cities with relatively large numbers of injecting drug users began low level needle exchange programmes as early as 1985. The most extensive programme, known as the ZIPP-AIDS project, was developed in the city of Zurich. During 1989, ZIPP-AIDS distributed close to 1.5 million syringes, about 90 per cent of which were returned.

The availability of sterile needles varies from canton to canton. Supplies are restricted in some of the more rural areas of the country.

An estimated 10–30 per cent of inmates of Swiss

prisons are believed to be drug dependent and, on average, some 10–15 per cent of inmates are also believed to be HIV positive. These figures are based on rough estimates since there is no compulsory testing in prisons. In 1992 it was suggested that syringes be distributed in prisons. While this proposal appeared to have the backing of the Federal Office of Public Health, the Conference of the Cantonal Chiefs of Police and Justice Departments objected to it on the grounds that it could result in increased drug injecting in prisons. While debate continues, some prisons have taken precautionary measures such as the distribution of bleach to enable prisoners to disinfect used needles and syringes; a pilot needle exchange scheme in one prison was due to begin in May 1994.

Condoms

Objections to campaigns urging condom use were voiced by some members of the medical community, who suggested that it could be misleading for the campaign to imply that condoms provided complete protection against infection. Partly in response to these concerns, the private Association for Quality Seals for Condoms, of which Switzerland's two largest consumer associations and the AHS are members, created a new Swiss standard and a quality seal for condoms. The standard was deemed even higher than that of the International Standard Organization. In 1993 the 'Stop AIDS' campaign produced a billboard reminding people of the importance of using condoms bearing the Swiss quality label.

Evaluation

Switzerland was among the first countries to institutionalize evaluation at the national level, and its evaluation programme is probably the most comprehensive in Europe. In the early stages of the campaign the FOPH invited the Institute of Social and Preventive Medicine at the University of Lausanne to conduct a thorough and systematic evaluation by conducting and commissioning research. The evaluation conducted by the Institute continuously measures the effects and effectiveness of the whole preventive strategy and so helps to contribute to its success by guiding the selection of subsequent strategies. The earliest evaluation was carried out immediately following the March 1986 leaflet drop, and attempted to gauge interest and acceptance. More than 30 further studies were carried out, including a survey which focused specifically on behaviour modification. Some of the studies were concerned with process evaluation (development of preventive programmes, role of opinion leaders and other 'multipliers' of prevention messages) and others on the results (modifying behaviour, condom use, etc.).

Country visit: Kaye Wellings and Claire Gibbons, 1990 and 1993

Report preparation: Renée Danziger and Kaye Wellings

Individuals and organizations contacted:

Martin Büechl, Andrea Keller, Therese Stutz Steiger, François Wasserfallen
Federal Office of Public Health, Berne

Dr Françoise Dubois-Arber, Dr Dominic Hausser, Andre Jeannin, Professor Fred Paccaud, Dr Erwin Zimmerman
University Institute of Social and Preventive Medicine, Lausanne

Bernard Gloor
AIDS-Hilfe Schweiz, Zurich

Iris Reutler
PWA Schweiz, Zurich

Peter Zeugin
Zurich

Bibliography

AIDS surveillance in Europe, quarterly report no. 44 31 December 1994, European Centre for the Epidemiological Monitoring of AIDS

Context of sexual behaviour in Europe, selected indices relating to demographic, social and cultural variables

May 1993, Becky Field and Kaye Wellings, EC Concerted Action 'Sexual behaviour and the risk of HIV infection'

The STOP AIDS Story 1987–1992 1993, Swiss AIDS Foundation and Federal Office for Public Health

UNITED KINGDOM

Context

Epidemiology

According to the European Centre for the Epidemiological Monitoring of AIDS, by 31 December 1994 the cumulative total of AIDS cases was 10,304 with an incidence rate (per million population) of 20.5 (n = 1,189). The cumulative total of AIDS cases, by transmission group (percentages in parentheses) was as follows: homo/bisexual male 7,463 (73.7); injecting drug user (IDU) 591 (5.8); homo/bisexual IDU 165 (1.6); haemophiliac/coagulation disorder 442 (4.4); transfusion recipient 90 (0.9); heterosexual contact 1,264 (12.5); other/undetermined 107 (1.1).

The first AIDS case in the UK was registered in December 1981, and the first death from the disease was recorded in the following year.

Social and political background

After a period of sexually liberalizing legislative reform in the 1960s (including the legalization of abortion and homosexuality, and the reform of divorce law), and an ensuing period of greater sexual freedom in the next decade, the 1980s saw a reversal of these trends. Attempts – although ultimately unsuccessful – were made during the course of the decade to restrict access to contraception (for those under the age of sexual consent), to tighten laws relating to abortion and to impose limitations on the expression of homosexuality.

In 1994 Parliament voted against the equalization of the age of consent for homosexual men with the heterosexual age of consent (16), the majority of MPs voting instead to lower the age of consent from 21 to 18.

Between December 1984 and March 1986 the mandate from the Department of Health to GPs to give contraceptive advice and treatment to young women without parental consent was withdrawn as the result of action by Victoria Gillick. The Department of Health and Social Security subsequently appealed to the House of Lords and the ruling was overturned. 1993 and 1994 government guidelines clarified that the principle of confidentiality applies equally to those under 16 as to those over the age of sexual consent.

The United Kingdom's gay movement is, however, powerful, broadly based and well organized, which had positive consequences for early attempts at AIDS education.

The UK is highly centralized politically, and the state plays a key role in the funding and delivery of health and welfare services, as epitomized by its National Health Service, subdivided hierarchically into regional and district health authorities. Mechanisms for coordinating between local and regional levels are elaborate and extensive, but generally policies emanate from the centre.

Health education

National health education in Britain is largely the responsibility of the Health Education Authority (HEA). Numerous other organizations with specific

Issue	Legislation	Date of legislation	Services provided
Homosexuality	Age of consent 18[1] for men (heterosexuals 16). Legal in non-public settings. No law for women	1994	Yes
Abortion	Legal on social, socio-medical socio-economic grounds <24 weeks. No time limit when risk of grave injury to woman's life/physical/mental health or foetal health or handicap. Consent of 2 doctors required. <16s need parental consent. Free under NHS	1967, 1990	Yes
Drug use (non-medicinal)	Trafficking and possession illegal; stricter penalties for class A (e.g. heroin/cocaine) than class B (e.g. cannabis). Maximum sentences are severe but 85 per cent of all drug offenders convicted of possession	1971	Yes
Prostitution	Soliciting, loitering with intent to solicit, kerb crawling are civil offences; keeping a brothel, encouragement, third-party involvement are criminal offences		Yes
Contraception	Family planning is incorporated into the NHS, all contraceptive advice and prescribed supplies free of charge	1974	Yes
Contraception for those under age of sexual consent	16 is the age of medical consent to treatment (including contraception and abortion), <16s can get contraception without parental consent, if young person is considered mature enough to understand the implications	1969, 1986[2]	Yes

[1]Previously 21 [2]A 1986 Law Lords ruling upheld existing Department of Health guidelines to doctors to provide contraceptive advice and supplies to under 16-year-old girls without parental permission in exceptional cases.

interests – the British Heart Foundation, Coronary Prevention Group, Action on Smoking and Health, and the Family Planning Association – also have prominent education, information and communication programmes. In the past there have been public education campaigns about heart disease, contraception, dental health, smoking, road accidents, STDs, infant health and pregnancy.

The HEA is responsible for health promotion in England. The Health Education Board for Scotland (HEBS), the Health Promotion Agency for Northern Ireland and Health Promotion Wales have corresponding roles for Scotland, Northern Ireland and Wales. However, for mass media work on AIDS/HIV, the HEA's remit is UK-wide.

Sex education

As a result of the 1986 Education Act, governors of all county and maintained schools have since 1987 been legally required to have a school sex education policy, and to make that policy available to parents. Policy makers have constantly to take account of a vociferous moral lobby who claim that sex education has a pernicious influence. A clause in this Act placed a requirement on local education authorities to ensure that schools conformed to 'family values' in their sex education classes, though careful wording of the clause permitted some latitude in the interpretation of what constituted a 'family'.

The 1993 Education Act (in force from August 1994) reaffirmed the responsibility of *primary* school governors to decide whether the school includes sex education in the curriculum. Governors of all state-maintained *secondary* schools are required to ensure that sex education, including AIDS/HIV and STD education, is provided for pupils, and to produce a sex education policy outlining the content and organization of the curriculum. Parents of both primary and secondary school pupils have the right to withdraw pupils (including those over 16) from any sex education other than that in any part of the National

Curriculum. National Curriculum guidelines for health education provide a progressive programme of sex education to help teachers and governors planning their programme.

The role of the media

Early media treatment of AIDS issues presented major difficulties for AIDS public education in the UK. Despite guidelines issued by the National Union of Journalists in 1984, AIDS was virtually synonymous with the term 'gay plague' in national press reportage in the UK. The tone of reporting was highly retributive, suggesting that this was a disease which was visited on deserving minorities.

This had two major consequences for the public education campaigns. It meant, firstly, that a good deal of investment was needed to counter the myths relating to casual transmission (e.g. the 'No catch' series of advertisements). Secondly, a consequence of the labelling of AIDS as a 'gay plague' in the early stages of the epidemic has been that mass media work had to reiterate constantly the message that everyone could be at risk (e.g. the 1986 Department of Health campaign, 'AIDS is not prejudiced', and the HEA's 1990 'experts' campaign).

AIDS/HIV public education

Aims and objectives

The objectives of the HEA's work include:
- the creation and maintenance of a well-informed public and a supportive climate of opinion;
- assistance to other workers and agencies;
- provision of advice to the Secretary of State for Health.

Structure and organization

Between March 1986 and October 1987, the Department of Health (DoH) was responsible for AIDS public education in the UK. An AIDS unit, specifically set up to establish policy and coordinate all AIDS preventive activities, was created within the DoH. Early public education campaigns, from spring 1986 until spring 1987, were conducted under the aegis of the DoH.

In October 1987, responsibility for all aspects of AIDS public education, with the exception of drugs, was transferred to the HEA and the remit for this area of work extended to the whole of the UK.

The statutory sector was strengthened in 1989 at local level by the creation of AIDS coordinator posts at district health authority level, when regional authorities were given budgets for AIDS work. The internal structure of the HEA was revised in 1989 so that AIDS took its place among other prevention programmes within the HEA's strategy, as opposed to being an autonomous division. This was inevitably seen by some as a downgrading of the importance of the disease, but was in part a necessary consequence of downward revisions of predictions of the expected scale of the epidemic. Justification for the continuation of initially high injection of funds into AIDS became more difficult as people realized that the worst possible scenario seemed unlikely to become a reality.

The UK has been characterized by high level political coordination of AIDS policies. A number of internal expert committees were set up to this end: the Expert Advisory Group on AIDS (EAGA), formed at the DoH in January 1985 and composed of experts from the medical, voluntary and statutory sectors advises UK chief medical officers on matters relating to AIDS policy; the Interdepartmental Group on AIDS (IDGA) coordinates policies among government departments; and a committee on AIDS Public Education coordinated AIDS public education. In addition, the Chief Scientist's Meeting was established to coordinate the programmes of research of the various scientific funding agencies. The National AIDS Trust was established by the Secretary of State for Social Services in May 1987 to raise funding for, and aid the coordination of, voluntary sector AIDS activities. The All Party Parliamentary Group on AIDS (APPGA) lobbies on issues of ethics and policy.

Development of campaigns

As in many other countries, the earliest responses to the epidemic came from the voluntary sector, in particular those organizations who served communities directly affected, and who could mobilize resources more rapidly than could the statutory bodies. Most notably, the Terrence Higgins Trust, born out of a conference organized by the then Greater London Council and Health Education Council in 1983, and named after the first man to die from AIDS in the UK, published a good deal of safer-sex literature and opened a telephone helpline in February 1984, with DoH funding. Other organizations prominent in preventive efforts included Body Positive, Frontliners, the Scottish AIDS Monitor, the Lesbian and Gay Switchboard and the Standing Conference on Drug Abuse.

This early phase was followed by a period of national priority and policy formation, as political and public fears about the threat of immediate spread in the general population grew. In early 1986, the DoH embarked on a national public education campaign through the mass media, organized by the government's Central Office of Information and developed by the advertising agency TBWA, the objectives of which were to educate people about the facts and myths of the disease; offer advice and reassurance; and influence the social climate in which the epidemic has occurred. In March 1986, full-page advertisements aimed at presenting the facts accurately to the British public appeared in the national press and continued throughout the next eight months. This relatively low profile campaign was intensified in impact and visibility in November 1986. From autumn 1986 to spring 1987, a high profile campaign was launched culminating in 'AIDS Week' at the end of February 1987, when unprecedented cooperation between TV and broadcasting networks and the statutory bodies aimed to bring the full facts and severity of the AIDS epidemic to the attention of the general public. A peak of activity was achieved through the use of multi-media including national posters and magazine advertising, radio, television and cinema commercials. A leaflet 'AIDS:

don't die of ignorance' was distributed to all 23 million households in Britain in January 1987, and to the armed forces, police and prisons, with further availability through general medical practitioners, citizens' advice bureaux, colleges, youth organizations and other outlets. The campaign was supported by a national telephone helpline, the number of which was extensively featured in advertising. This campaign achieved great success in terms of raising awareness although it also attracted criticism for being too heavily dependent on alarmist tactics.

Tone and style

Early interventions in the UK campaign were characterized by and criticized for a heavy reliance on the use of fear to motivate the general public. The earliest TV advertisements transmitted in the autumn of 1986 contained imagery linking death with sexuality. Images of volcanoes erupting were juxtaposed with lilies falling on to tombstones, while icebergs served to show that far more of the problem lay hidden than had yet been exposed. These ads succeeded in generating widespread awareness of AIDS.

Responsibility for campaign management passed to the HEA in the autumn of 1987; in spring 1988 a series of magazine advertisements appeared, showing possible excuses people resorted to in avoiding condom use. The TV advertisements showed situations in which young people needed to make decisions relating to acceptable risks ('You know the risks, the decision is yours'). These ads represented attempts to introduce greater realism into the campaign and to move away from the apocalyptic approach.

In common with those in other countries, campaigns in the UK have become progressively more light-hearted.

Messages

Twofold messages relating to risk reduction have featured in public education campaigns: to restrict numbers of sexual partners, and to use a condom. Decisions relating to the inclusion of messages were

Campaign chronology

Date and agency	Campaign theme/title	Aims	Media	Main message/endline	Target groups	Tone and style
Spring 1986 DoH/ TBWA[1]	Government press campaign	Provide the general public with the facts about AIDS and the means by which risk could be reduced	Press, posters	'AIDS: don't die of ignorance'	General public	Informational (close text)
Autumn 1986– spring 1987 DoH/TBWA	First government TV campaign 'AIDS Week' February– March 1987	Raise awareness of AIDS, provide basic information (i.e. transmission routes and means of prevention)	TV, cinema, national press, youth magazines, posters, leaflet drop (January 1987)	'AIDS: don't die of ignorance'	General public	High profile, alarmist
1988 HEA	'No catch'	Correct myths of transmission	Press, magazines, posters	'You don't get AIDS by …' (e.g. shaking hands)	General public	Informative
February 1988– September 1988 HEA/TBWA	'Stay' and 'Disco' (TV), women's campaign, holiday campaign	Inform young people about the risks of HIV; provide information on protection	TV, press, posters	'AIDS: you know the risks, the decision is yours'	General public, travellers	Realistic
December 1988– March 1989 HEA/BMP[1]		Reiterate the facts about AIDS/HIV; encourage young people to discuss and use condoms	Press (national and youth), posters, radio	'AIDS: you're as safe as you want to be'	General public, opinion formers, young people[2]	Informational
December 1989– March 1990 HEA/BMP	Experts campaign	Provide authoritative factual information on spread of HIV; clarify confusion surrounding heterosexual transmission	TV, national press	'AIDS: you're as safe as you want to be'	General public, opinion formers, young people[2]	Authoritative
July– September 1990 HEA	Inhibitions campaign	Remind young people of the risks of HIV infection; encourage them to take and use condoms on holiday	Posters, radio	Use condoms on holiday	Young people[2]	Pragmatic
December 1990– March 1991 HEA/BMP	Personal testimony I	Emphasize reality of AIDS/HIV	TV	Ordinary people can get HIV	General public, young people[2]	Documentary, serious
	Condom normalization I (Mrs Dawson)	Normalize condom use and break down some of the embarrassment associated with condoms (which act as a barrier to use)	Cinema	Condoms are an everyday practice		Light-hearted, supportive
July 1991– September 1992 HEA/BMP	Personal testimony II	Emphasize reality of AIDS/HIV, especially over summer months	TV, radio,	Ordinary people can get HIV	Young people[2]	As above

Date/Agency[1]	Campaign component	Objective	Media	Message	Target audience	Tone
	Condom normalization II (Mrs Dawson)	Continue to normalize condom use and break down some of the embarrassments associated with condoms	Cinema	Condoms are an everyday practice		
December 1991–February 1992 HEA/BMP	Personal testimony III	Reiterate reality of AIDS/HIV	TV	Ordinary people can get HIV	Young people,[2] gay men	As above
	Condom normalization III (Mrs Dawson, Mr Brewster, Casanova)	Familiarize people with condoms (breaking down the embarrassment which may prevent use); demonstrate modern condoms are acceptable	Mrs Dawson – TV, Mr Brewster – cinema, Casanova – male interest press and magazines	Condoms are an everyday practice		
July–September 1992 HEA/BMP	Personal testimony IV	Remind people of reality of AIDS/HIV, especially over summer months	Radio	Ordinary people can get HIV	Young people[2]	As above
	Condom normalization IV (Mr Brewster)	Continue to familiarize people with condoms and counter embarrassment/'myths' which act as barriers to use	Cinema	Condoms are an everyday practice		
July 1992–March 1993 HEA	Young people's press campaign	Give advice about best time to mention condoms to a sexual partner	Young women's press and magazines	'How far will you go before you mention condoms?'	Young people	Pragmatic
		Demonstrate that modern condoms are acceptable	Male interest press and magazines	'Casanova'		
December 1992–March 1993 HEA/BMP	Condom normalization V (Mrs Dawson, Mr Brewster)	Encourage a climate which is positive and open about condoms, in order to permit unembarrassed discussion about sex and protection and talking about 'sexual health'	TV, (Mrs Dawson after 21.00, Mr Brewster after 22.30)	Condoms are an everyday practice	General public, young people	Light-hearted, supportive
July–September 1993 HEA/BMP	Holiday travel campaign, lessons 68, have a safe journey	Keep AIDS on the public agenda; encourage safer sex	Radio, posters at airports	Use a condom; buy a condom before you travel	Young people, travellers	Minimalist, action-prompting

[1]TBWA and BMP are advertising agencies. [2]Sexually active outside a long-term or monogamous relationship.

at times made difficult by the competing claims from different interest groups on the content of the campaign materials. Tension between the demands of the moral lobby (who wanted to stress the message to practise monogamy, and who exerted a strong and vociferous influence on health ministers) and health education workers (who wanted to see pragmatic and realistic messages) made it difficult for those responsible for executing campaign components to produce universally acceptable advertisements.

The campaign components which have been most successful in terms of both public recall and external recognition were those which contained a simple single message. Advertisements which featured as part of the yearly holiday campaign, for example, simply showing a condom with such captions as 'Don't go too far without one' or 'Life insurance at 50p' were well received.

Heightened controversy over whether or not HIV was efficiently transmitted heterosexually resulted in a campaign launched in spring 1990, featuring 'AIDS experts' speaking authoritatively about the continuing risk to the general population. The message that everyone was at risk continued in the next campaign, via the testimonies of people from diverse regional backgrounds, sexual orientations and routes of infection.

As yet there have been no campaigns run by the HEA carrying specific messages urging solidarity with those affected. However, a secondary objective of the personal testimony campaigns was to encourage tolerance and sympathy for those infected with HIV. Post-campaign evaluation showed positive improvements in these measures.

Target groups

In addition to the general population, AIDS information campaigns have been directed towards young people (especially those who are sexually active outside a long-term or monogamous relationship), men who have sex with men, travellers (holiday and work), professional and community workers in the field of AIDS/HIV, opinion formers, and black and minority ethnic groups.

Other measures of prevention and control

HIV surveillance and testing

Screening of donated blood was introduced in July 1985. An AIDS (Control) Act was passed in 1987, laying a requirement on health authorities to provide annual reports detailing the prevalence of AIDS within their area and the steps they are taking in response. General public health legislation has been extended specifically to cover AIDS. AIDS has not been made a notifiable disease but certain control powers can be used, such as the power (in exceptional cases) to confine compulsorily to hospital someone whose behaviour and infectious condition endangers public health. This measure has only been used once.

Anonymous testing was an issue of debate; original advice was that it was not legally possible. However, an unlinked anonymous prevalence monitoring programme was established in January 1990 which has led to increased confidence in predicting the future course of the epidemic. The National Health Service (Venereal Diseases) Act Regulations 1974 prohibit National Health Service employees from communicating information about an HIV test which might identify an individual concerned.

Needle exchange schemes

The first needle exchange schemes were established in 1986 as a way of reducing the transmission of HIV, although not without some controversy. In Scotland, the establishment of such schemes has encountered strong local opposition, and the needle exchange in Dundee had to be closed down as a result. There is a marked reduction in projected new cases in the UK among injecting drug users. The reasons for the sharp decline in infection in this exposure category during the second part of the 1980s are unclear, but the success may be partly due to early implementation of needle exchange schemes.

Condoms

Considerable progress has been made in reducing public resistance to open discussion of condoms. Regulations previously prohibiting the commercial advertising of condoms were lifted in March 1987, a move which was given Home Office approval four months later. The first commercial condom advertisements, featuring the products of the London Rubber Company, were seen on British television screens in July 1987. Unlike other forms of contraception, there is no mandate to provide condoms free of charge, although they are often free at family planning and genito-urinary medicine clinics. They have nevertheless been liberally dispensed as prophylactics – in student information packs, in AIDS promotional materials, etc. – and their correct usage encouraged as a risk-reduction strategy since the start of the AIDS public education campaign.

Evaluation

The main instrument for the evaluation of the UK AIDS campaign has been the AIDS Strategic Monitor, used by the British Market Research Bureau to investigate knowledge, attitudes and behaviour relating to AIDS in the UK population. This was first commissioned in 1986 by the Department of Health. When responsibility for AIDS public education (and hence its evaluation) passed from the DoH to the HEA in October 1987, the design of the Monitor was altered slightly in order to meet new needs. Changes to the questionnaire were kept to a minimum in order to ensure comparability over time. The system of successive 'waves' of fieldwork was however abandoned in favour of continuous data collection, because continuous monitoring reflected the change of emphasis of the new campaign – from one of intensive short-term impact to a more sustained approach aimed at maintaining AIDS awareness in the public consciousness. Continuous monitoring also provided a more flexible approach to monitoring public response than had previously been possible, facilitating more accurate synchronization between specific campaign initiatives and the measurement of their impact and effect. In addition, this method of fieldwork made possible retrospective monitoring of interventions implemented by other than official agencies (voluntary agencies, mass media, etc.). The timing of such interventions, as well as unforeseen media events (e.g. Freddie Mercury's death) was not necessarily coordinated with HEA campaigns.

Since 1987 the HEA has been monitoring the knowledge, attitudes and behaviour of men attending gay bars in Britain. One of the objectives of this work is to assess the response to campaign initiatives.

In addition to the AIDS Strategic Monitor surveys a number of studies of the more sexually active younger population were conducted between 1989 and 1991.

Scotland

In Scotland the Health Education Board for Scotland (HEBS) provides initiatives which complement the UK-wide campaign. Activities have regard to Scotland's special circumstances, notably the significance of injecting drug use and the problem of vertical transmission from mother to baby. HEBS has embarked on initiatives with statutory and voluntary agencies. Health boards, local authorities and voluntary agencies are all active at local level, the most extensive programmes being (as expected) in areas of Scotland where prevalence is highest. A range of different advertising methods are used locally, including local press and radio, billboard sites and messages on buses. In July 1991 the Minister of State at the Scottish Office set up a taskforce to review current prevention activities in order to consider what further practical measures might be taken and to assess the effectiveness of the present arrangements for coordination of action at national and local level. One result of this was the establishment by HEBS of SHAIR (Scottish HIV/AIDS Initiatives Register), a database of information about current and planned initiatives – media campaigns, needle exchanges, training courses, HIV testing and research work. This service (calls are charged at local rates) is aimed at workers in health boards, education and social work departments, voluntary and religious organizations. The service is intended to be of practical use in helping these workers to develop projects and to make contact with others carrying out similar kinds of activities. The database contains details of approximately 800 initiatives and is being distributed to various local sites throughout Scotland.

Northern Ireland

In Northern Ireland the age of sexual consent is 17, one year higher than the rest of the UK. The 1967 Abortion Act does not extend to Northern Ireland, and except in exceptional circumstances (such as to save the mother's life) abortion is not available.

Health education is one of six crosscurricular themes in the Northern Irish curriculum; since September 1992 schools have been legally required to ensure that their curriculum promotes health education. The framework for sex education is further set by the Department of Education NI circular (1987/45), which advises schools to have a sex education policy, but leaves it to the discretion of headteachers in consultation with the school's governors and parents.

The Health Promotion Agency for Northern Ireland is funded by central government, as an independent regional organization, with a remit to promote health.

The Agency's sexual health programme attempts to address issues of sex education, family planning and the prevention of STDs, including AIDS/HIV. In its work, and in considering the needs of young people in particular, the Agency has been collaborating with Convenience Advertising, a commercial company which specializes in reaching tightly defined sections of the population who may be difficult to reach by more conventional means of communication.

Wales

In Wales, Health Promotion Wales (HPW) complements the work of the UK-wide mass media campaign through a range of research activities and community-based education projects. HPW was closely involved in the development of strategic directions for HIV prevention work in Wales set out in the 1993 Warwick Report commissioned by the Welsh Office, and in the protocol on 'Healthy living' produced by the Welsh Health Planning Forum in 1993. HPW's approach is to address AIDS education issues in the context of broader sexual health concerns, including unplanned pregnancies and other STDs.

In 1995 HPW published an analysis of the Welsh data from the UK National Survey of Sexual Attitudes and Lifestyles, which highlighted aspects of sexual risk taking among the Welsh population and gave recommendations for future sexual health promotion work. In the same year data were collected from 1,400 15- to 16-year-olds in Wales on their sexual knowledge, attitudes and practices, using the WHO Health Behaviour in School-aged Children protocol; it is hoped to repeat this survey biennially, in order to provide trend data on young people's AIDS-related knowledge, attitudes and sexual behaviour. HPW has also implemented and evaluated a number of community-based AIDS education projects in collaboration with local health and education services and voluntary agencies such as the Family Planning Association. Groups targeted through these projects have included young people in schools, youth clubs and further education settings; parents; and women prostitutes and their clients. The need to provide AIDS education materials in the Welsh language is also an important priority for HPW. Current projects include a Welsh language translation of a sex education resource pack for use in schools and youth clubs, and an HIV prevention leaflet for gay and bisexual men.

Fieldwork: Kaye Wellings 1990 and 1993

Report preparation: Kaye Wellings and Becky Field

Individuals and organizations contacted:

Joanna Goodrich, Dr Mukesh Kapila, Dominic McVey, Lindsay Neil, Susan Perl
Health Education Authority, London

Carmel Kelly
Health Promotion Agency for Northern Ireland, Belfast, Northern Ireland

Nick Partridge
Terrence Higgins Trust, London

Dr Steve Platt, Clive Powell
Health Education Board for Scotland, Edinburgh, Scotland

Bibliography

AIDS surveillance in Europe, quarterly report no. 44 31 December 1994, European Centre for the Epidemiological Monitoring of AIDS
A Brief History of Recent Sex Education Legislation

and Guidance January 1994, Sex Education Forum

Health Education Authority public education campaigns part 1: an overview of progress 1994 (draft) Kaye Wellings, London School of Hygiene and Tropical Medicine

Health Education Authority HIV/AIDS mass media activity 1986–1993 Health Education Authority, London

Sex education in schools: changes in legislation 1993/94 November 1993, Dilys Went

Index

Note: references in bold denote country reports